The Augmented Breast: Radiologic and Clinical Perspectives

The Augmented Breast: Radiologic and Clinical Perspectives

Edited by

David P. Gorczyca, M.D.
Radiology Specialists, LTD.
Director of Breast Imaging
Columbia Sunrise Hospital & Medical Center
Columbia Sunrise Mountain View Hospital
Las Vegas, NV

R. James Brenner, M.D., J.D.
Associate Clinical Professor
Iris Cantor Center for Breast Imaging
Department of Radiological Sciences
University of California, Los Angeles
Los Angeles, California

1997

Thieme
New York · Stuttgart

Thieme Medical Publishers, Inc.
381 Park Avenue South
New York, NY 10016

The Augmented Breast:
Radiological and Clinical Perspectives
David P. Gorczyca, M.D.
R. James Brenner, M.D.

Library of Congress Cataloging-in-Publication Data

The augmented breast : radiologic and clinical perspectives / edited
by David P. Gorczyca, R. James Brenner.
p. cm.
Includes bibliographical references and index.
ISBN 0-86577-612-1. — ISBN 0-86577-612-1
1. Augmentation mammaplasty. 2. Breast implants—Complications.
3. Breast—Imaging. I. Gorczyca, David P. II. Brenner, R. James.
[DNLM: 1. Mammaplasty. 2. Breast Implants—Adverse effects.
3. Silicones—adverse effects. 4. Prosthesis Failure.
5. Diagnostic Imaging. WP 910 A921 1997]
RD539.8.A94 1997
618.1′90592—dc21
DNLM/DLC
for Library of Congress 96-44700
CIP

Important note: Medical knowledge is ever-changing. As new research and clinical experience broaden our knowledge, changes in treatment and drug therapy may be required. The authors and editors of the material herein have consulted sources believed to be reliable in their efforts to provide information that is complete and in accord with the standards accepted at the time of publication. However, in view of the possibility of human error by the authors, editors, or publisher of the work herein, or changes in medical knowledge, neither the authors, editors, publisher, or any other party who has been involved in the preparation of this work, warrants that the information contained herein is in every respect accurate or complete, and they are not responsible for any errors or omissions or for the results obtained from use of such information. Readers are encouraged to confirm the information contained herein with other sources. For example, readers are advised to check the product information sheet included in the package of each drug they plan to administer to be certain that the information contained in this publication is accurate and that changes have not been made in the recommended dose or in the contraindications for administration. This recommendation is of particular importance in connection with new or infrequently used drugs.

Some of the product names, patents, and registered designs referred to in this book are in fact registered trademarks or proprietary names even though specific reference to this fact is not always made in the text. Therefore, the appearance of a name without designation as proprietary is not to be construed as a representation by the publisher that it is in the public domain.

Printed in the United States of America

5 4 3 2 1

TMP ISBN 0-86577-612-1
GTV ISBN 3-13-103881-0

To my wife, Pamela, the love of my life,
and our daughters
Stephanie and Kathryn,
who add so much to the joy of life.

To my parents, Casimir and Lorraine,
who taught me the rewards of self-discipline
and hard work.

David P. Gorczyca

This work is dedicated to my wife Barbara
who stands patiently with me as my free time is devoted
to research and community causes,
with acknowledgments to John, Dorothy, Danny, Robby,
Maryann, Tom, Armand, and Ed,
the memory of Max, Stacy, and Cheim,
and those courageous women who grapple with the uncertainty
of breast cancer and silicone on a daily basis.

R. James Brenner

Contents

Contributors

Christina Ahn, M.D.
Plastic and Reconstructive Surgery
University of California, Los Angeles
School of Medicine
Los Angeles, CA

Lawrence W. Bassett, M.D.
Department of Radiological Sciences
Iris Cantor Center for Breast Imaging
University of California, Los Angeles
Los Angeles, CA

Nachman Brautbar, M.D.
Clinical Professor of Medicine
Department of Medicine
University of Southern California School of Medicine
Costa Mesa, CA

R. James Brenner, M.D., J.D.
Director of Breast Imaging
Eisenberg Keefer Breast Center
John Wayne Cancer Institute
St. Johns Hospital and Health Center
Associate Clinical Professor
Department of Radiological Sciences
University of California, Los Angeles
Los Angeles, CA

Gilda Cardenosa, M.D.
The Susan G. Koman Breast Center
St. Francis Medical Center
Peoria, IL

Nanette D. DeBruhl, M.D.
Department of Radiological Sciences
Iris Cantor Center for Breast Imaging
University of California, Los Angeles
Los Angeles, CA

G.W. Eklund, M.D.
The Susan G. Koman Breast Center
St. Francis Medical Center
Peoria, IL

Lenore I. Everson, M.D.
Assistant Professor
Director of Breast Imaging
University of Minnesota
Minneapolis, MN

Armando E. Giuliano, M.D.
Chief of Surgical Oncology
John Wayne Cancer Institute at
Saint John's Hospital and Health Center
Santa Monica, CA

David P. Gorczyca, M.D.
Radiology Specialists, LTD.
Director of Breast Imaging
Columbia Sunrise Hospital & Medical Center
Columbia Sunrise Mountain View Hospital
Las Vegas, NV
Assistant Clinical Professor
Iris Cantor Center for Breast Imaging
University of California, Los Angeles
Los Angeles, CA

J. Michael Guenther, M.D.
Attending Staff, Surgical Oncology
Assistant Director, Surgical Residency
Kaiser Permanente
Los Angeles, CA

Kathleen M. Harris, M.D.
Associate Professor of Radiology
Chief of Breast Imaging
University of Pittsburgh Medical Center
Medical Director Breast Imaging
Magee-Womens Hospital Breast Centers
Comprehensive Breast Center of Pittsburgh Cancer Institute
Pittsburgh, PA

Daniel J. Herling, J.D.
Gordon & Rees
San Francisco, CA

Nir Kossovsky, M.D.
Associate Professor
Department of Pathology and Laboratory Medicine
University of California, Los Angeles
Los Angeles, CA

M.S. Middleton, Ph.D., M.D.
Department of Radiology
University of California, San Diego Medical Center
San Diego, CA

Debra L. Monticciolo, M.D.
Director, Division of Breast Imaging
Emory University Hospital
Atlanta, GA

William Shaw, M.D.
Plastic and Reconstructive Surgery
University of California, Los Angeles
Los Angeles, CA

James Watson, M.D.
Plastic and Reconstructive Surgery
University of California, Los Angeles,
Los Angeles, CA

David K. Wellisch, Ph.D.
Professor-in-Residence
Department of Psychiatry
University of California, Los Angeles,
School of Medicine
Los Angeles, CA

Aristo Vojdani, Ph.D.
Drew University School of Medicine and Science
Madison, NJ

Preface

Silicone. A product as ubiquitous in every day life as is the earth element silicone from which it is derived. A substance which serves as a paradigm for the combined efforts between modern medicine and industry. A topic in which the worlds of science and business and politics collide.

The emergence of cosmetic procedures to afford women breast augmentation has been a pioneering effort that has brought great personal satisfaction to more than 2 million women in this country. Much of this work has employed silicone breast implants. Such implants, like any medical devise, are subject to failure. When failure occurs under circumstances that are both difficult to detect and of unknown significance, the history of a product's development is reviewed. When that history is obscured by both the process and substance of development, then fears of misconduct arise.

The fear of circumstances surrounding the augmented breast is a very real one in society today. Concerns about rupture and leakage, pain and paresthesia, psychological trauma and autoimmune disease have challenged both the medical community and the courts to find answers and accountability.

There are several areas in medicine today that invite strong emotional responses from those within and outside the profession. Whenever issues of health are at stake, public scrutiny of the scientific process should be expected. The public depends on rigorous protection in medicine, which includes prescribed processes of ongoing peer review and regulation of industry. If that process is either untested or abridged, fears emerge that may or may not be justified. The fear itself is an unwelcomed component of any public discussion.

Our most powerful weapon against fear is knowledge. In this book, we have brought reviews of experts from all medical disciplines together in an attempt to define what is and what is not known regarding the augmented breast. Imaging experts have helped define the potentials and limitations of mammography, ultrasonography, computed tomography, and magnetic resonance imaging in detecting integrity of the multitude of different implants, and even their relationship to detecting tumors. General and reconstructive surgeons discuss operations regarding the augmented breast and pathologists consider the physiology of tissue response. Immunologists consider the body's physical reaction to augmentation and psychiatrists focus on the emotional reactions. Finally, legal commentary is provided to place the concepts of science and the law into perspective. Each author has provided a thorough overview of the respective subject with conclusions necessarily extended from their own perspectives.

The publishing of a text on a subject matter in which definitive answers will not be known for years is a task which invites criticism. We believe that the absence of a text, where expert opinions are brought into one forum for reference by physicians of all disciplines (i.e., radiologists, surgeons, internists) and the lay public, is a far greater dilemma. In a field where many questions cannot be answered, those involved in public discussion need to be as informed as possible about all the aspects of the augmented breast if that discourse is to be constructive.

Foreword

LAWRENCE W. BASSETT, M.D.

It is estimated that between 1 and 2 million women have undergone breast augmentation. The great majority of breast implants are of the silicone gel type. Breast implants are subject to a variety of complications, including hardening and rupture. Implants also limit the ability to detect breast cancers with mammography. Recently, it has been postulated that silicone implants may increase the risk for connective tissue diseases and some other systemic illnesses. Motivated by increasing concerns about the safety of silicone implants, the Food and Drug Administration has imposed a ban on their use, except under specific conditions. Coverage of these issues by the mass media has sparked unparalleled anxiety, fear, and anger among women with implants.

These patients have many questions for radiologists and other clinicians, such as whether mammography could damage their implants. A variety of imaging modalities have been employed to evaluate the integrity of breast implants. Thus, it has become important to learn everything we can about breast implants and implant imaging. Unfortunately, the information that is available is dispersed in a large number of journals from several different specialties. Furthermore, published data about implants is not always correct, conclusions are not always based on scientific evidence, and some studies have reported divergent findings. Because of these obstacles, there is a real need for a comprehensive resource that covers the full range of issues concerning breast implants, critically evaluates the literature, and provides appropriate imaging strategies and diagnostic criteria.

This textbook meets the challenge. Chapters 1 through 4 provide the reader with an excellent overview of breast augmentation, including an introduction to the psychosocial aspects of breast implantation, surgical approaches to breast augmentation and explantation, and the types and classifications of implants that are encountered in clinical practice. Chapters 5 through 10 provide an exhaustive review of each of the imaging modalities that are used to evaluate the augmented breast (mammography, ultrasonography, computed tomography, and magnetic resonance imaging), including comparisons of the effectiveness of each of these modalities. Chapters 11 and 12 address tumor detection and treatment in the augmented breast. In these two chapters the authors carefully delineate the potential successes and pitfalls of breast cancer detection and the surgical treatment of patients with breast augmentation. Chapters 13 and 14 review pathology and immunology specific to breast implants. I particularly appreciated the review of basic principles of pathophysiology and immunology prior to the presentation of the relevant literature. Chapter 15 is a primer on the medical–legal aspects of breast implants. Public alarm has been accompanied by widespread lawsuits against individual physicians, as well as product liability suits against the corporations that produce silicone implants. Therefore, this chapter is important reading for all physicians who are now involved in delivering medical care to patients with breast implants.

The Augmented Breast: Radiological and Clinical Perspectives is unique in its breadth and scope, thoroughness, and clear writing. Every chapter in this book has been written by recognized experts in their field. The result is a long-awaited, comprehensive, and definitive textbook on this very timely subject.

1

The Silicone Controversy: A Brief History of the Problem

R. JAMES BRENNER AND DAVID P. GORCZYCA

Two years after undergoing a mastectomy and an 8-week course of radiation therapy for cancer of the right breast, a young woman elected breast reconstruction. Five years later, on the advice of another physician, she elected to undergo a second reconstruction involving a breast implant and autologous tissue. The surgery was uneventful, but shortly thereafter she suffered complications of the wound including infection and tissue necrosis. During this time, she claimed to have made repeated attempts to discuss the clinical circumstances with her surgeon. The patient sued, but her lawsuit was dismissed by the trial court. A federal appeals court in New Mexico reversed the trial court decision, and reinstated the case.[1] The lawsuit was not alleging defect in or rupture of the breast implant, or delay in diagnosis of breast cancer, or pain associated with the first reconstruction, or improper informed consent, or development of autoimmune disease. The lawsuit was for the negligent infliction of mental distress.

Since 1992 when the United States Food and Drug Administration (FDA) issued its recommendations on the future use and monitoring of women with breast silicone implants, an intense and focused discussion has emerged regarding the ramifications of breast reconstruction and augmentation. Almost inseparable from the national (international) priority given to prevention, early detection, and treatment of breast cancer, concern by and for women with breast implants continues to increase in the scientific community, the lay community, and in the courts, with far-reaching ramifications.

The sense of well-being, for both the woman who has undergone cancer therapy and seeks to normalize her life with reconstruction as well as the woman whose self-image is improved with augmentation, is a complex psychological dynamic that cannot be reduced to simple terms. The availability of such surgery has been a welcomed technology for many women. As with any medical intervention, potential risks and complications may result. Decisions based on available scientific information and knowledge of the potentials and limitations of monitoring the consequences of such surgery are the essence of informed personal choice.

Breast augmentation and reconstruction is not a recent phenomenon. In 1895 Czerny transplanted a patient's lipoma (encapsulated fatty tissue) from one portion of her body to her breast in helping to resolve a surgical defect created by the removal of a benign adenoma.[2] Beginning in the early 1900s, liquid paraffin was injected directly into the breast for purposes of augmentation, the complications of which were reported as early as 1912 by Hollander. Mixtures of petroleum jelly and olive oil created hard masses or "knots" sometimes called paraffinomas, in addition to inflammation, tissue necrosis, draining sinus tracts, and even pulmonary embolism. In the 1950s similar injections of liquid silicone (polydimethylsiloxane) were performed, first in Japan and then in the United States. Silicone injections were used with the assumption that the desired cosmetic enlargement of the breast could be accomplished uneventfully by what was considered to be a new, chemically inert derivative of sand (silica). However, the same hard masses (siliconomas) and inflammatory sequelae that occurred with paraffin injections also occurred with silicone injections. Subsequently, reports from Japan of women undergoing liquid silicone injections and suffering autoimmune symptoms led the FDA to ban such injections in 1965. By then, many women had undergone silicone injections, and the silicone could not be removed. The women were suffering painful hardening sometimes referred to as "silicone mastopathy."

The number of women with known silicone injections is virtually impossible to reckon. It has been estimated, as one indicator, that over 10,000 women in the entertainment-oriented city of Las Vegas, Nevada, have undergone silicone injections.[3]

Interest in placement of prostheses instead of free injection of foreign material began to emerge in the early 1950s. Sponge prostheses of ivalon or polyvinyl alcohol, as well as polystan tapes rolled into a ball, polyurethane, polypropylene, and polytef (Teflon) were considered as candidates for prostheses. However, clinical observations of infection, shrinkage, and tissue necrosis prompted early removal of such implants.

In 1962 Cronin at Baylor College of Medicine in Houston developed the first silicone prosthesis, and together with Gerow who had completed similar work, found that a hardened form of silicone could be chemically developed from longer chains of the basic polymer (poly)dimethylsiloxane to enclose the liquid form of silicone. The first silicone prostheses were manufactured for general use by Dow Corning Wright, a subsidiary in Arlington, Tennessee of Dow Corning, which is headquartered in Midland, Michigan. As a foreign body, the implant was expected to elicit a fibrous scar or capsule that would surround the silicone shell and contain its contents, preventing migration. However, implants were found to migrate, to rupture, and to cause in some individuals a fibrous reaction sufficient to deform the implant and elicit pain (capsule contraction).

Design modifications by various manufacturers followed. Earliest implants included gels, which were more viscous and easier to remove from an implant pocket if ruptured. These are described later in the text. However, to provide a more natural feeling, implant "responsive" gels containing shorter-chained diluent became available in the 1970s.[4] To provide a more stable anatomic relationship, Dacron patches were added on the posterior surface of the implants placed in the subglandular location abutting the pectoral muscle. To abate the complications of leakage of silicone and its sequelae, Jenny and the Heyer-Schulte Corporation began to market in 1968 an implant with a silicone envelope but filled instead with saline. To provide the firmness and texture of silicone but the presumed safety of saline, a double-lumen implant was developed, originally with a 9 : 1 ratio of silicone to saline, but with manufacturer-dependent specifications. Further variations included an inner saline component with an outer silicone component. To reduce the risk of capsular contracture, some models of silicone envelopes were coated with polyurethane foam. However, following the observation that such coating could be chemically broken down under laboratory conditions with the release of 2,4-toluene diamine (TDA), which has been implicated as a mammalian carcinogen, production of these implants was terminated. Approximately 10% of women with gel-filled implants received ones with polyurethane foam.

Modifications were also developed for the placement of breast implants. Preferred locations included the subglandular space superficial to the pectoral muscle, the subpectoral location, and sometimes the compartment deep to the latissimus dorsi. Both the number of implants (eg, "stacked implants") as well as the operative entrance site varied. For reconstruction and even cosmesis, implants were developed with injectable valves located in different locations. Many women were either not told or incorrectly informed as to both the type and location of their implants.[5]

It is estimated that nearly 2 million women currently have prosthetic breast implants, including more than 700 varieties. About 80% of these implants have been placed for cosmetic reasons.[6] Autologous reconstruction is technically difficult and expensive and approximately 400,000 women (20% of those with implants) who have undergone mastectomy have elected to have implant reconstruction instead of autologous flap reconstruction. Of more than 130,000 women who underwent breast augmentation in 1990, 65% were under the age of 35.[7] Whether filled with silicone gel or saline, prosthetic breast implants, as mentioned, are surrounded by a silicone polymer, a "foreign body" that has prompted a reevaluation of the manufacturing of silicone, its known and suspected biologic implications, and its regulation in the marketplace.

Until 1976 no governmental agency assumed jurisdiction in the regulation of medical devices, and thus manufacturing entities maintained internal research and development responsibility for their safety and use. Although the FDA was granted authorization to regulate such devices at that time, it was not until 1988 that Commissioner Frank Young requested safety data from implant makers. In 1990 the agency under Acting Commissioner James Benson asked manufacturers of breast implants to file for FDA approval. In November 1991 the FDA's General and Plastic Surgery Devices Panel conducted three days of public hearings and found that no sponsor had met the statutory requirements for safety and effectiveness. The panel recommended that the devices remain on the market while clinical tests be conducted to address safety concerns. The panel also recommended that manufacturers provide data on preclinical studies that were either inadequate or missing in the submission process of premarket approval applications. In addition, a registry of these devices was recommended, together with a process of informed consent to fully indicate to patients the potential risks and benefits.

On January 6, 1992 FDA Commissioner David A. Kessler requested a voluntary moratorium on further use of silicone gel breast implants, pending additional FDA advisory panel hearings. In March an internal Public Health Service Breast Task Force on Silicone Breast Implants was established by the US Department of Health and Human Services. Following extensive testimony and considerable public attention in the lay media, and coincident with emerging lawsuits against manufacturers regarding breast implants, the FDA announced its guidelines and restrictions regarding the use of silicone gel-filled breast implants on April 16, 1992. In January 1992 the Canadian Department of National Health and Welfare suspended distribution of implants.

Not addressing saline-filled implants, which are surrounded by a silicone envelope, the FDA provided for the use of silicone gel implants under selected circumstances with the intent that all future implants would be subjected to clinical studies. Indicating a public health benefit of gel implants to women who have undergone mastectomy due to treatment for cancer, trauma, and developmental malformation, silicone gel implants would be permitted for reconstructive purposes under three circumstances or stages, the last stage including some women desiring implants for cosmetic purposes.[8]

Stage I, Urgent Need Exemption, permitted immediate access to implants if the woman's physician certified that she was appropriately assigned to one of three categories: women with temporary tissue expanders due to be replaced by gel implants; women with gel implants who require replacement for medical reasons such as rupture, gel leakage, or severe contracture; and women having mastectomies before clinical studies were in place and for whom immediate reconstruction at the time of mastectomy was medically and surgically more appropriate than delayed implantation, with additional documentation by the physician that saline-filled implants were not a satisfactory alternative. Stage I patients were required to sign a special form certifying that they had been told about the risks of implants, and that they agreed to enroll in a registry in order to be notified in the future, if necessary, about new information regarding their implants.

Stage II, Adjunct Clinical Protocol, included any woman who required gel-filled implants for reconstruction under studies established by implant manufacturers and approved by the FDA. This category included women who had breast cancer surgery, severe injury to the breast, or a medical condition causing severe anatomic abnormalities, in addition to women who required an existing implant replaced for medical reasons. The indications were similar to those in stage I, but were less urgent, and included provisions for similar disclosure of risks, informed consent, and registry enrollment. Stage II was distinguished from stage I by its design to include women only after deliberate clinical trials had been established and approved.

Stage III, Core Clinical Protocol, includes patients for both reconstruction and augmentation procedures and is designed to prospectively study each specific model of silicone implant that manufacturers wish to keep on the market. More detailed safety questions will be investigated, such as the incidence of rupture, contracture, psychological benefits of implant, and impact of explantation. In addition to manufacturer-sponsored studies, a study is being conducted under the sponsorship of the National Cancer Institute (NCI), part of the National Institutes of Health (NIH). Funding for research and clinical investigation and explantation is also provided by other manufacturers, in part a response to legal settlements.[9] Stage III also requires information regarding risks, enrollment in a registry, and informed consent.

In 1992 the FDA received 21,968 adverse Medical Device Reports from companies, and in 1993 more than 20,000 reports were filed. Over the two years, patients and clinicians filed an additional 2000 reports.[10] While the safety of implants will now be the subject of investigation, a large number of lawsuits have emerged regarding their development and use. By 1994 more than 6000 lawsuits were filed in this country by women who claimed injury related to silicone implants, including issues of breast cancer, birth defects, and autoimmune disease.[11] Most of these suits were filed against manufacturers, but a significant portion were also filed against physicians. The extent to which class-action lawsuits and negotiated settlements will mitigate individual legal actions is difficult to predict.

More than 100 medical devices include silicone, such as artificial joints, blood-vessel grafts, and heart valves. First synthesized in 1938, silicone has found extensive practical value as a lubricant, sealant, insulator, and coolant. One of Dow Corning's first silicone products, Silly Putty, was widely marketed for children in the 1950s. Forms of silicone are used to coat hypodermic needles and plastic syringes for ease of injection and as antiflatulents in over-the-counter medications (eg, simethicone). Silicone gel used in implants, however, differs from other silicone products, and a brief consideration of its chemistry is useful to understand some of the controversies regarding its safety. A more detailed analysis of the chemical properties of various forms may be found elsewhere.[12]

The element silicon is ubiquitous, existing in many forms. Silicates are found in beer, and usually remain water soluble. Crystalline silicon dioxide—also known as silica—is a major component of sand, and can be found in a large percentage of the earth's crust. Silicone dioxide may act as an adjuvant and has been implicated in autoimmune disorders suffered by individuals suffering increased exposure to this material, such as sand blasters. Most commercial silicone is produced by reducing silica (sand) to elemental silicon and allowing it to react with methyl chloride and water to produce linear or cyclic low-molecular-weight methyl siloxanes, a simple example being dimethylsiloxane (dimethicone). The most prevalent siloxane of this process, octamethylcyclotetrasiloxane, is treated with silanoate catalysts to form high-molecular-weight polydimethylsiloxane linear polymers, the silicone that is used in silicone gel implants.

Thus, silicone polymers are characterized by carbon (usually methyl groups) to silicon (organosilicon) bonds or linkages and silicon-oxygen-silicone (siloxane) bonds, although other groups may be substituted for the methyl group to alter chemical and physical properties (eg, resistance to solvent).

Platinum and hydride-containing polymers may be added to the gel.[13] Silicone envelopes contain chains where some of the methyl groups may be replaced by trifluoropropyl and phenyl groups supplemented with the addition of fumed silica of an amorphous or particulate (10–15 μm) type.

Depending on the length of the chain and type of cross-linking, organosiloxanes may be produced as fluid, gel, gum (elastomer or rubber), foam, or resin. Viscosity is a function of average molecular weight and molecular number distribution of the polymer, with lower chain lengths producing a less viscous oil.

Silicone gel is found in breast, chin, testicular, and hiatal hernia implants. The gel fluid is contained in but not bound to the envelope, which contains a loose network of cross-linked chains. Components of the fluid or the fluid itself are capable of diffusing into and through the elastomeric envelope or shell, a phenomenon known as "bleed." The phenyl and trifluoropropyl organosilicon components of the implant envelope are designed to minimize gel bleed, but they do not eliminate the process. In 1978 Barker and colleagues[14] concluded that all silicone gel implants underwent gel bleed, regardless of molecular weight. In addition to gel bleed, silicone particles may shed from envelope surfaces.[15] Thus silicone implants that have not ruptured may still be associated with silicone beyond the fibrous capsule, accounting for its image-defined or palpable presence in lymph nodes (intramammary or axillary) as well as in other parts of the body to which it has been transported.

The considerable variability of silicone polymers precludes a universal determination of their safety. Rather, each compound requires individual evaluation of its properties with respect to biologic mobility and activity.[12] The presumption that silicone is chemically "inert" is likely based on the obtuse bond angle between carbon and oxygen permitting freer rotation of the organic groups on silicon and making the siloxane bond environment less accessible for chemical reactivity.[16] Silicone implants (or injected silicone) by definition are not biologically inert because as a foreign body an inflammatory response is both anticipated and created, leading to the fibrous capsule that surrounds the implant. The extent to which both chemical and biologic reactivity of both implanted silicone and possible breakdown products exists is the subject of much investigation and will be discussed in later chapters.[17]

Much of the research and many of the FDA criteria for enrollment in its protocols is concerned with the presence of free silicone in the breast. The ability therefore to identify silicone beyond the confines of the envelope preoperatively has been the subject of much investigation in the imaging community. Identification of free silicone in the breast, in a patient who has not had a prior implant removed or undergone silicone injections, is presumptive evidence for a ruptured implant envelope and capsule. Identification of silicone within the capsule but beyond the envelope may represent gel bleed or a ruptured envelope. Detection of silicone within lymph nodes may reflect different processes in different individuals.

Determining the location of silicone provides an important anatomic parameter in evaluating a woman with implants. The significance of imaging findings are reckoned by combining such information with clinical and psychosocial information. If reactivity to silicone is a universal phenomenon secondary to gel bleed, then the extent of exposure must be assessed, especially if there exists a relationship between biologic response and exposed silicone that is quantitative in nature (eg, dose-response relationship). Imaging of silicone provides a basis for analysis. Deliberate use of imaging requires an understanding of the potentials and limitations of different methods. Because of the large numbers of women involved, a form of cost-benefit analysis in the context of the clinical situation is prudent. It should be recalled that imaging remains of paramount importance in such patients—as in all women—in the detection of nonpalpable malignancies.

On the other hand, evaluation of the individual patient depends on more than simply defining the presence and location of silicone gel. The development of capsular contraction, the risk of relieving the pain associated with such contraction by manual manipulation (closed capsulotomy), and the possibility of identifiable disease secondary to silicone exposure are parameters that need to be assessed in addition to the image-defined presence of silicone.

Both the clinical and imaging parameters of silicone exposure need to be considered in the context of the woman's sense of well-being, a condition that is the basis upon which implantation is usually predicated. Even this parameter is complicated when that decision is modified by emerging information regarding the potential complications of silicone. The degree to which new information affects the initial decision to undergo implantation is only now emerging as an area for investigation. In addition, newfound interest in evaluation of both corporate and political forces in the development and regulation of implants is being generated from many interested parties.

As is inferred from the FDA protocols, the "failing" implant may be defined by clinical, imaging, and social parameters. The history of surgical augmentation of the breast for either reconstructive or cosmetic reasons, and the sequelae following implantation reflect the interactions involving all three parameters, combined with issues of regulation, research, and development. The importance of self-image is one that cannot easily be measured, and decisions by the individual woman regarding risks and benefits of interventions that have impact on well-being are not easily subjected to a standardized frame of reference. Nonetheless, both public discussion and personal decision making is served by informed opinion. It is to this purpose that this book has brought together expert authorities in the field to assist in the evaluation of the augmented breast.

Women experiencing problems with their breast that they feel are related to implants or women seeking further information should contact the United States Pharmacopeia (UPO), which is under contract to FDA to collect and organize problems. The address is 12601 Twinbrook Parkway, Rockville, MD 20852, Attn: Dr. Joseph Valentino.

REFERENCES

1. Whalley v Sakura, 804 F.2d 580 (C.A.10, N.M., Oct 19, 1986).
2. Letterman G, Schurter M. History of aesthetic breast surgery. In: Goldwyn RM, ed. *Plastic and Reconstructive Surgery of the Breast.* Boston: Little, Brown; 1976:3–36.
3. Vinnik CA. Silicone mastopathy. In: Owsley JQ Jr, Peterson RA, eds. *Symposium on Aesthetic Surgery of the Breast,* vol. 18. St. Louis: CV Mosby; 1978:151–155.
4. Grody GS. Silicone technology for the plastic surgeon. *Clin Plast Surg.* 1988;15:517–525.
5. Berg WA, Caskey CI, Hamper UM. Single- and double-lumen silicone breast implant integrity: prospective evaluation of MR and US criteria. *Radiology.* 1995;197:45–52.
6. Stinback B, Sisson Hardt N. Breast implants, common complications, and concurrent breast disease. *Radiographics.* 1993;13:95–105.
7. Sanchez-Guerrero J, Schur PH, Sergent JS, et al. *Arthritis Rheum.* 1994;37:158–168.
8. *Update on Silicone Gel-Filled Breast Implants.* Rockville, MD: Department of Health and Human Services, Food and Drug Administration; May 25, 1992.
9. Roan S. Time not on their side, say women with implants. *Los Angeles Times,* May 18, 1993, pp. E1, E8.
10. Kessler DA, Merkatz RB, Shapiro R. A call for higher standards for breast implants (commentary). *JAMA.* 1993;270: 2607–2608.
11. McCormick B. Physicians insurers fear flood of implant liability suits. *AMA News,* July 19, 1993, pp. 3, 27.
12. Council on Scientific Affairs, American Medical Association. Silicone gel breast implants. *JAMA.* 1993;270:2602–2606.
13. Claman HN, Robertson AD. Antinuclear antibodies and breast implants. *West J Med.* 1994;160:225–228.
14. Barker PE, Retshy MI, Schultz S. "Bleeding" of silicone from bag-gel breast implants and its clinical relation to fibrous capsule reaction. *Plast Reconstr Surg.* 1978;61:836–841.
15. Teuber SS, Yoshida H, Gershwin ME. Immunopathologic effects of silicone breast implants. *West J Med.* 1995;162: 418–425.
16. Chedd G. *Half-Way Elements: The Technology of Metalloids.* Garden City, NY: Doubleday; 1969:117–148.
17. The breast implant controversy: an interview with Dow Corning scientists. *Epidemiol Monitor.* 1992;13:1–14.

2

Psychosocial Aspects of Breast Implantation

DAVID K. WELLISCH

This chapter explores the complex interaction of psychological factors with regard to breast augmentation for cosmesis, and in the case of breast reconstruction postmastectomy. The chapter addresses six main areas: (1) motivation factors for breast augmentation; (2) psychological outcomes/impacts of augmentation; (3) assessment of psychopathology in patients prior to surgery, including areas for evaluation, potential contraindications for surgery, and psychopathology of the body experience; (4) the collaboration of plastic surgeons and mental health professionals; (5) psychological issues in breast reconstruction postmastectomy; and (6) psychological issues in explantation.

The nexus of the interface between these psychological factors and the breast augmentation experience is the patient's body image. This writer is in substantial agreement with Pruzinsky and Cash[1] as to the importance of several of their thematic concepts about body image: (1) "Body images are multifaceted." These may include aspects such as perceptions and attitudes about one's appearance, body size estimations, body competence, and gender-linked aspects. Breast implant surgeries may have impact on any or all of these aspects. (2) "Body image experiences are intertwined with feelings about the self." The development of the self and self-image is fundamentally influenced by identification with, and internalizations from, significant others, especially parents. Thus, physical features shared with parents and conflicts with or about parents become amalgamated into body image perceptions. This may lead to difficulties in changing body image perceptions in a satisfactory fashion for the patient even after surgery is performed. (3) "Body images are socially determined." Beyond parental attitudes about bodies and body functions are societal attitudes and impacts. These societal standards, which are by no means static or unchanging, have powerful influences on motivations, attitudes, and perceptions around body image. Thus, breast surgery and the psychological experience are mediated by the body image, which is made up by both conscious and unconscious experiences.

■ MOTIVATIONAL FACTORS TO UNDERGO BREAST AUGMENTATION

A series of studies has directly addressed this issue in the period of the 1960s to 1990s. In one uncontrolled study, in a series of women seeking augmentation mammoplasty, 60% were viewed to have depression, low self-esteem, and hysterical traits.[2] Another such study, based on scores on psychological tests, reported breast augmentation patient-subjects to be insecure, inadequate, and prone to impulsive behavior.[3] Several problems may exist with these earlier evaluations: (1) lack of evaluators being blind to knowledge that all patient-subjects were seeking augmentation; (2) lack of ability to make diagnoses from psychological test data; (3) problems with validity and reliability of psychiatric diagnostic classification systems—these systems have had three major revisions since the 1960s; and (4) most importantly, lack of appropriate control groups.

In a systematic study done in the United States that compared women seeking augmentation mammoplasty with two control groups (one, a group of women with average bust size not seeking surgery; two, a group of women with small bust size not seeking surgery), several significant differences differentiated the augmentation group. The most powerful and consistent included lower evaluation of breast in general, higher body self-consciousness, and a perception of their breasts as less potent than the average-breasted women but not different from the small-breasted women. Almost none of the purely psychological variables were significantly different among the three groups.[4] A second controlled study done in Sweden compared women seeking augmentation mammoplasty with women from general surgery ear, nose, and throat clinics. The groups were closely matched on age. Data were gathered by interview and one psychological test. Several significant differences emerged differentiating the augmentation group: (1) significantly more negative attitudes toward relationships to both mothers and fathers, with fathers being the most significantly negative; (2) significantly more indifferent or negative perceptions of their relationships to spouses; (3) very significant self-consciousness about the unclothed bodies with husbands, children, and other women; and (4) significantly more visits to a psychiatrist (51% vs. 21%).[5] A third controlled study in South Africa randomly selected 20 augmentation mammoplasty patients and 20 patient controls from the general medical wards. Controls who were dissatisfied with their breasts were not included. Groups were matched for age and socioeconomic status. Data were collected via interview plus one projective psychological test. Again, several significant differences emerged differentiating the augmentation mammoplasty group: (1) lower evaluations of childhood relationships with parents; (2) poorer body image evaluation; (3) significantly higher evaluation of sexual dysfunction in the self; and (4) avoidance of nudity with the partner.[6]

A more recent study in England compared three groups of women. One group was on a waiting list for augmentation mammoplasty, one group was on a waiting list for breast reduction, and one group was demographically similar but requesting no breast cosmetic surgery. Data were collected by means of a mailed questionnaire. Response rates were very good for mail-out surveys by all groups. As previously, several significant differences differentiated the augmentation group: (1) a significantly higher rate of divorce than the other two groups; (2) a greater wish to feel feminine as a motivation for surgery; (3) a greater wish to be less shy with men as a motivation for surgery; and (4) a greater sense of embarrassment undressing as a motivation for surgery.[7] The common factors from these controlled studies are as follows:

- Higher body self-consciousness
- Lower evaluation of breast attractiveness
- Avoidance of nudity, especially with partner/spouse
- Suggestion of childhood relational problems with parents where patient may have felt inadequate or disappointing.

These four controlled studies cannot be accepted as conclusive given the overall modest number of patients studied. However, the similarity of conclusions in the light of the wide geographic, cultural, and patient differences is striking. Some of the common themes such as self-consciousness and lower evaluations of breast attractiveness are obvious and would be expected. The findings on parent-child alienation are less obvious and are provocative. The notion of lack of parental validation and acceptance becoming integrated into the child's self-image and ultimately body image appears worthy of further investigation. The step from this to an adult searching for an intervention to elevate a sense of self and other acceptability seems logical and therefore predictable.

■ IMPACTS ON PSYCHOLOGICAL FUNCTIONING/OUTCOME

Table 2–1 reflects methodologic, medical, and psychosocial outcomes in four studies of augmentation mammoplasty.[8–11] These four studies, two American and two Swedish, report on a total of 346 patients. Follow-up among the four studies ranges from 3 months to 60 months, with an overall average follow-up period of approximately 19 months across the four studies. The methodology of these follow-up studies varies from face-to-face interviews to mail-out questionnaires. It was not clear if in some instances the interviewer/assessor was the operating surgeon. This could possibly bias the data in the direction of the patient inflating positive ratings to try to please the surgeon. Another important methodologic issue is percentage of follow-up response from the augmented population, which ranged from 94% of the original surgically augmented population[10] to only 30% of the original population.[11] It is fair to assume in the latter study that among the 70% of patients unable to be followed up, negative feelings and outcomes might well exist. However, regardless of these methodologic problems and differences, the outcomes, even across these very different cultural groups, bear a striking similarity. Satisfaction with the procedures ranges from 84 to 96%, either in the form of willingness to do it again, or in direct ratings of satisfaction. This was in spite of variable percentages of implant hardening, which varied across studies from 17% to 59%.[8,10] These variations in hardening, as pointed out by Hetter,[9] may result from differences in implants (gel vs. saline) or surgical techniques (inframammary vs. periareolar). The uniformly high levels of satisfaction appear to override the medical complications even when the complications are at a relatively high level as in the Ohlsen et al[8] study. An important issue that was addressed in two of the studies was psychiatric symptomatology and the needs for psychiatric intervention. In the Meyer and Ringberg[10] study the finding of 33% with brief postoperative depression should not be confused with pathologic reactivity to the procedure or increased needs for psychiatric intervention. Alternatively this can be viewed as expected and normal reactive depression to a surgical proce-

Table 2–1. Psychosocial Outcomes of Augmentation Mammaplasty

Study	*Number Followed*	*Length of Follow-up*	*Assessment Measures*	*Results*
Ohlsen, Ponten, and Hambert, 1978	71 (82% of original sample)	1–5 years	1. Ratings of surgery by surgeon, RN, aide, photographer 2. 37 chosen at random for psychiatric interviews 3. All interviewed about physical problems,	59% had implant hardening 84% "very satisfied" (highest rating) with outcome 11% "doubtful" or "dissatisfied" with results Gross discrepancies between surgeons' evaluations of results and evaluations of other raters (surgeon more likely to rate "very good" (48% vs 13%) Postoperative need for psychiatric treatment diminished
Hetter, 1979	165 (69% of original sample)	17–29 months (average 22.5 months)	Mailed questionnaire	40% had implant hardening 91% had improved self-image 53% rated sex life as improved, 2.5% rated sex life as worsened 47% rated self as more outgoing 96.5% would repeat procedure 96% met expectations
Meyer & Ringberg, 1987	36 (94% of original sample) 33 matched surgical controls	12 months	Interview	17% had implant hardening 86% satisfied with result of surgery 43% now accepted sexual breast touch (0% preoperatively) 36% had more frequent coitus Short-term postoperative depression in 33% (median duration 7 days)
Kilmann, Sattler, and Taylor, 1987	75 (30% of original sample)	3–36 months	Mailed questionnaire	Women in same relationship pre/post (group I) surgery reported positive effects of surgery on relationships, but less than expected Group I women reported significantly elevated effects of surgery on self-image, sense of attractiveness, and estimation of body Women *not* in same relationship pre/post surgery (group II), reported positive (nonsignificant) effects of surgery on self-esteem, sense of attractiveness, and estimation of body

dure. This surgery can have acute sequelae including gradual metabalization of anesthesia, pain, use of narcotics for pain, and sleep disruption secondary to pain. All of these factors can singly or jointly contribute to transient postoperative depressive symptoms. These symptoms will usually remit with biologic restabilization and standard emotional support. The fact that this was noted and reported reflects a sensitivity in this research group that is noteworthy.

Another interesting and important outcome variable is that of sexuality and sexual activity. The figures for improvement in frequency of sexual intercourse, accepting breast-oriented sexual fondling, and general rating of sexual life range from 36 to 53%.[9,10] Thus, augmentation mammoplasty appears more prone to change self-image than sexual behavior or evaluation of the sexual relationship. The Kilmann et al[11] study makes an important distinction between impact on the longer-term ongoing relationship and impact on the individual who is either dating or in a newly formed or shorter-term relationship. It appears that augmentation mammoplasty may be synergistic with a long-term sexual and emotional relationship, where anxiety is low regarding commitment. However, the data in the Kilmann et al study appear to show that augmentation mammoplasty cannot bolster the anxiety and insecurity so often present in dating or newly found relationships in terms of increasing estimations or ratings of sexual quality of life. Even for the group with long-term relationships, however, the effects of the surgery on the relationship were less than expected.

As previously noted, four studies on 346 patients may not present a complete picture of outcome. However, the findings, regardless of methodology of investigation, national setting, or length of time (short vs. medium term), appear to point in the direction of satisfaction. This satisfaction is present in spite of medical complications and seems to more greatly influence body image than sexual behavior or the quality of one's sexual relationship. While expected, transient psychiatric adjustment reactions may be present, psychiatric decompensation and increased utilization of psychiatric services postmammoplasty does not appear to be part of the outcome picture.

■ ASSESSMENT OF PSYCHOSOCIAL FACTORS IN PATIENTS PRIOR TO AUGMENTATION MAMMOPLASTY

In a fundamental article in this area, Edgerton et al[12] present the basic reality that most patients requesting plastic surgery, in this case augmentation mammoplasty, will present with symptoms such as self-consciousness, social inhibition, anxiety, and depression. The question then becomes how to sort out those that are significantly more psychologically disturbed, and what to do or not to do with these patients. After surgical experiences with 87 significantly psychiatrically disturbed patients with an average of 6.2 years follow-up, the Edgerton group recommends four basic psychosocial issues to evaluate presurgically:

1. What are the patient's motivations for surgery? Edgerton et al differentiate *internal* motivations from *external* motivations. An example of an internal motivation for augmentation mammoplasty would be improvement of a long-term feeling of self-consciousness over being extremely small-breasted. An example of an external motivation would be the desire to improve a dull marriage, or to engage the attention of a chronically "workaholic" spouse. The internally motivated patient is viewed as more likely to achieve her expectations with such a surgery. Our own research in the area of postmastectomy breast reconstruction would also validate this finding, with internal motivations (eg, "to feel more balanced," "to feel more feminine") being much more frequent motivations than external motivations (eg, "to improve my marital relationship").[13]
2. What are the patient's expectations regarding surgery? Edgerton et al point out that patient expectations extend on a continuum from realistic to unrealistic to frankly delusional. They note that patients with delusional expectations cling to these expectations in spite of education and confrontation. This is to be expected with delusions, which have both defensive aspects as well as psychotic distortions of reality. An example of a delusion around augmentation mammoplasty would be a woman with lifelong and chronic self-image and psychological problems expecting she will be discovered and become a film star after surgery. This would represent a defense against the pain of the ordinariness of her life as well as a gross distortion of the realities of her personality, life situation, and fundamental physical presence. Edgerton et al point out such delusional expectations become a criterion for rejection for surgery.
3. What is the patient's level of psychological functioning? The Edgerton group placed their 87 patients in a triadic distribution ranging from moderate to mid-level to severe psychological disturbance of personality organization and functioning. The moderately disturbed group had evidence of psychological symptoms (anxiety, depression, self-consciousness) at a level to influence but not control or disable their work and social lives. They would be most likely to be classified in the neurotic range of personality organization and functioning. There is little doubt they would be helped by surgery.

The mid-range group, as perceived by the Edgerton group, had psychological disturbances at a level sufficient to dominate their lives in relation to their sense of deformity. Edgerton et al viewed them as maintaining limited occupational and social functioning. They would be most likely to be classified in the borderline range of personality organization and functioning. This writer would view this group as most difficult to assess and most volatile to manage for the plastic surgeon in the augmentation mammoplasty context. This population is not always easy to characterize or diagnose in the first meeting or even series of meetings. They may, especially with certain subtypes of borderline personality disorders, have a history of occupational achievements that are extremely impressive. This can be in contrast to the Edgerton group's finding of uniformly low occupational functioning.[12] This may be especially true for the narcissistic personality disordered patient who may, in fact, be a high-frequency candidate for breast surgery. Several key variables in the basic borderline personality disorder present potential pitfalls for the plastic surgeon: (a) a pattern of unstable and intense interpersonal relationships characterized by alternating between extremes of idealization and devaluation—this pattern can easily and quickly extend to the doctor-patient relationship; (b) identity disturbance—markedly and persistently unstable self-image or sense of self; who you see and know on one occasion can seem profoundly different on another visit or occasion; (c) affective instability due to a marked reactivity of mood (eg, intense episodic dysphoria, irritability, or anxiety); (d) inappropriate anger or difficulty controlling anger; and (e) transient, stress-related paranoid ideation or severe dissociative symptoms. These can effectively extinguish a working doctor-patient alliance.[14] Many or all of these factors can be latent and only stimulated by episodes of stress. Unfortunately, the plastic surgery context can be laden with many interpersonal and physical stresses. What may be tolerable and unnoticed by the neurotic patient may be provocative and overwhelming for the borderline patient. The pattern of psychological decompensation by the borderline patient is extremely rapid. The difference between the borderline and the psychotic patient is that the borderline will just as rapidly *recompensate* while the psychotic will not recompensate rapidly.

The severely disturbed group was characterized by Edgerton et al[12 (p 596)] as having "their entire lives dominated by their delusional sense of deformity." Body dysmorphic disorder will be discussed in the next section. Edgerton et al viewed them as alienated, schizoid, and without ability to manage employment. They would be most likely to be classified in the psychotic range of personality organization and functioning. Of note in the Edgerton series, those 36 patients in this range had no greater negative psychological impact and just as much marked psychological improvement postsurgery as did the patients in the other two ranges of psychological adjustment.[12]

Thus, patients in the upper third and lower third of psychological adjustment are relatively easy to classify and predict. Patients in the middle third are relatively difficult to predict and classify.

4. Will the patient allow the time and number of sessions necessary to be intensively evaluated psychosocially, and also to develop therapeutic rapport with the prospective plastic surgeon and, *if necessary,* mental health professional? The patient who the surgeon feels requires this kind of evaluation and alliance building who cannot settle down and effectively participate probably is not a viable candidate for surgery. If an alliance cannot be developed prior to surgery, it is doubtful one can be built during and after surgery. The Edgerton group needed up to ten evaluation sessions, sometimes exceeding over a period of 2 years, to deal with patients in the more disturbed groups.[12]

■ CONTRAINDICATIONS FOR SURGERY

Seven potential psychosocial issues might either be "red flags" or contraindications for surgery (five are suggested by the Edgerton group, and two by this writer):

1. The noncompliant patient.[12] This is the patient in too great a hurry to comply with needed presurgical evaluations.
2. The noncommunicating patient.[12] This is the patient unable/unwilling to communicate the nature of her anatomical concerns. In addition, this is the patient with whom the surgeon and/or mental health professional perceives through nonverbal cues that what is felt or thought is not being communicated. Fear of rejection for surgery may underlie such hesitancy to articulate on the part of such patients.
3. The unrealistic patient.[12] This is the patient who has expectations that cannot be modified to mesh with what is realistically possible for surgery to provide as an outcome.
4. The overidealizing patient. This is a variant of the unrealistic patients. This is the patient who is flattering to the prospective surgeon in a fashion that is beyond reason, but may disguise unrealistic to delusional expectations. As related in the previous discussion of the patient with borderline personality dynamics, this overidealization can quickly boomerang into devaluation and paranoid rage with stress or disappointment.
5. The ambivalent patient. This is the patient who "just cannot make up my mind" no matter how intensive or broad a discussion is held. This patient may in a subtle or overt fashion pressure the surgeon to make a decision to proceed. Psychologically such a patient is not ready or able to proceed with surgery. This kind of ambivalence is usually a symptom of severe underlying anxiety, or a severe personality disorder such as dependent personality disorder or obsessive-compulsive personality disorder, or may reflect an underlying thought disorder reflected by incapacitating ambivalence.
6. The obsessively perfectionistic patient.[12] This is the patient who challenges the surgeon beyond his/her realistic skill level. This is a covariant of the unrealistic patient. Such patients make impossible demands on themselves and therefore will transfer such impossible demands onto the surgeon. Such obsessive perfectionism can be a defense against substantial underlying hostility and rage. Frequently in childhood such people have been required to meet impossible standards with substantial internalized frustration as a result.

7. The economically or geographically restricted patient.[12] This is the patient who cannot hope to meet the surgeon's needs for evaluation or fee because of sociodemographic factors. If the surgeon's needs are not met, this will almost certainly have impact on the doctor-patient alliance.

■ PSYCHOPATHOLOGY OF THE BODY EXPERIENCE

Psychopathology of the body experience is best defined in two major subgroups: (1) patients whose body image problem is *central* to the psychopathologic disorder, such as somatization disorder, conversion disorder, and body dismorphic disorder; and (2) patients whose body image disorder is *associated with* but not central to the psychopathology, such as patients with depression and sexual dysfunction.[15]

Disorders Where Body Image is Central

SOMATIZATION DISORDER

Somatization disorder now includes and integrates Briquet's syndrome (hysteria), formerly a separate diagnosis. Like all somatoform disorders, it is identified by the presence of physical symptoms that suggest a general medical condition, but is not explained satisfactorily by a general medical condition. Somatoform disorders are not reflective of malingering or factitious (self-caused) disorders, in that they are not intentional or under voluntary control.[16] Somatization disorder has as its essential feature recurring, clinically significant somatic complaints. Physical examination is remarkable in the absence of objective findings to substantiate these somatic complaints. The lifetime prevalence rates of somatization disorder in females ranges from 0.2 to 2.0%.[16] A crucial feature, both clinically and diagnostically, is a history of such complaints beginning prior to age 30, often long prior. Thus, it has become a "way of life" as termed by one authority on the somatizing disorders.[17] Somatization disorder to be diagnosed must include a history of such complaints before age 30, four pain symptoms, two gastrointestinal symptoms, one sexual symptom, and one pseudoneurologic symptom. These must not be intentionally produced, and cannot be fully explained by a known medical condition.[16] One issue of particular interest to plastic surgeons is the correlation between this disorder and polysurgery and polysurgical addiction. Several studies have shown this population to be far more likely than a control population (up to seven times more likely) to have undergone a minor or especially gynecologic surgical procedure.[18,19] A second issue of particular importance to the plastic surgeon is the drug seeking and drug dependence of patients with this diagnosis. This would involve drugs such as narcotic analgesics, hypnotics, and minor tranquilizers.[17]

CONVERSION DISORDER

Conversion disorder has as its essential feature the presence of symptoms or deficits affecting voluntary motor or sensory function that suggest a neurologic condition, but that are actually "psychoneurologic." The symptoms of a conversion disorder do not follow known anatomical pathways or physiologic mechanisms. Instead, they are inconsistent and follow what a patient might think a condition might reflect.[16] The basic notion of conversion implies the somatic symptom is a symbolized representation and resolution of an unconscious conflict. Such a symptomatic resolution binds or reduces anxiety, and shifts the focus out of psychological awareness toward a somatic focus ("primary gain"). Conversion symptoms also present the possibilities of honorable releases from work and sexual relations, and may present monetary benefits ("secondary gain"). A subgroup of patients with conversion symptoms may exhibit *la belle indifference,* meaning a lack of appropriate concern or emotional reactivity that would normally be associated with a disabling symptom such as a paralysis. Reported rates of conversion disorder range from 11/100,000 to 300/100,000 in the general population. It represents 1 to 3% of outpatient referrals to mental health clinics.[16] Conversion disorder to be diagnosed must include (1) one or more symptoms or deficits affecting voluntary motor or sensory function, suggesting a neurologic condition; (2) initiation or exacerbation of symptoms closely preceding or associated with conflicts or other stressors; (3) the symptoms or deficit is not intentionally produced or feigned; (4) the symptoms or deficit cannot, after appropriate investigation, be fully explained by a general medical condition, the direct effects of a substance, or as a culturally sanctioned behavior; (5) the symptoms or deficit causes clinically significant distress or impairment in social, occupation, or other important areas of functioning, or warrants medical evaluation; and (6) the symptom or deficit is not limited to pain or sexual dysfunction, does not occur exclusively during the course of somatization disorder, and is not better accounted for by another mental disorder.[16] Of particular importance to the plastic surgeon is that conversion symptoms may remit quickly, *without* resolution of underlying emotional problems that may result in other symptoms ("symptom substitution"). The concern here is that breast augmentation may be sought by such a patient as an external intervention for an underlying conflict around sexuality that may historically have generated conversion symptomatology.

BODY DYSMORPHIC DISORDER

Body dysmorphic disorder (BDD) is a somatoform disorder of particular importance to plastic surgeons. Patients with this disorder can be expected to repeatedly seek consultations with plastic surgeons and/or dermatologists.[20] The essential feature of BDD is a preoccupation with a defect in appearance that is either imagined or slight. The individual's concern and focus is markedly excessive. Such preoccupations usually become so excessive as to significantly impair most areas of functioning. Feelings of self-consciousness may lead to social avoidance. This led historically to this disorder being termed "dysmorphophobia."[21] This reflects the phobic avoidance associated with the core problem. Thus, BDD is a diagnostic label that addresses the core of the problem which lies in distorted self-appraisal of (an aspect of) body image. At a behavioral level such individuals can become "trapped" in rituals of self-checking, whether in mirrors, store windows, or with magnifying glasses in bathrooms. The distress associated with this disorder can lead to suicidal ideation, hospitalization, suicide attempts, and completed suicide.[16] Data on the prevalence of BDD are not available.[16]

In a well-performed empirical study of 30 patients with BDD there were several key findings: 97% avoided usual social and occupational activities, 17% had made suicide attempts, 33% had a psychotic disorder, and 93% had an associated lifetime diagnosis of major mood disorder. Of particular importance in this study was an evaluation of the treatment histories of these 30 patients with BDD. Treatments ranged from surgery (in 25 of 30 patients) to psychotherapy (24 of 30) to pharmacotherapy (28 of 30 patients had undergone a total of 187 adequate medication trials). The only intervention modality that showed any significant results was pharmacotherapy, with surgery and psychotherapy reflecting essentially no impact whatsoever. Of most important note, 80% of the BDD sample were evaluated as "worse" after surgery. The major type of pharmacologic intervention that reflected improvements were medications in the family of serotonin specific reuptake inhibitors (SRRIs).[22] These drugs presented "remissions" in a range from 21 to 29%, and combined ''remissions" plus "partial improvements" in a range from 53 to 72%. The two specific medications in this group that reflected these results were fluoxetine (Prozac) and clomipramine (Anafranil). Both of these medications are known to be important agents for obsessive-compulsive disorder symptoms as well as mood disorder symptoms.[22] As described, BDD has important features of obsessive-compulsive symptoms and ritualistic behaviors.

Body dysmorphic disorder may be diagnosed if the following criteria are present: (1) preoccupation with an imagined defect in appearance—if a slight physical anomaly is present, the person's concern is markedly excessive; (2) the preoccupation causes clinically significant distress or impairment in social, occupation, or other important areas of functioning; and (3) the preoccupation is not better accounted for by another mental disorder (e.g., anorexia nervosa–generated dissatisfaction with body shape/size).[16] Two final points are of particular interest to plastic surgeons involved in breast augmentation. First, in the Phillips et al[23] study, 10% of the patients' imagined effects were located in the breast area. Second, to quote directly from the *Diagnostic and Statistical Manual of Mental Disorders*' (DSM-IV) subsections on BDD:

> Individuals with body dysmorphic disorder often pursue and receive general medical, dental, and surgical procedures to rectify their imagined defects. Such treatments may cause the disorder to worsen, leading to intensified or new preoccupations which may in turn lend to further unsuccessful procedures so that individuals may eventually possess "synthetic" noses, ears, breasts, and lips which they are still dissatisfied with.[16 (p 467)]

Disorders Where Body Image is Associated

Depression can be associated with body image disturbance ranging from low self-esteem affecting self-appraisal to hypochondriacal preoccupations that include delusions about body image. An extensive literature links depression and body image problems.[24,25] The key finding of this literature is that depressed people view their appearance more negatively than nondepressed people.[25] This is in spite of lack of objectively evaluated differences in physical presentation and appearance.[26] Of importance to plastic surgeons is the finding that depression and requests for plastic surgery show a positive correlation in several studies, specifically including augmentation mammoplasty patients.[27,28] These findings argue for routine evaluation of depressive symptomatology prior to plastic surgery being performed.

Sexual dysfunction can be intrinsically associated with body image and the bodily experience. The DSM-IV offers several diagnoses that would address such an interaction of factors: (1) sexual aversion disorder, where body image may be aversive and anxiety producing; (2) hypoactive sexual desire disorder, due to psychological factors; or (3) female sexual arousal disorder.[29] Body image problems interface with sexual dysfunction with symptomatology such as sexual anxiety, arousal problems, and orgasm problems. These kinds of symptoms are frequently long-term, chronic, and deeply seated. The hope and fantasy of breast augmentation mammoplasty candidates can be to "short-circuit" such symptoms, which may be unrealistic. It is possible for the patient to have an improved body image and still have these symptoms, as was related earlier in the chapter on impacts of augmentation mammoplasty on sexual outcomes.[9,10] This area, like depressive symptoms, warrants clinical evaluation and exploration prior to surgical intervention. If these feelings and symptoms stem from a lifelong history of shame, parental nonvalidation as an attractive female, and phobic anxiety about sex leading to avoidance, then sex therapy and psychotherapy might be strongly considered as adjuncts to surgery, prior to surgery.

■ COLLABORATION OF PLASTIC SURGEONS AND MENTAL HEALTH PROFESSIONALS

Two key issues must be carefully considered by the plastic surgeon in selecting a potential mental health professional (MHP) for collaboration: (1) knowledge base, and (2) functional availability, which includes flexibility. In regard to knowledge base, there are important questions to consider: (1) Does the MHP have a functional working knowledge of the surgical procedures and biomedical issues involved in plastic surgery, in this case augmentation mammaplasties? This would include issues such as expected pain levels, drug effects, postoperative delirium, and metabolic impacts on mood and anxiety levels. (2) Does the MHP have a functional working knowledge of the psychological aspects, steps, and stages in the plastic surgery procedure that enables him/her to predict where the patient is headed, and to effectively gauge reactions within expected limits and outside expected limits? (3) Has the MHP done at least a rotation on a psychiatric consultation-liaison service, and thus learned the routines of psychological work and interventions in a surgical ward? Both psychiatrists and clinical psychologists can have access to such training. Ideally, the MHP will specialize in work in the medical hospital such that he/she will be very familiar with every aspect of the environment. The plastic surgeon has every right to assess the knowledge and experience of the prospective MHP in these areas. A qualified MHP will deal with such an assessment with a high level of comfort and ease.

In regard to functional availability/flexibility, important questions to consider are: (1) Does the MHP have the time to assess the plastic surgeon's patients, or is he/she fitting them in at odd hours outside of regular practice times? (2) Does the MHP respond in a timely fashion to the plastic surgeon's needs for consultations? Can the patient be seen within 1 to 3 days, or does it take 14 days to see the patient and a month to receive a report? An additional question with such reports is, Do they make sense to the plastic surgeon? Are they so jargon-laden and obscure as to be useless and undecipherable? The MHP who is highly skilled communicates in jargon-free terms, both to the surgeon and to the patient. If the plastic surgeon cannot understand what the MHP is saying, it is almost certain the patient and her family also cannot either. (3) Does the MHP have the flexibility to leave his/her office and come to see the patient in the hospital, especially in a crisis? This can be especially crucial within the immediate preoperative, intraoperative, and postoperative periods.[30] These periods may present patient management issues such as anxiety or panic attacks, transient delirium, transient depression, and posttraumatic stress disorder due to unexpected traumatization from surgery. Organic delirium can be a genuine psychiatric-medical emergency, and life threatening in nature.[31]

This writer agrees with the goals presented by Pruzinsky[30] as to the MHP's role in assisting the plastic surgeon: (1) to aid in the *prevention* of postsurgical traumas and decompensations, and (2) to *provide services* to the patient to enable her to successfully undergo surgery and realize benefits from that surgery. This writer would add a third goal, which is to aid in the *prediction* of adjustment of the patient to the procedures. MHPs are not able to make absolute predictions of behavior, but can aid in making generalized prediction as to outcomes. Such predictions can come from (1) careful examination of the patient's past history and behavioral adjustments; (2) systematic psychological testing of the patient's present symptomatology, personality organization, and coping styles; and (3) careful interviewing of the patient's present status, potentially over more than one session to detect shifts, deeper feelings, and formal disorders in thinking. Standard assessments of psychological status can be especially helpful in screening for depression, body dysmorphia disorder, or somatic delusions.[30] Standard assessments can now also screen for borderline personality disorder, which can alert and sensitize the surgeon as to behavioral/emotional possibilities.

The interaction of the MHP and patient presurgically can set the stage for a therapeutic alliance in the period long after the surgery, if necessary. This can be most important if the patient has a negative reaction or outcome from the surgery, or if the patient has a positive surgical outcome only to discover augmentation mammoplasty did not alter her life to the degree she anticipated.

■ PSYCHOLOGICAL ISSUES IN BREAST RECONSTRUCTION POSTMASTECTOMY

Issues for patients undergoing postmastectomy breast reconstruction differ, by definition, from those of patients electing augmentation mammoplasty. It is difficult to separate the intertwining emotional impacts of diagnosis, mastectomy, and breast reconstruction. Breast reconstruction comes at the end of a series of unfolding, usually traumatic, medical and surgical decisions.

Five studies in the 1980s reported psychological data for two or more patient groups who underwent postmastectomy breast reconstruction.[32–36] One study compared psychological status of a group of mastectomy patients with reconstruction with a control group of mastectomy patients without reconstruction.[32] Three studies compared reconstructed groups in relation to timing of reconstruction, immediate or delayed.[33–35] One study compared reconstructed patients in regard to subgroups of those with and without nipple reconstruction.[36] Each of these five studies reported psychological benefits of breast reconstruction, with benefits heavily outweighing negative outcomes. Benefits included reduced sense of deformity, improved self-concept, improved body image, and access to a wider variety of clothing styles.

Satisfaction with outcome of breast reconstruction postmastectomy was reported in at least six studies in the 1980s, and has ranged from 63 to 93%.[37–42] Rates of dissatisfaction with results tend to be much lower, in the range of 1 to 4%.[37,38,43]

Four studies have reported psychological data for two or more patient groups who underwent postmastectomy breast reconstruction in the 1990s. These studies are abstracted and results presented in Table 2–2.[44–47] Two of the four studies reflect the fact that the technology of breast reconstruction changed considerably between the 1970s–1980s and the 1990s. None of the studies published in the 1980s (data presumably collected in the 1970s and early 1980s) compared implants with autologous tissue reconstruction. The contradictory results of the two studies published in the 1990s are noteworthy.[44,47] In one, implants had the best impact on body image and in the other transverse rectus abdominus myocutaneous (TRAM) flaps had the best impact on body image. More data is needed to clarify this contradiction, but surgical skill and number of procedures done with TRAM flaps may figure heavily in patient satisfaction. The other two studies published in the 1990s also reflect important psychosocial issues. The Reaby and Hart[45] 1995 study appears to reflect the reality that not all women need or desire reconstruction to recover psychologically from mastectomy. Why some women feel they need reconstruction and others do not is still not well described in terms of depth psychological dynamics in the literature. The Schover et al[46] 1995 study appears to validate an earlier finding by Wellisch et al[48] that postmastectomy breast reconstruction facilitates women who have had mastectomies to perceive themselves as more like women who have had lumpectomies.

■ PSYCHOSOCIAL ISSUES IN EXPLANTATION

A very modest amount of psychosocial data exists in print at present in regard to this subject. This is in sharp contrast to the number of biomedical articles in print regarding implant removal and medical problems suspected to be associated with silicone implants. A computerized literature search in 1991 yielded 71 biomedical articles in this area. A similar search in 1995 on psychosocial issues and explantation yielded five databased studies that in some way addressed this issue.[49–53] Of these five studies, four deal with the impacts of media reports on women's psychological concerns and thoughts about explantation,[49–52] while only one assessed women psychologically prior to explantation.[53] The impact of the media surveys assess a range of patient groupings including two samples who underwent augmentation mammoplasty,[49] a sample who underwent reconstruction postmastectomy,[50] and a sample of both these conditions.[51,52] In a sample of only augmentation mammoplasty patients all had heard media reports and 90% perceived these reports to be negative. Prior to the negative media reports, 1% had wanted their implants removed. This shifted to 6% after the media reports. However, 75% were concerned about implant safety. This study systematically measured anxiety and depression symptoms. These did not appear adversely affected by the media reports and were, on average, well within normal ranges.[49] In a sample of postmastectomy breast reconstruction patients, all had heard negative media reports, and 55% were concerned about implant safety. Of this population, 13% were considering implant removal as a result of the controversy.[50] In a study focusing on patient anxiety, it was concluded that patients who experienced difficulty with their reconstruction reported more anxiety associated with media coverage.[51]

As previously mentioned, only one study reports on psychological and biomedical parameters in a sample of women (n =52) actually seeking explantation.[53] On a psychological test measuring nine symptom areas, only two showed the majority of the patients to be in the range where they would meet the criteria for psychiatric "caseness." These were somatization (67% in range of caseness) and obsessive-com-

Table 2–2. Psychosocial Outcomes of Postmastectomy Breast Reconstruction in the 1990s

Study	*Number Followed*	*Groupings*	*Satisfaction with Outcomes*	*Rates of Dissatisfaction*
Franchelli, Leone, Berino,et al, 1995	102	Implants, $n = 52$ autologous tissues, $n = 50$	Better body image with implants than with TRAM flaps	Low for all 102 patients
Reaby and Hart, 1995	95	Mastectomy with reconstruction, $n = 64$ Mastectomy without reconstruction, $n = 31$	Body image ratings equivalent between groups	Not described
Schover, Yetman, Tuason, et al, 1995	218	Breast reconstruction postmastectomy, $n = 146$ Partial mastectomy, $n = 72$	Sexual satisfaction and psychological adjustment adjustment equivalent between groups	Under 20% for both groups in areas of body image, sexual functioning and psychological adjustment
Garbay, Rietjens, and Petit, 1992	323	Prosthesis, $n = 223$ Latissimus dorsi flaps, $n = 36$; TRAM flaps, $n = 64$	TRAM flap best for body image, latissimus dorsi worst Significantly greater satisfaction with delayed reconstruction	Not described

pulsive (62% in range of caseness). On a test measuring depressive symptomatology, 24% had moderate to severe depression and 10% had severe depression. The average number of rheumatologic symptoms (total possible was 23) was 11.9 per patient. There was a high and statistically significant correlation between global psychological symptoms (as measured by one of the tests in the study) and number of rheumatologic symptoms endorsed ($r = .39$, $p = .01$). This would follow given the high rates of somatization and obsessive-compulsive symptomatic caseness found in this study.

Few conclusions are possible with so few psychological studies and so little data regarding psychological aspects of explantation. The available data appear to suggest that most women wish to keep their implants regardless of the existence of negative media reports and regardless of their concerns about safety in relation to those reports. Studies are needed in this area measuring the effect of explantation on later psychological symptomatology and quality of life. This remains unknown at present. The data from the preexplantation study may suggest that women more prone to obsessive-compulsive patterns and somatization may become more decompensated secondary to concerns about implant safety.[53]

■ CONCLUSION

This chapter has been a broad survey in the area of psychological issues with the patient who is contemplating or who has undergone breast augmentation. Certain areas have been studied more than others. For example, data on motivations for augmentation mammoplasty and on expected outcomes are relatively consistent and predictable, but data on psychosocial outcomes for breast reconstruction postmastectomy is less consistent and offers less predictability given the rapidly changing medical technology and procedures in the area within the last decade. The advisability of some form of presurgical psychosocial assessment of the augmentation mammoplasty patient is a firm conclusion of the chapter given the multiplicity of psychiatric syndromes potentially present in this population. The key here is not excluding patients for psychiatric reasons, but rather engaging the resources to effectively bring them through such surgery. Finally, explantation remains an area of the future in terms of psychological understanding of the women who present for and are given this highly impactful procedure.

REFERENCES

1. Pruzinsky T, Cash TF. Integrative themes in body image development, deviance, and change. In: Cash TF, Pruzinsky T, eds. *Body Images: Development, Deviance, and Change.* New York: Guilford; 1990:337–349.
2. Edgerton JT, Meyer E, Jacobson WE. Augmentation mammoplasty. II. Further surgical and psychiatric evaluation. *Plast Reconstr Surg.* 1961;27:297–302.
3. Baker JL, Kollin IS, Bartlett ES. Psychosexual dynamics of patients undergoing mammary augmentation. *Plast Reconstr Surg.* 1974;53:652–659.
4. Shipley RH, O'Donnell JM, Bader KF. Personality characteristics of women seeking breast augmentation: comparison to small-busted and average-busted controls. *Plast Reconstr Surg.* 1977;60(3):369–376.
5. Beale S, Lisper HO, Palm B. A psychological study of patients seeking augmentation mammoplasty. *Br J Psychiatry.* 1980; 136:133–138.
6. Schlebusch L, Levin A. A psychological profile of women selected for augmentation mammoplasty. *S Afr Med J.* 1983; 64:481–483.
7. Birtchnell S, Whitfield P, Lacey JH. Motivational factors in women requesting augmentation and reduction mammoplasty. *J Psychosom Res.* 1990;34(5):509–514.
8. Ohlsen L, Ponten B, Hambert G. Augmentation mammoplasty: a surgical and psychiatric evaluation of the results. *Ann Plast Surg.* 1979;2:42–52.
9. Hetter GP. Satisfactions and dissatisfactions of patients with augmentation mammoplasty. *Plast Reconstr Surg.* 1979;64(2): 151–155.
10. Meyer L, Ringberg A. Augmentation mammoplasty—psychiatric and psychosocial characteristics and outcome in a group of Swedish women. *Scand J Plast Reconstr Surg.* 1987;21: 199–208.
11. Kilmann PR, Sattler JI, Taylor J. The impact of augmentation mammoplasty: a follow-up study. *Plast Reconstr Surg.* 1987; 80(3):374–378.
12. Edgerton MT, Longman MA, Pruzinsky T. Plastic surgery and psychotherapy in the treatment of 100 psychologically disturbed patients. *Plast Reconstr Surg.* 1991;88(4):594–608.
13. Schain WS, Wellisch DK, Pasnau RO, Landsverk J. The sooner the better: a study of psychological factors in women undergoing immediate versus delayed breast reconstruction. *Am J Psychiatry.* 1985;142(1):40–47.
14. First MB, ed. *Diagnostic and Statistical Manual of Mental Disorders,* 4th ed. Washington, DC: American Psychiatric Press; 1994:629–673.
15. Pruzinsky T. Psychopathology of body experience: expanded perspectives. In: Cash TF, Pruzinsky T, eds. *Body Images: Development, Deviance, and Change.* New York: Guilford; 1990: 170–189.
16. First MB, ed. Somatoform disorders. In: *Diagnostic and Statistical Manual of Mental Disorders,* 4th ed. Washington, DC: American Psychiatric Press; 1994:445–470.
17. Ford CV. *The Somatizing Disorders: Illness as a Way of Life.* New York: Elsevier Biomedical; 1983.
18. Lindberg BJ, Lindegard B. Studies of the hysterical personality attitude. *Acta Psychiatr Scand.* 1963;39:170–180.
19. Bibb RC, Guze SB. Hysteria in a psychiatric hospital. *Am J Psychiatry.* 1972;129:224–228.
20. Thomas CS. Dysmorphobia: a question of definition. *Br Psychiatry.* 1984;144:513–516.
21. Andreasen NC, Bardach J. Dysmorphobia: symptom or disease? *Am J Psychiatry.* 1977;134:673–676.
22. Kaplan HI, Sadock BJ. *Pocket Handbook of Psychiatric Drug Treatment,* 2nd ed. Baltimore: Williams and Wilkins; 1996: 146–156.
23. Phillips KA, McElroy SL, Keck PE, et al. Body dysmorphic disorder: 30 cases of imagined ugliness. *Am J Psychiatry.* 1993; 150:302–308.

24. Taylor MJ, Cooper PJ. Body size overestimation and depressed mood. *Br J Clin Psychol.* 1986;25:153–154.
25. Marsella AJ, Shizuru L, Brennan J, et al. Depression and body image satisfaction. *J Cross Cultural Psychol.* 1981;12: 360–371.
26. Noles SW, Cash TF, Winstead BA. Body image, physical attractiveness, and depression. *J Consult Clin Psychol.* 1985;53: 88–94.
27. Cash TF, Horton CE. Aesthetic surgery: effects of rhinoplasty on social perception of patients by others. *Plast Reconstr Surg.* 1983;72:543–548.
28. Schlebusch L. Negative bodily experience and prevalence of depression in patients who request augmentation mammoplasty. *S Afr Med J.* 1989;75:323–326.
29. First MB, ed. Sexual and gender identity disorders. In: *Diagnostic and Statistical Manual of Mental Disorders,* 4th ed. Washington, DC: American Psychiatric Press; 1994:493–538.
30. Pruzinsky T. Collaboration of plastic surgeon and medical psychotherapist: elective cosmetic surgery. *Med Psychother.* 1988; 1:1–13.
31. Fleishman S, Lesko LM. Delirium and dementia. In: Holland JC, Rowland JH, eds. *Handbook of Psychooncology.* New York: Oxford Press; 1989:342–355.
32. Goldberg P, Stolzman M, Goldberg HM. Psychological considerations in breast reconstruction. *Ann Plast Surg.* 1984;13: 38–43.
33. Dean C, Chetty U, Forrest AP. Effects of immediate breast reconstruction on psychological morbidity after mastectomy. *Lancet.* 1983;1:459–462.
34. Stevens LA, McGrath MH, Druss RG, et al. The psychological impact of immediate breast reconstruction for women with early breast cancer. *Plast Reconstr Surg.* 1984;73:619–628.
35. Schain WS, Wellisch DK, Pasnau RO, et al. The sooner the better: a study of psychological factors in women undergoing immediate versus delayed breast reconstruction. *Am J Psychiatry.* 1985;142:40–46.
36. Wellisch DK, Schain WS, Noone RB, et al. The psychological contribution of nipple addition in breast reconstruction. *Plast Reconstr Surg.* 1987;80:699–704.
37. Asplund O, Korlof B. Late results following mastectomy for cancer and breast reconstruction. *Scand J Plast Reconstr Surg.* 1984;18:221–225.
38. Van Dam FS, Bergman RB. Psychosocial and surgical aspects of breast reconstruction. *Eur J Surg Oncol.* 1988;14: 141–149.
39. Teimourian B, Adham MN. Survey of patients' responses to breast reconstruction. *Ann Plast Surg.* 1982;9:321–325.
40. Cooper GG, Webster MH, Bell G. The results of breast construction following mastectomy. *Br J Plast Surg.* 1984;37: 369–372.
41. Filiberti A, Tamburini M, Murru L, et al. Psychological effects and esthetic results of breast reconstruction. *Tumori.* 1986;72: 585–588.
42. Noone RB, Frazier TG, Hayward CZ, et al. Patient acceptance of immediate reconstruction following mastectomy. *Plast Reconstr Surg.* 1982;69:632–638.
43. Berkowitch S. Psychological results of reconstructed patients. *Acta Chir Belg.* 1980;79:165–167.
44. Franchelli S, Leone MS, Berrino P, et al. Psychological evaluation of patients undergoing breast reconstruction using two different methods: autologous tissues versus prostheses. *Plast Reconstr Surg.* 1995;95(7):1213–1218.
45. Reaby LL, Hart LK. Postmastectomy attitudes in women who wear external breast prostheses compared to those who have undergone breast reconstructions. *J Behav Med.* 1995; 18(1):55–67.
46. Schover LR, Yetman RJ, Tuason LJ, et al. Partial mastectomy and breast reconstruction. A comparison of their effects on psychosocial adjustment, body image, and sexuality. *Cancer.* 1995; 75(1):54–64.
47. Garbay JR, Rietjens M, Petit JY. Esthetic results of breast reconstruction after amputation for cancer. 323 cases. *J Gynecol Obstet Biol Reprod (Paris).* 1992;21(4):405–412.
48. Wellisch DK, DiMatteo R, Silverstein MJ, et al. Psychosocial outcomes of breast cancer therapies: lumpectomy versus mastectomy. *Psychosomatics.* 1989;30(4):365–373.
49. Handel N, Wellisch DK, Silverstein MJ, et al. Knowledge, concern, and satisfaction among augmentation mammoplasty patients. *Ann Plast Surg.* 1993;30:13–22.
50. Winer EP, Fee-Fulkerson K, Fulkerson CC, et al. Silicone controversy: a survey of women with breast cancer and silicone implants. *J Natl Cancer Inst.* 1993;85(17):1407–1411.
51. Anderson RC, Larson DL. Reconstruction and augmentation patients' reaction to the media coverage of silicone gel filled implants: anxiety evaluated. *Psychol Rep.* 1995;76(3 pt2): 1323–1330.
52. Palcheff-Wiemer M, Concannon MJ, Conn VS, et al. The impact of the media on women with breast implants. *Plast Reconstr Surg.* 1993;92(5):779–785.
53. Wells KE, Roberts C, Daniels SM, et al. Psychological and rheumatic symptoms of women requesting silicone breast implant removal. *Ann Plast Surg.* 1995;34:572–577.

3

Surgical Approach to Breast Augmentation and Implant Removal: Procedures, Clinical Evaluations, and Complications

JAMES WATSON, WILLIAM SHAW, AND CHRISTINA AHN

Clinicians who are involved in the management of breast implant patients need to have a basic understanding of implant types, implant placement, and implant removal. Because of the many manufacturing and design modifications that have been made, the term *breast implant* is a nebulous one, describing a constellation of devices filled with saline, colloid, silicone gel, or peanut oil. The implants are covered with a solid silicone shell that may be smooth, texturized, or coated with polyurethane.[1–15] Over ten manufacturers have made these devices and labeled them with various trade names. For this reason, practitioners must pay close attention to patients when they describe their breast implant by its filler, coating, brand name, or manufacturer.

Indications for breast implants include both reconstructive and aesthetic reasons.[1,5,11] In aesthetic cases, implants are used to enlarge breast size or correct ptosis. In reconstructive cases, implants are used to correct breast asymmetry and acquired absence of the breast (postmastectomy reconstruction). Regardless of the indication, complications of breast implants occur and include capsular contracture, displacement, rupture, infection, extrusion, and other problems.[16–20] Physicians caring for these patients must know how to examine these patients and know when to refer patients for treatment.

■ HISTORY

Although attempts at breast augmentation can be traced back to 1895, the first sealed shell breast prosthesis was a silicone gel–filled implant made by Dow-Corning. This was first reported by Cronin and Gerow in 1962.[6] The first saline-filled prosthesis was made by Simaplast and reported by Arion in 1965. Although both implants were met with initial enthusiasm, a decline in saline implant use occurred. This was largely attributed to implant unreliability and the more natural "feel" of the gel-filled prosthesis. Saline-filled implant deflation rates from 1.2% to 84% were reported in the literature.[3]

Despite having a more natural feel, silicone gel implants still had significant problems with capsular contractures.[21–32] In an attempt to prevent this complication, a polyurethane coating was added (Natural Y) and first reported by Ashley in 1972.[23] Although this polyurethane coating unquestionably reduced capsular contracture rates, the polyurethane-coated implants were taken off the market in 1987 by the Food and Drug Administration (FDA), due to concerns that polyurethane could theoretically biodegrade into toluene diisocyanate (TDI) and its potentially carcinogenic amine form, toluenediamine (TDA). The silicone shells of breast implants were also texturized by many manufacturers in another attempt to combat capsular contracture. This modification was used by many companies for both saline-filled and gel-filled implants in the late 1980s.

Over the years the number of breast augmentation surgeries continued to rise, reaching a high of 130,000 patients per year by 1989. During the same period of time, the FDA requested safety data from the breast implant manufacturers, due to safety concerns about silicone gel implants. The experimental data were submitted to the FDA over the next 2 to 3 years; however, some of the experimental data were not disclosed, and later came to light during a product liability suit against Dow Corning in 1991. In January 1992 the FDA called for a voluntary moratorium on the use of silicone gel–filled breast implants. In April 1992 the FDA announced that silicone gel–filled implants would be available only under controlled clinical studies.[33] Since 1992 only saline-filled implants have been available for breast augmentation, outside of a clinical trial. Today, there are clinical trials being conducted to evaluate silicone gel–filled implants (Mentor and McGhan Corp.) and peanut oil–filled implants (Lipomatrix Corp.).

▪ IMPLANT TYPES

Many companies manufactured and sold more than one type of implant, making the implant brand name ambiguous as well. To avoid these problems, breast implants have been descriptively classified based on their filler material, the number of lumina, and surface characteristics of the shell. No universally accepted classification system has been adopted, however, so we will simply describe different breast implants based on these three characteristics (Table 3–1).

▪ IMPLANT FILLER TYPES

Gel-Filled Implants

An estimated 1.6 to 2 million patients have undergone breast implantation in the United States. The majority of these have been silicone gel–filled implants done for aesthetic purposes. Silicone gel is a polymer of dimethylsiloxane that is heat stable (from −54°C to +54°C) and slightly heavier than water (specific gravity of 1.13).[7,9] The viscosity of the gel depends on its molecular weight (length of the polymers). The original Dow-Corning gel-filled implant was a smooth-walled, teardrop-shaped bag with Dacron patches on the posterior wall to anchor the implant to the chest wall. A number of subsequent modifications were made in an attempt to reduce capsular contracture problems, including thinning the implant walls. These thin-walled implants were noted to become sticky after several days, and laboratory analysis confirmed that this was due to gel leaching through the envelope. This is how the terms *gel bleed* and *gel leaching* originated.[34] In response, Dow Corning developed a "low bleed" shell (Silastic II) that was claimed to have a leaching capacity of one tenth that of the earlier shells. Despite this improvement, most surgeons agree that all silicone gel implants bleed and many studies have confirmed evidence of silicone in the tissues surrounding intact gel-filled implants after long-term placement.

Table 3–1. Breast Implant Characteristics

Filler Material	*Shell Surface*	*Number of Lumens*
Saline	Smooth	Single
Silicone gel	Textured	Double
Colloid	Polyurethane	
Peanut oil		

Granuloma formation around silicone gel implants has often been attributed to this gel bleed and many hypothesize that this may contribute to capsular contracture. Of even greater concern is the incidence of implant rupture with silicone gel implants (Figs. 3–1 and 3–2).[35] Reported rupture rates vary widely in the scientific literature, but most long-term studies suggest an increasing rupture rate as the implant ages. The health concerns related to implant rupture are very controversial today, due to court claims and media reports of individual cases of illnesses attributed to implant rupture. Despite epidemiologic studies that do not support any correlation between silicone gel and autoimmune disease, this issue has not been completely resolved and is beyond the scope of this chapter.

Saline-Filled Implants

Because silicone gel–filled implants are gradually being removed and new implants placed since 1992 are saline filled, the percentage of patients with saline-filled implants is gradually increasing. Saline implants are often called "inflatable implants" because manufacturers distribute them as empty, solid, silicone shells. This feature allows these implants to be placed through smaller incisions, which gives them an aesthetic advantage over silicone gel–filled implants, which come prefilled and sealed. The primary disadvantage of these implants is their tendency to leak, which results in implant deflation, implant removal, and replacement. Reported leak rates vary widely (0.5–84%) and have been attributed to a large number of causes, including iatrogenic puncture, faulty filler valves, and thin shells.[3] Most experts today believe that the majority of late-occurring leaks are due to folds in the implant wall, which produce "stress cracking" of the shell. Common patient complaints with saline implants are that they do not "feel natural," that they cause "skin rippling" over subglandular implants, and that the patients hear and feel the saline "sloshing" with exercise. Today, saline-

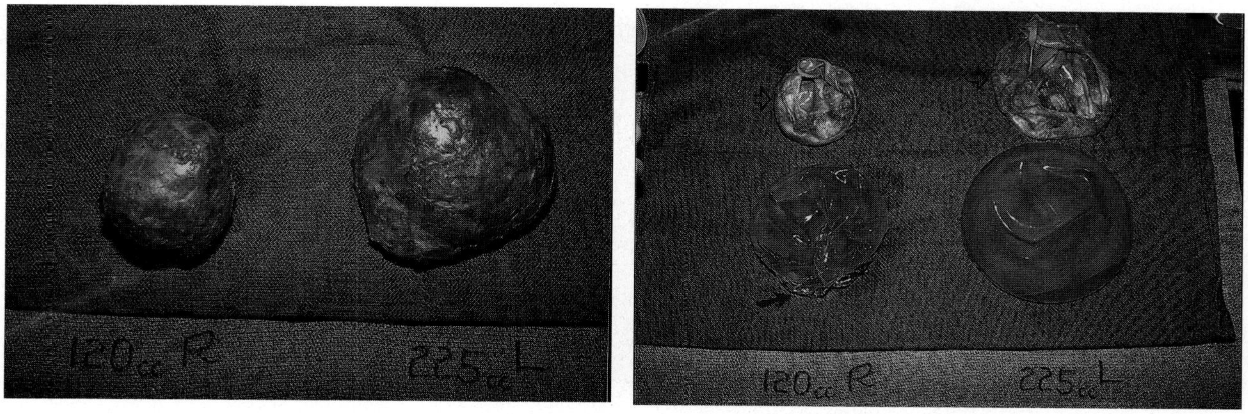

A B

Figure 3–1. Ruptured and intact silicone gel–filled implant from the same patient. (**A**) Periprosthetic fibrous capsules surrounding the ruptured right implant and the intact left implant. (**B**) The periprosthetic capsules have been removed from the silicone implants (open arrows). The ruptured right implant has free silicone outside the implant shell (arrow). This patient had different size implants in her breasts; a 120-cc implant had been placed in her right breast and a 225-cc implant had been placed in her left breast. See Plates IA and IB.

filled implants are currently "allowed" but not "approved" by the FDA. The agency has called on the manufacturers to provide safety data to address these issues. Isolated case reports of saline-filled implants causing systemic health risks have appeared in the media, the courts, and the scientific literature; however, large epidemiologic studies have not confirmed these claims.

Colloid-Filled and Oil-Filled Implants

Several attempts have been made to find a new biodegradable, radiolucent, implant filler with a natural feel. A bio-oncotic, radiolucent gel implant (MISTI Gold) was introduced in 1990 that reportedly would be metabolized and excreted. The implant was voluntarily taken off the market by its manufacturer (Bioplasty) in 1991, however, due to FDA action.

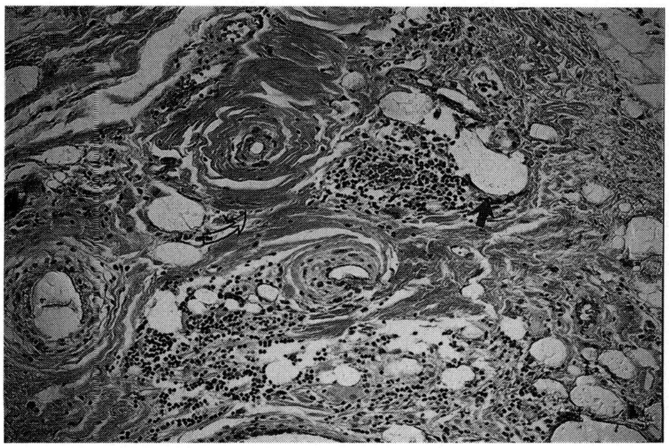

Figure 3–2. Microscopic histology of periprosthetic capsule showing silicone granuloma (arrow) and dense irregular collagen fibrils (open arrow). See Plate II.

More recently, soybean oil–filled implants have been developed and clinically used in Europe (Lipomatrix). The vegetable oil is biodegradable, radiolucent, and has been reported to have a more natural feel when compared with saline implants. Clinical trials in the United States are under way.

■ IMPLANT SHELLS

All implant shells that have been clinically used in the United States are made of solid silicone, regardless of their filler, shell surface characteristics, or number of lumina.

Smooth-Walled Shells

All implants made in the 1960s were smooth implants with a thin silicone shell. Early attempts to reduce capsular contractures were directed toward creating thinner walls. These thin-walled implants leaked, however, prompting a reevaluation of this theory of capsular contracture. As implant walls were made thicker, leak rates decreased, but contracture rates did not significantly change. This prompted the development of the polyurethane coat.

Polyurethane-Coated Shells

In 1970 Ashley[4] introduced a silicone gel–filled implant with a textured polyurethane coating. Subsequent reports extolled the low incidence of capsular contractures using this implant. Although the implants would form thick capsules, the spongy fibrotic tissue capsule surrounding these implants appeared to randomly disperse the normal contractive forces, with little loss of compressibility of the breast. Concern over polyurethane biodegradation was sparked by a report of an in vitro experiment in which polyurethane hydrolysis yielded a toxic by-product, toluene diisocyanate (TDI).[23,36] TDI's amine form, toluenediamine (TDA) is a potential carcinogen in animals. This prompted the FDA to take the polyurethane implant off the market.

Texturized Shells

The impetus to texturize the surface of the solid silicone shell followed the research on the polyurethane-coated implants that showed less organized and less dense collagen around rough-textured silicone implants. Small, prospective, controlled studies have demonstrated a decrease in clinical contracture rates with these shells, but not all studies agree.[21,22] Despite the ongoing controversy, most surgeons today use textured shell saline-filled implants.

■ DOUBLE-LUMEN IMPLANTS

Double-lumen implants were developed in an attempt to combine the best features of silicone gel– and saline-filled prostheses. Some double-lumen implants were designed with a silicone gel–prefilled inner lumen and an inflatable outer lumen. Other double-lumen implants were developed with the opposite configuration: a saline-filled inner lumen and a gel-filled outer lumen (Becker). Each design had certain advantages; however, both double-lumen designs are no longer available.[1,11]

■ IMPLANT MANUFACTURERS

Many breast implant patients know the manufacturer or the implant trade name, yet they may not know what type of implant they have. For this reason, physicians should have access to a reference list of implant manufacturers (Table 3–2). Although ten implant manufacturers were operating in the 1980s, only two are still manufacturing implants that are being used today (Mentor and McGhan). Implants made by all these manufacturers are presumably still implanted in patients today. Historically speaking, the largest implant manufacturers were Dow Corning, Baxter, and Surgitek. Lipomatrix has FDA approval only for clinical trials at this time.

In addition to implant augmentation, breast augmentation with injections of free silicone gel and fat have been reported worldwide, despite opposition by the American Society of Plastic and Reconstructive Surgeons (ASPRS). Mammographic artifacts due to necrosis of injected fat may make cancer surveillance more difficult. Free silicone oil injection into any area of the body has been condemned by the ASPRS and banned by the FDA, due to health concerns.

Table 3–2. Implant Manufacturers in the United States

Manufacturer (Parent Corp)	*Implant (Trade Name)*	*Characteristics (Filler)*
Bioplasty[3]	MISTI	Gel, colloid filled
Cox-Uphoff[2,5]		Saline filled
Dow Corning[3,4] (Dow Chemical)	Silastic II Silastic MSI	Gel, saline
Heyer-Schulte[3]		Gel, saline
Lipomatrix[1]		Soybean oil
McGhan[1]	RTV, UHP, BIOCELL	Gel, saline
Mentor[1,5]	Siltex, Becker	Gel, saline
Porex[2,5]		Gel
Simaplast[2,5]	Mammaplast	Saline filled
Surgitek[2,4] (Bristol-Meyers)	Replicon, Meme Optimam, SCL	Gel, polyurethane coated
V. Mueller[2,4] (Baxter)		Gel

[1]Still manufacturing.
[2]No longer manufacturing.
[3]Bankrupt.
[4]Participated in global settlement.
[5]Did not participate in global settlement.

■ PERIPROSTHETIC CAPSULES

All foreign bodies implanted in humans form a surrounding fibrous tissue. With breast implants, this tissue has been termed a *periprosthetic capsule,* or just *capsule* (Fig. 3–1). If this periprosthetic capsule becomes firm, this complication is called a "capsular contracture." The etiology behind this phenomenon still remains a mystery and its incidence unpredictable.[29] Unilateral capsular contractures often occur in patients with identical implants placed by the same surgeon. Many hypotheses have been proposed. The two main theories point to noninfectious stimuli (hematoma, granuloma, and hereditary factors) and infectious stimuli (subclinical infection) as the cause for these contractures. Capsular thickness per se does not correlate with capsular contracture. Capsular contracture does correlate with implant position (higher in subglandular vs. submuscular pocket) and time (long follow-ups have higher rates). Attempts to minimize capsular contractures include implant massage exercises, steroids, vitamin E, antibiotics, and implant texturization (polyurethane coat or textured silicone surface). Some of these factors have statistically decreased contracture rates, but no method has yet been developed to eliminate capsular contractures.[29]

Capsular firmness varies in severity. Many mechanical devices have been described to quantitate contractures including tonometers and calipers. Only Baker's classification, which is based on clinical findings, has gained widespread clinical acceptance and is considered the standard for evaluating and reporting contracture rates (Fig. 3–3)[1,11,31] (Table 3–3).

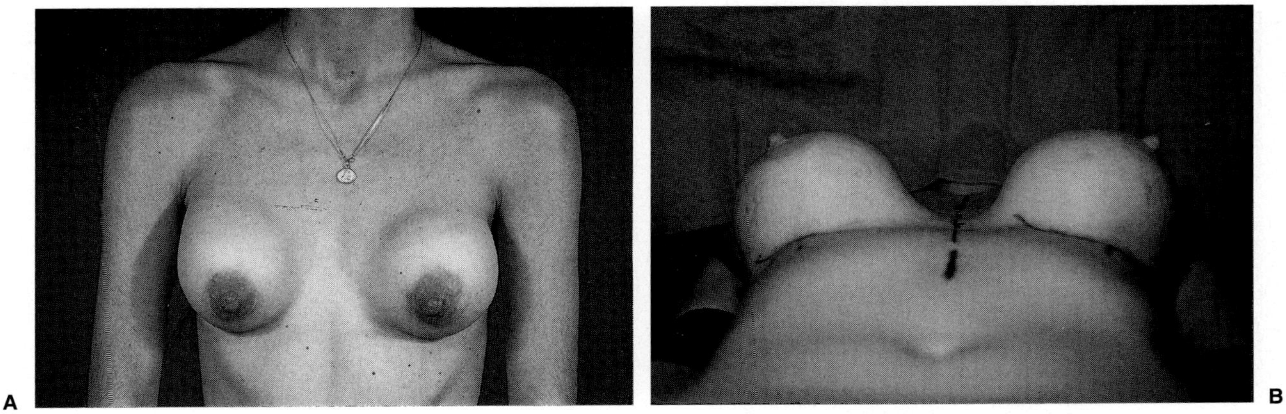

Figure 3–3. Patients with Baker IV capsular contractures. (**A**) Front view—patient has distorted, unnatural-appearing breasts. The clinical examination demonstrated hard, tender, and cold breasts. (**B**) Supine view—preoperative view in a different patient shows the unnatural-appearing breasts that stand upright when the patient is supine.

■ AUGMENTATION SURGERY

Indications and Contraindications

In aesthetic cases, breast implants are used to enlarge breast size and/or correct breast ptosis. The most common indication for aesthetic augmentation is to treat developmentally small breasts or breasts that are small due to postpartum involutional changes (Fig. 3–4). In both cases, the primary goal is to increase volume. In patients with postpartum involutional changes, however, a second goal is to correct breast ptosis (sagging of the skin and breast parenchyma). Although moderate to severe ptosis may require other surgery, such as a mastopexy, mild cases of ptosis can often be corrected with breast implants alone.

In reconstructive cases, implants are used to correct congenital or acquired breast asymmetries and to treat acquired absence of the breast (ie, postmastectomy reconstruction). Examples include idiopathic congenital asymmetry, Poland's syndrome, and tuberous breast deformities. Acquired breast asymmetries following breast reconstruction occasionally require implant placement in the contralateral breast to achieve symmetric size and shape. Relative contraindications to breast implant placement include a radiated chest wall, the presence of local infection, bleeding disorders, and unrealistic patient expectations. These factors may be associated with a prohibitively high incidence of implant failures and complications.

Table 3–3. Baker's Classification of Capsular Contracture

Grade	*Findings on Physical Examination*
I	Soft, no palpable capsule
II	Capsule palpable, but not visible
III	Capsule palpable and visible
IV	Hard, tender, painful, cold, and distorted

Patient Evaluation

Many medical and psychosocial issues need to be addressed when evaluating a patient for breast augmentation. The evaluation must include current breast size, desired breast size, patient expectations, motivation for surgery, lifestyle, future plans for pregnancy, previous history of breast disease, and an evaluation of breast cancer risk factors (Table 3–4). Physical examination must include a thorough breast examination for parenchymal pathology as well as an assessment of breast volume, ptosis, asymmetry, and chest wall deformities. For patients over 35 to 40 years of age, a preoperative baseline screening mammogram is also recommended.

Patient education must include a thorough discussion about the risks and complications of breast implants, including bleeding, infection, anesthesia, nipple sensation loss, capsular contracture, implant rupture, secondary chest wall deformities, and the need for revisional surgery (Table 3–5). Although systemic symptoms that may represent autoimmune disease have been reported in the literature, long-term definitive scientific research has yet to conclusively determine a cause and effect relationship between implants and autoimmune disease.

■ SURGICAL TECHNIQUE

After the patient is evaluated and determined to be an acceptable candidate for augmentation mammoplasty, the technical issues that the surgeon must address include surgical incisions, implant pocket position, anesthesia, as well as implant type and size. These factors should be discussed

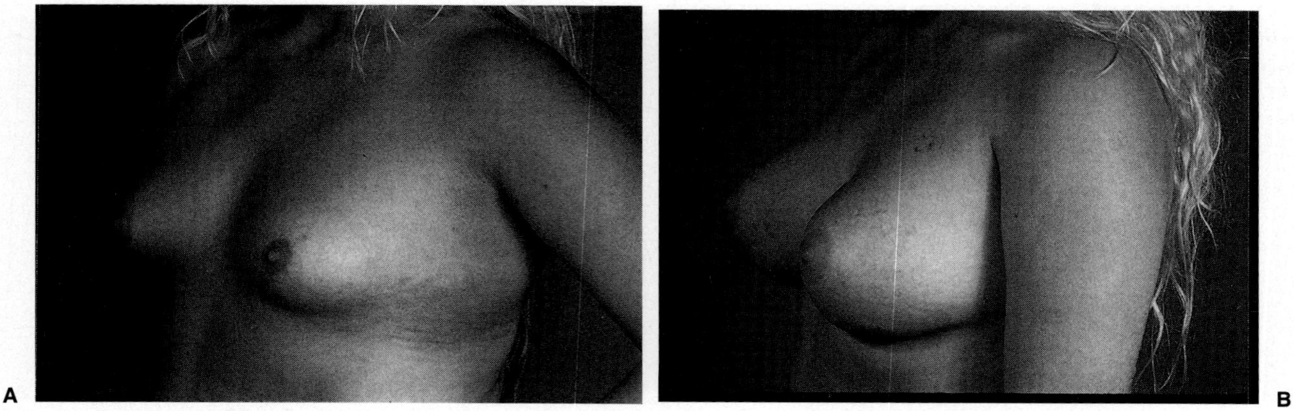

Figure 3–4. Pre- and postoperative patient for breast augmentation. Preoperative photograph (**A**) and postoperative photograph (**B**) showing good aesthetic results.

with the patient preoperatively, especially the factors that may affect the patient's lifestyle and capsular contracture risk.

Technical Factors Affecting Capsular Contracture

Because capsular contractures are the most common complication of breast augmentation, technical factors that reduce capsular contracture rates must be explained to the patient. The most important capsular contracture factor that the surgeon can alter is the surgical pocket location (subglandular vs. submuscular). Reported studies of capsular contracture rates almost all conclude that there is a lower rate of capsular contracture with implants placed in the submuscular position.[37] In the past 10 years, many studies have suggested that textured surface implants also lower the capsular contracture rate, when compared with smooth surface implants, although this issue has not conclusively been proven.[21,22] Subclinical periprosthetic infection has also been suggested as a cause for contracture (see Periprosthetic Capsules, above), although this has not been conclusively proven either. Nevertheless, most surgeons believe that the best way to minimize capsular contractures is to place a textured surface implant in a submuscular pocket, irrigating the pocket with antibiotics, and using strict sterile technique.

Surgical Incisions

Three incisions for implant placement are commonly used: periareolar, inframammary, and transaxillary.[1,11] Endoscopically placed implants via an umbilical incision have also been reported, but this is beyond the scope of this chapter. Each approach has its own unique advantages and each patient often has her own opinion as to where she wishes to have the scar. For this reason, these options must be discussed with the patient preoperatively.

Anesthesia

Anesthetic options for breast augmentation include local anesthesia with IV sedation, intercostal nerve blocks, and general anesthesia. Because submuscular implant placement requires good pectoralis muscle relaxation, this technique is usually done under general anesthesia. Subglandular augmentation can be done under either general anesthesia or local anesthesia with IV sedation. Intercostal nerve blocks can

Table 3–4. Augmentation Patient Evaluation

Indication for Surgery	*Psychosocial History Issues*	*Examination*	*Risks*	*Complications*	*Technical Factors*
Micromastia Ptosis Asymmetry Poland's syndrome Implant syndrome Tuberous breast	Expectations Motivation Compliance Exercise Lifestyle	Cancer risk Breast size Desired size Future pregnancy?	Pathology Volume Ptosis Asymmetry Chest wall deformity	Bleeding Infection Anesthesia Sensation loss Contracture Deflation Further surgery	Incisions Position Anesthesia type Implant size

Table 3–5. Patient Education

Implant Types	*Implant Complications*	*Surgical Complications*	*Technical Factors*	*Long-term Risks*
Smooth vs. textured Gel vs. Saline Future implants	Rupture Contracture Infection Mammography Skin rippling Extrusion Displacement Distortion	Nipple sensation changes Asymmetry Bleeding Infection Anesthesia	Incision options Implant position Revision surgery	Capsular contracture issues Deflation Chest wall deformities

be used to augment local anesthesia or for early postoperative pain relief with general anesthesia.

Subglandular Augmentation

Subglandular augmentation is the technique that places the breast implant behind the breast parenchyma, directly on the surface of the pectoralis major muscle. The advantages of this approach are that it can be done under local anesthesia with IV sedation, it may be more effective than the submuscular technique for ptosis correction, and it may cause less functional impairment in patients involved in sports that depend heavily on pectoralis muscle function (body building, tennis, swimming, etc.). Disadvantages of this approach include higher capsular contracture rates, rippling of the overlying skin, and implants that are palpable (and more firm, with saline implants).[21,22] These disadvantages seem to be magnified in patients with minimal breast parenchyma and thin skin, making this technique less desirable in these patients. Many surgeons prefer to use the subglandular approach primarily for patients with larger breasts who request ptosis correction without a mastopexy (for postpartum involutional changes). In most other patients, this technique is reserved as a second choice.

Submuscular Augmentation

Because of the lower capsular contracture rate, submuscular augmentation is usually considered the first choice for implant placement in most patients. With this technique, the breast implant is placed under the pectoralis major muscle and over the pectoralis minor muscle. Although the pectoralis muscle effectively covers the implant superiorly and medially, the implant may be only partially covered inferiorly and laterally. To help cover the implant, some surgeons mobilize the serratus anterior muscle laterally and the rectus fascia inferiorly. The most important advantage of submuscular augmentation is the lower capsular contracture rate.[21,22] The added soft tissue decreases the skin rippling over the implant and makes the implant less palpable. For this reason, the submuscular approach is the best technique in patients with minimal breast parenchyma. Disadvantages of this approach include potential weakening of the pectoralis muscle, implant movement with exercise (pectoralis muscular contraction), and difficulty in correcting the ptotic breast.

Complications of Breast Implants

The controversy about breast implants has centered around the safety of implants, not the safety of the surgical technique. Complications can be grouped into early and late complications. Early complications are mostly related to surgical technique, whereas late complications are mostly related to the breast implants. Early complications are much less common than late complications. Although there have been reports of autoimmune symptoms occurring in patients with breast implants, large epidemiologic studies have failed to show statistically significant cause and effect relationships between them. Because of these concerns about implant safety, however, much has been published recently regarding implant complications.[38–41]

EARLY COMPLICATIONS

Technical errors in implant positioning may result in asymmetric breasts. Coagulation disorders or poor hemostasis may result in hematoma formation, which has been associated with a higher risk of capsular contracture. Nipple-areolar sensation can occur due to injury to the lateral cutaneous rami of the fourth intercostal nerve. Temporary loss of sensation is relatively common, whereas permanent sensation loss is rare, except in patients who have had multiple reoperations. Infections are uncommon with strict sterile technique and the use of perioperative antibiotics. If a purulent periprosthetic infection occurs, however, the implant must usually be removed and replaced after the infection has resolved. Pneumothorax following breast augmentation is rare, but has been reported. Complications related to anesthesia as drug reactions, atelectasis, and pneumonia may occur as in other surgeries.[1,11]

LATE COMPLICATIONS

Late complications are common and their incidence increases with time. For this reason, breast implant studies

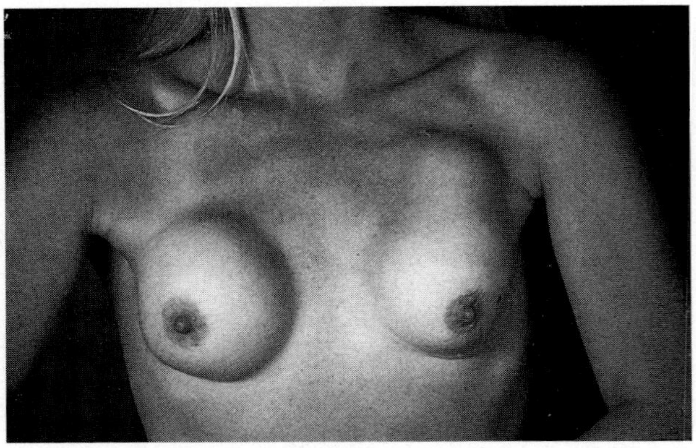

Figure 3–5. Patient with Baker grade IV contracture with displaced left silicone implant.

with short-term follow-up are likely to report much lower complication rates than those with long-term follow-up. The most common complication, overall, is capsular contracture (Fig. 3–3)[1,11] Symptoms of breast pain, tenderness, and hardness associated with Baker grade IV capsular contractures are usually the most disturbing complaint of patients. Implant displacement and breast distortion with resulting asymmetry can also occur due to capsular contracture formation (Fig. 3–5). In patients with minimal overlying breast soft tissue, rippling of the skin may occur, especially with saline-filled textured implants. Implant extrusion has also been reported to occur, which invariably leads to an infected prosthesis. Secondary chest wall depressions with rib remodeling have been reported and are well documented radiologically. These changes are attributed to long-standing implant pressure on the rib cage and are largely asymptomatic occurrences. Occult periprosthetic calcifications also occur and must be well documented on mammography.[42] Although isolated incidents of periprosthetic cancer have been reported, large epidemiologic studies have confirmed that breast implants are not associated with any increased risk of breast cancer, despite the fact that implants do mask breast parenchyma on screening mammograms.

Much of the interest in implant safety has focused on the issue of implant leak and rupture (Fig. 3–6). All implants appear to decrease their wall tensile strength and malleability with time.

Current theory suggests that the shell is maximally stressed at a fold or ripple, resulting in "fracture fatigue" of the wall and a resultant leak (or rupture). For saline-filled implants, a leak (or rupture) usually results in implant deflation, which patients and their physician can easily detect. More disturbing, however, is the fact that silicone gel implants gradually undergo gel bleed and may rupture without being detected by the patient or the physician. Although many patients can detect changes in their breast with implant rupture, others may have no signs or symptoms of implant rupture. A thorough history and physical examination may provide clues to such an occurrence, but their accuracy is too low to be reliable (see Implant Removal, below). This fact has probably been the major reason for the recent interest in magnetic resonance imaging (MRI) of the augmented breast.

Implant Removal and Reconstruction

Although the correlation between patient symptoms and implant rupture is unclear, all scientific studies have correlated an increasing implant rupture rate with increasing age of the breast implant. Most studies suggest a statistically significant increase in rupture risk once the implant is 10 years old.

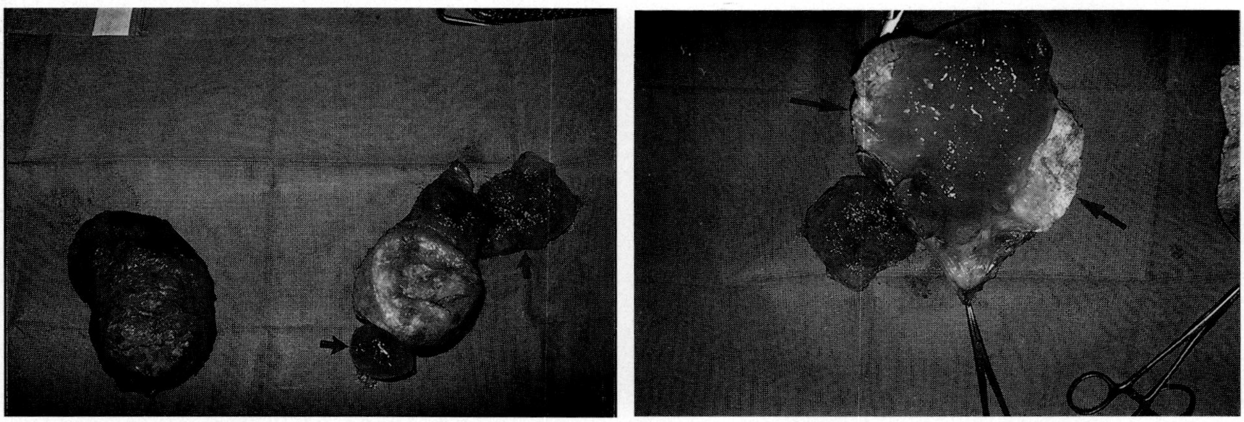

A B

Figure 3–6. Ruptured and intact gel-filled silicone implant. (**A**) The ruptured left implant demonstrates extruded free silicone (arrows) extending from the calcific periprosthetic capsule. The right implant was intact. (**B**) Close-up photograph of the ruptured left implant with a partially calcified periprosthetic capsule (arrows). See Plates IIIA and IIIB.

Because the highest number of silicone gel breast implantations occurred in the 1980s, it is likely that the 1990s will result in a wave of implant removals. For this reason, it is imperative that physicians be familiar with managing these patients.

PATIENT EVALUATION

Patients presenting with breast implants have their own unique circumstances and concerns about their current health, their future health, and their appearance. Each patient evaluation must be individualized and must start with objective information gathering. In addition to the usual history, all the relevant information regarding implants and implant surgery must be obtained (Table 3–6).

A thorough examination must also be done, including an examination for breast masses, axillary adenopathy, nipple-areolar sensation, and breast asymmetry. Using the information about the patients prior bra size, current bra size, implant size, and physical examination, an estimate of the volume that is breast tissue (%) and that is implant (%) should be made. The degree of ptosis (grade I, II, or III) and capsular contracture (Baker I, II, III, or IV) should also be assessed and recorded. Any history or physical clues to possible implant rupture should also be elicited. For instance, a patient who previously had a hard, painful breast that suddenly turned into a soft, Baker I capsule may have had an implant rupture. Likewise, a patient presenting with a positive squeeze test on examination may also be suspect for an implant rupture. The squeeze test involves compressing the augmented breast and identifying extravasated silicone gel filling the axilla or upper pole of the breast when the implant can still be palpated under the examiner's hands. This sign, if present, is highly suggestive of implant rupture. Although diagnosing of silicone gel implant rupture by history and physical examination is highly inaccurate, an astute clinician may be able to screen out those patients requiring further radiologic testing.

DECISION MAKING

Once an objective evaluation has been completed, all options for breast implant treatment need to be explained to the patient, along with the benefits and risks. These options include no surgery (follow-up), implant removal only, removal and replacement with saline implants, removal with mastopexy, removal with adjacent tissue transfer, and removal with autologous flap reconstruction. In patients with no evidence of rupture, no symptoms, mild capsular contractures, no breast deformity, and implants that were recently placed, the best option may be observation alone. In patients with evidence of rupture, breast pain and tenderness, and severe capsular contractures with breast deformities, surgery is probably a better option. Because many factors are involved in the decision-making process, each patient treatment must be individualized based on the objective evaluation. Once a decision has been made to proceed with surgery, then the surgical options must be addressed.

IMPLANT REMOVAL

Implant removal entails much more than simply removing the implant. Although each patient's treatment must be individualized, there are some generally accepted principles. The implant should be removed intact, whenever possible, without rupturing the implant shell. Because all implants undergo gel bleed and some implants may be ruptured at the time of removal, the safest way to minimize gel extravasation is to remove the surrounding periprosthetic capsule with the implant with an en bloc technique. The periprosthetic capsule can then be opened and the implant inspected after it has been removed from the breast. After implant removal, the remaining breast tissue should be palpated for breast tumors, silicone granulomas, and scar tissue. The axilla should also be palpated intraoperatively for adenopathy and extravasated silicone.

ADJUNCTIVE PROCEDURES

Implant removal alone often produces unacceptable secondary deformities, such as a wrinkled breast (excess skin, inverted or depressed nipple) with an irregular breast contour (asymmetry, skin dimpling, etc.) (Fig. 3–7). Surgical planning must anticipate these secondary deformities and include surgery to treat or minimize them. Preoperative breast ptosis and parenchymal volume (as a function of augmented breast volume) information can be used to predict whether the patient will have an acceptable cosmetic result from implant removal alone. In general, patients with large implants, minimal breast parenchyma, and significant ptosis are more

Table 3–6. Implant Patient Evaluation

Patient Information	*Implant Information*	*Implant Surgery*	*Examination*
Patient age	Implant manufacturer	Date of surgeries	Masses?
Hx of breast dz	Implant model/type	Implant position	Sensation?
Adenopathy?	Implant size	Surgical incision	Asymmetry?
Family hx of breast cancer	Implant filler	Prior capsulectomies?	Ptosis?
Bra size prior to augmentation	Implant coating?	Prior exchanges?	Breast vol?
Current bra size	Mammograms?	Prior closed capsulotomies?	Contracture?
Symptoms?	MRIs?		Squeeze test?

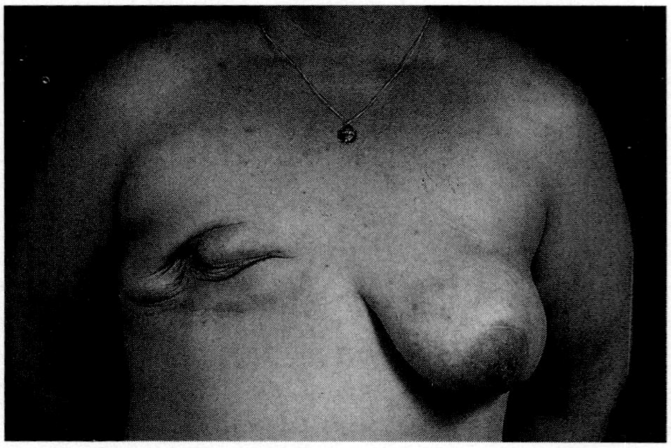

Figure 3–7. Implant removal patient with a poor aesthetic result of the right breast with skin retraction and asymmetry. The left implant was not removed.

likely to have an unacceptable result from implant removal alone. In these patients, adjunctive procedures should be explained to the patient. These procedures include implant replacement (submuscular or subglandular), mastopexy (nipple and parenchymal repositioning, skin excision), adjacent tissue transfer, and autologous tissue reconstruction (Fig. 3–8). A discussion of these options is beyond the scope of this book.

■ CURRENT AND FUTURE STATUS OF IMPLANTS

The current status of breast implants in the United States is as follows. Silicone gel implants may only be placed in FDA-approved protocols, being carried out by the Mentor Corporation. Saline-filled implants are FDA allowed but not officially FDA approved. The FDA has requested premarket approvals (PMAs) for saline-filled implants from all implant manufacturers. Soybean oil implants are being studied in an FDA-approved protocol, carried out by the Lipomatrix Corporation. The current position of the American College of Rheumatology is that there is "compelling evidence that silicone implants expose patients to no demonstrable additional risk for connective tissue or rheumatic disease." The issues of product liability and patient injury have not been settled in the courts yet.

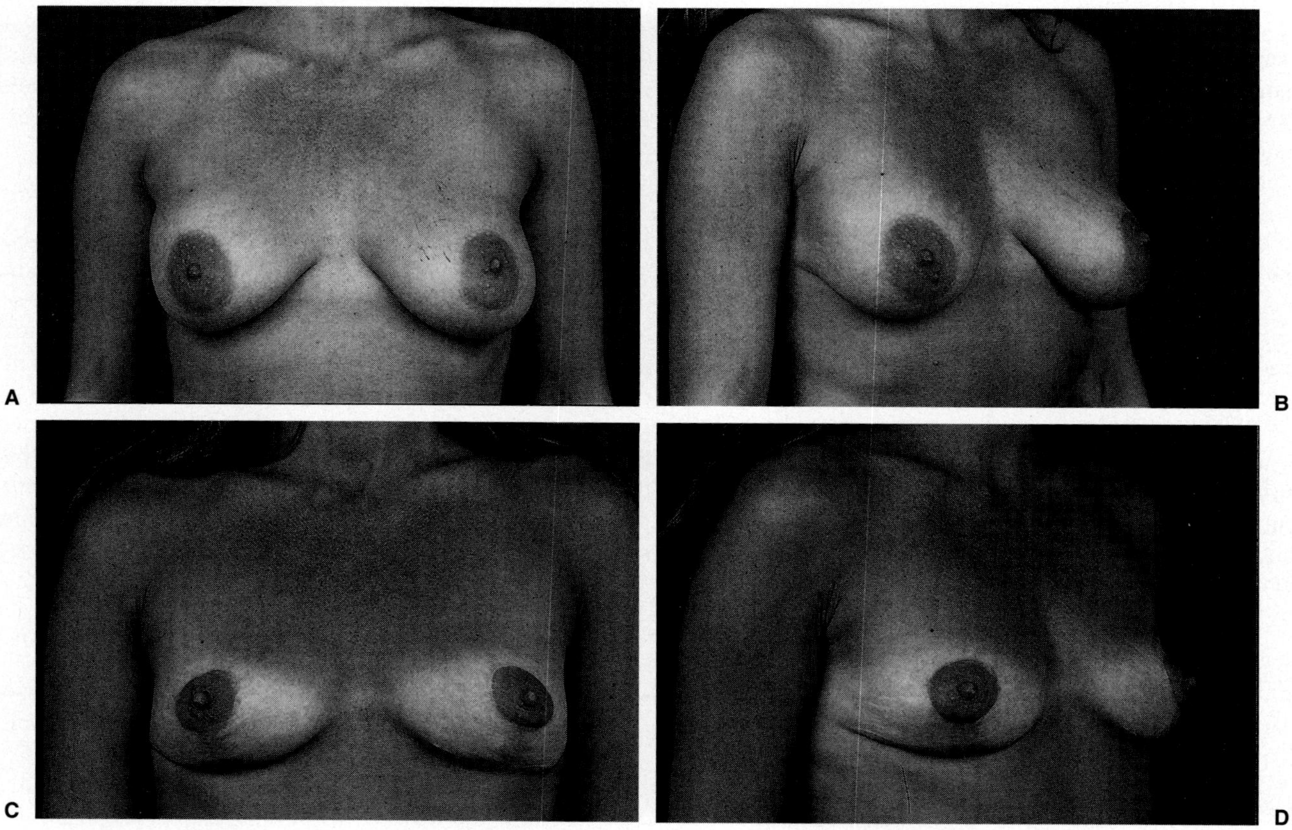

Figure 3–8. Preoperative implant removal photograph of patient in frontal (**A**) and oblique (**B**) view. Post-operative implant removal and mastopexy in same patient with good aesthetic results in frontal (**C**) and oblique (**D**) view.

The future of breast implants and their role in aesthetic and reconstructive surgery is still unclear. Although many studies are currently under way to scientifically evaluate the health risks of implants, other factors such as public opinion, the FDA, the media, and the legal system may ultimately determine the future role of breast implants.

REFERENCES

1. Letterman G, Schurter M. History of aesthetic breast surgery. In: Lewis JR, ed. *The art of aesthetic plastic surgery.* Vol. 1. Boston, Mass: Little, Brown, 1989;21–27.
2. Biggs TM, Cukier J, Worthing LF. Augmentation mammaplasty: a review of 18 years. *Plast Reconstr Surg.* 1982;69:445.
3. Lavine DM. Saline inflatable prostheses: 14 years' experience. *Aesthetic Plast Surg.* 1993;17:325.
4. Vasquez B, Given KS, Houston GC. Breast augmentation: a review of subglandular and submuscular implantation. *Aesthetic Plast Surg.* 1987;11:101.
5. Broadbent TR, Woolf RM. Augmentation mammaplasty. *Plast Reconstr Surg.* 1967;40:517.
6. Cronin TD, Gerow F. Augmentation mammaplasty: a new "natural fell" prosthesis. In: Transactions Third International Congress Plastic Surgery. *Excerpta Medica.* Amsterdam, 1964. pp. 41–49.
7. Rees TD, Guy CL, Coburn RJ. The use of inflatable breast implants. *Plast Reconstr Surg.* 1973;52:609.
8. Bridges AJ, Vasey FB. Silicone breast implants: history, safety, and potential complications. *Arch Intern Med.* 1993;153:2638–2644.
9. Habal MB. The biologic basis for the clinical application of the silicones. *Arch Surg.* 1984;119:843–848.
10. Shapiro MA. Smooth versus rough: An 8-year survey of mammary prostheses. *Plast Reconstr Surg.* 1989;84:449.
11. McInnis WD. Plastic surgery of the breast. In: Mitchell GW, Bassett LW, eds. *The female breast and its disorders.* Baltimore: Williams & Wilkins, 1990;203–210.
12. Dukes CE, Mitchley MI. Polyvinyl sponge implants: experimental and clinical observations. *Br J Plast Surg.* 1962;15:225.
13. Radlauer CB, Bowers DG. Treatment of severe breast asymmetry. *Plast Reconstr Surg.* 1971;47:347.
14. Snyderman RK, Guthrie RH. Reconstruction of the female breast following radical mastectomy. *Plast Reconstr Surg.* 1971;47:565.
15. Strombeck JG. Mammaplasty: Report of a new technique based on the two-pedicle procedure. *Br J Plast Surg.* 1960;13:79.
16. Scheflan M, Kalisman M. Complications of breast reconstruction. *Clin Plast Surg.* 1984;11:343.
17. Woods JE. Unusual complications of submuscular placement of implants in breast surgery. *Plast Reconstr Surg.* 1984;73:972.
18. Cronin TD, Persoff MM, Upton J. Augmentation mammaplasty: complications and etiology. In: Owsley JQ, Peterson RA, eds. *Symposium on aesthetic surgery.* St. Louis: Mosby, 1978.
19. McIndoe AH, Rees TD. Mammaplasty: inications, technique and complications. *Br J Plast Surg.* 1958;10:397.
20. Burkhardt BR. Comparing contracture rates: probability theory and the unilateral contracture. *Plast Reconstr Surg.* 1984;74:527.
21. Pollock H. Breast capsular contracture: a retrospective study of textured versus smooth-silicone implants. *Plast Reconstr Surg.* 1993;91:404.
22. Hakelius L, Ohlsen L. A clinical comparison of the tendency to capsular contracture between smooth and textured gel-filled silicone mammary implants. *Plast Reconstr Surg.* 1992;90:247.
23. Hester TR, Nahai F, Bostwick J, et al. A 5-year experience with polyurethane-covered mammary prostheses for treatment of capsular contracture, primary augmentation mammaplasty and breast reconstruction. *Clin Plast Surg.* 1988;15:569.
24. Ersek RA. Rate and incidence of capsular contracture: a comparison of smooth and textured silicone double-lumen breast prostheses. *Plast Reconstr Surg.* 1991;87:879.
25. Cairns TS, De Villiers W. Capsular contracture after breast augmentation: a comparison between gel and saline-filled prostheses. *S Afr Med J.* 1980;57:951.
26. Gylbert L, Asplund O, Jurell G. Capsular contracture after breast reconstruction with silicone-gel and saline-filled implants: a 6-year follow-up. *Plast Reconstr Surg.* 1990;85:373.
27. Puckett CL, Croll GH, Reichel CA, et al. A critical look at capsule contracture in subglandular versus subpectoral mammary augmentation. *Aesthetic Plast Surg.* 1987;11:23.
28. Burkhardt BR, Dempsye PD, Schnur PL, et al. Capsular contracture: a prospective study of effect of local antibacterial agents. *Plast Reconstr Surg.* 1986;77:919.
29. Burkhardt BR. Capsular contracture: hard breasts, soft data. *Clin Plast Surg.* 1988;15:521.
30. Williams JE. Experiences with a large series of silastic breast implants. *Plast Reconstr Surg.* 1972;49:253.
31. Baker JL, Bartels RJ, Douglas WM. Closed compression technique for rupturing a contracted capsule around a breast implant. *Plast Reconstr Surg.* 1976;58:137–141.
32. Gruber RP, Jones HW. Review of closed capsulotomy complications. *Ann Plast Surg.* 1981;6:271–275.
33. Kessler DA. The basis of the FDA's decision on breast implants. *N Engl J Med.* 1992;326:1713–1715.
34. Brody GS. Fact and fiction about breast implant "bleed." *Plast Reconstr Surg.* 1977;60:615–616.
35. Ahn CY, Shaw WW, Narayanan K, et al. Definitive diagnosis of breast implant rupture using magnetic resonance imaging. *Plast Reconstr Surg.* 1993;94(4):681–691.
36. Berkel H, Birdsell DC, Jenkins H. Breast augmentation: a risk factor for breast cancer? *N Engl J Med.* 1992;326:1649–1653.
37. Dempsey WC, Latham WD. Subpectoral implants in augmentation mammaplasty. *Plast Reconstr Surg.* 1968;42:515.
38. Marik PE, Kark AL, Zambakides A. Scleroderma after silicone augmentation mammoplasty: A report of two cases. *S Afr Med J.* 1990;77:212–213.
39. Spiera H. Scleroderma after silicone augmentation mammoplasty. *JAMA.* 1988;260:236–238.
40. Steinbach BG, Hardt NS, Abbitt PL, et al. Breast implants, common complications, and concurrent breast disease. *Radiographics.* 1993;13:95–118.
41. Weiner SR. Silicone augmentation mammoplasty and rheumatic disease. In: Stratmeyer ME, ed. *Silicone in medical devices: proceedings of a conference held in Baltimore, MD, Feb 1–2, 1991.* Bethesda, MD: Department of Health and Human Services (Publication FDA 92-4249), 1991:81–102.
42. Young VL, Bartell T, Destouet JM, Monsees B, Logan SE. Calcification of breast implant capsule. *South Med J.* 1989;82:1171–1173.

4

Breast Implant Classification

M. S. MIDDLETON

Silicone gel–filled breast implants were first placed in a patient by Dr. Frank Gerow in 1962, and were later provided on a commercial basis by Dow Corning in 1964. At first there was only one style in one size. Additional styles of implants were made available initially by Dow Corning, and then by many other manufacturers. We have noted a cumulative total of more than 240 styles of breast implants and tissue expanders since 1962 from American breast implant manufacturers alone. Even within individual styles from a given manufacturer there is variability, and so the number of design variations is actually far greater. In addition to catalogued implants, manufacturers provided special order implants only slightly different from catalogued items (i.e., specially overfilled or underfilled), as well as custom implants by prescription designed especially for individual patients.

An early history of breast implants was provided by Braley[1] in 1973. In 1976[2] and then again in 1978[3] Gerow provided an update of that information containing photographs of several early implant types. Examples of various implant types have been illustrated in recent publications, showing their magnetic resonance (MR) imaging and mammographic appearances.[4,5] Demand for implant evaluation over the past 5 years, together with the success of MR and ultrasound imaging in evaluating breast implants, have engendered a need to understand better the various types of breast implants. For this reason we proposed a breast implant classification scheme consisting of 14 categories,[6–7] which will be described in this chapter. An increased understanding of breast implants will aid radiologists in implant imaging, and will minimize misinterpretation resulting from unfamiliarity with the various implant types. Stratification by data by implant type and style will also be useful in research regarding breast implants.

SOURCES OF INFORMATION

The following sources of information were used to understand better the variety of breast implant design and construction:

1. Medical records from over 1200 of our patients who have or had breast implants, who had a breast MR scan at our institution, and direct visual implant examination at explantation surgery for over 190 of those patients.
2. Medical records from over 150 outside breast implant MR evaluations of patients imaged elsewhere.
3. Medical records and direct visual observations of implants *after* explantation for more than 600 other patients.
4. Breast implant product data sheets, product inserts, and other materials provided to us by breast implant manufacturers, the Breast Implant Litigation Plaintiff Steering Committee, and plaintiff attorneys.
5. Formal meetings with representatives of Dow Corning concerning their breast implant products.
6. Informal feedback from representatives of Bioplasty, Cox Uphoff International (CUI), McGhan, Mentor, and Surgitek with regard to their individual products.
7. Published accounts of breast implant styles and types.

MR images shown in this chapter were obtained with a General Electric (Milwaukee, WI) 1.5 T scanner (4.8x software) using a dedicated bilateral breast surface coil. The imaging parameters have included field of view 15 to 20 cm, matrix size 256 ×256, and slice thickness 3 to 4 mm. Most images were T2 weighted obtained using a water suppression fast spin echo (FSE) pulse sequence (TE =208 or 304 msec, TR >3000 msec, bandwidth 16 kHz, Echo Train Length (ETL) =8 or 16).

■ BREAST IMPLANT CLASSIFICATION

A summary of our breast implant classification scheme is contained in Table 4–1, the various categories of which are described here. We based this scheme on differences in implant construction, together with the appearance of implants on MR images. Saline-filled, dextran-filled, and polyvinyl pyrrolidone–filled implants are in one category because they all have similar appearances on MR images. A brief description of the features that distinguish the various breast implant types and styles is contained in Table 4–2. A summary of the various types of polyurethane-coated breast implants is contained in Table 4–3. A summary of breast implant valve types is contained in Table 4–4.

Single-Lumen Silicone Gel–Filled Implants

NONPOLYURETHANE COATED IMPLANTS

Just over 80% of the breast implants we have imaged are single lumen silicone gel filled. Most have a smooth silicone elastomer shell (Figs. 4–1 and 4–2), but other more recent implants have a textured elastomer shell (Figs. 4–3 through 4–5). The implant shell is usually closed at time of manufacture by a patch (usually on the posterior surface of the implant), the appearance of which can be distinctive. Some rare gel inflatable implants from the 1970's have a fill hole closed with a plug. Although the manufacturer's name is sometimes marked on the back patch, nearly all of the older implants and some more recent ones are not so marked. Despite this, implant identification based on a careful direct visual inspection of the implant, back patch, and any markings on the implant shell is still possible in most cases because of differences in the appearance of these features from one manufacturer to the next, as described in Table 4–2.

POLYURETHANE COATED IMPLANTS

About 10% of the single-lumen silicone gel–filled breast implants we have imaged are coated with a layer of adhesive and polyurethane foam, intended to promote tissue ingrowth and reduce capsular contracture. Silicone gel is contained within a silicone elastomer shell that is most often closed with a back patch, and that is coated with an adhesive and a layer of polyurethane foam. Some of the silicone elastomer shells (Même implants) were reportedly manufactured to begin with by coating the preformed gel one side at a time with silicone and then vulcanizing and curing in an oven, as opposed to filling a manufactured shell with gel. The major styles of polyurethane-coated implants are described in Table 4–3.

Single-Lumen Gel-Saline "Adjustable" Implants

Fewer than 2% of the silicone gel–filled breast implants we have imaged are of this type. Gel-saline implants consist of a silicone elastomer shell prefilled by the manufacturer with silicone gel, which can then have saline added directly to the

Table 4–1. Types of Implants

Implant Type	*Description*	*Approximate Percentage of Implants**
Single lumen	Silicone gel filled	82%
Single lumen adjustable	Silicone gel filled, to which can be added variable amount saline at time of placement	<2%
Saline, dextran, or polyvinyl pyrrolidone filled	Mostly saline filled, some early implants were dextran filled, and some more recent implants are polyvinyl pyrrolidone (PVP) filled	Not applicable
"Standard" double lumen	Silicone gel inner lumen, saline outer lumen	15%
"Reverse" double lumen	Saline inner lumen, silicone gel outer lumen	<1%
"Reverse adjustable" double lumen	Silicone gel inner and outer lumen, variable amount saline added to inner lumen at time of placement.	<1%
"Gel-gel" double lumen	Silicone gel inner lumen, silicone gel outer lumen	<1%
Triple lumen	Silicone gel inner and middle lumen, saline outer lumen	<1%
Cavon	More cohesive gel, no shell	<1%
Custom	Nonstandard type, size, shape—individualized	<1%
Pectus	Solid implant to replace pectus muscle(s)	Not applicable
Sponge	Etheron (polyurethane) or Ivalon	Not applicable
Sponge adjustable	Silicone elastomer shell, sponge inside, dextran or saline filled, polyurethane coated	Not applicable
Other	Soy Bean Oil, etc.	<1%

*Not including saline, dextran, PVP, pectus, sponge, or sponge adjustable.

**Percentages are in reference to the total number of silicone gel–filled breast implants seen for breast MR scans at our institution, together with those seen in formal consultation for breast MR scans performed elsewhere. This table is based upon a table from Middleton et al.[7]

Table 4–2. Features of Breast Implants*

Feature	*Description*
Shape, size, and profile	Breast implants can have a round, oval, teardrop, contoured, or custom shape. For a given capacity shell, they can be very underfilled with silicone gel (sometimes called "special fill"), low profile, moderate profile, or high profile. In addition, for any given combination of the above factors, multiple sizes are usually available.
Back patch design	Implant back patches can vary considerably between styles, and also between manufacturers. For example, they can (a) be centrally or peripherally placed on the posterior surface of the implant; (b) be of different shape, diameter, or thickness; (c) be located inside or outside the implant shell, (d) have beveled edges (Surgitek); (e) be made of silicone elastomer alone, or be Dacron reinforced with netting that comes mainly in one of two patterns; (f) be smooth, textured, roughened, or have a multicircle or spiral (Heyer Schulte or Mentor) design imprinted upon them; (g) be multiple, with, for example, one back patch placed inside and another placed outside the implant shell; or (h) have the gel fill point (if present) located either centrally, peripherally on the patch, or placed outside the patch.
Shell and back patch markings	The name of the manufacturer is often placed on the implant back patch for more recent implants (CUI, Dow Corning, Koken, McGhan, and McGhan/3M). The implant size can be marked on the back patch or shell. For some "standard" double lumen implants, the name or other identifying lettering is only on the inner lumen back patch (CUI and Dow Corning). Other markings indicating manufacturer, size, profile, or style can often be found. In some cases, markings can be found indicating which mandrel was used to form the shell. Some McGhan and McGhan/3M implants have a white dot centrally (or rarely peripherally) placed on the outer surface of the back patch. The size of the implant in beveled radio-opaque numerals can be seen for some recent Surgitek implants on the internal surface of the back patch. The implant shells can vary in thickness from extremely thin, in the late 1970s and early 1980s, to quite thick in the oldest and some of the most recent implants. The shells can be manufactured in one, two, or three layers, and can appear clear, slightly opaque, or completely opaque and cream colored.
Textured surface	Some recent non–polyurethane-coated breast implants have a textured rather than a smooth implant shell outer surface, intended to reduce capsular contracture. The textured surface can promote tissue ingrowth. The pattern and method of producing the texturing varied between manufacturers (i.e., Biocell® for McGhan, MISTI® for Bioplasty, MSI® for Dow Corning, and Siltex® for Mentor).
Fixation/orientation	Older breast implants, in addition to the back patch closing the implant shell, can also have an additional patch or patches also attached to the implant shell for the purpose of providing fixation to surrounding tissues. Two common mechanisms of fixation have been Dacron mesh, and fenestrated silicone elastomer. Fixation tags and loops can also be used. Bars and external disks are occasionally attached to the back patch or shell.
Internal disks	Dow Corning placed an approximately 12 mm silicone elastomer disk on the internal surface of some of their breast implants from about 1971 to 1984, the purpose of which was to help seal the hole through which silicone gel was introduced into the implant. With adequate MR technique, this disk can often be visualized on T2-weighted images in which silicone is bright. Other manufacturers used disks inside and outside their implants, but none that we know of was of 12-mm diameter centered on the back patch internally.
Silicone gel and elastomer	The cohesiveness of the silicone gel can vary from runny to extremely cohesive. This is at least in part because of the ratio of cross-linked to non–cross-linked silicone used to formulate the gel. It may also be that the silicone is no longer a gel, owing in part to a combination of what was once a gel with proteinaceous body fluids, if the implants have ruptured. The gel (and implant shell) color can vary from clear and glassy to a deep bronze yellow even in implants that have never been implanted. One suggestion for these changes in color is continued slow reaction catalyzed by the platinum catalyst (zero oxidation state) used in the original formulation of the gel. Some implant back patches that we have seen (McGhan/3M and Heyer Schulte) can be considerably darkened or blackened compared to the implant shell.
Valve construction	For the six types of breast implant that have a valve or valves (saline, gel-saline, "standard" double lumen, "reverse" double lumen, "reverse adjustable" double lumen, and triple lumen), the appearance and construction of the valves themselves can be sufficiently distinctive so as to allow identification not only of the implant type and manufacturer, but also often of the specific implant style.

*The implant features, taken individually or in combination, can often be used as a basis for breast implant classification and identification.

Table 4–3. Types of Polyurethane-Coated Implants

Style	*Description*
Natural Y	The earliest polyurethane-coated silicone gel–filled breast implants (starting in about 1968) were contoured in shape, and were called "Natural Y" because of the presence of a Y-shaped baffle internally.
Optimam	Successor to the early "Natural Y" style, starting in about 1982.
Vogue	Low profile implant, starting in about 1982, with or without a baffle.
Même	Round low profile version of the Optimam without a baffle, very thin shell, starting in about 1982.
Replicon	Contoured high profile implant, no baffle, starting in about 1983.
Même Moderate Profile	Round moderate profile version of the Même, increased shell thickness, starting in about 1985.

gel at the time of surgery through a valve provided for that purpose (Figs. 4–6 and 4–7). A rare early polyurethane-coated gel-saline implant had no valve, with the saline being added by a needle placed directly through the implant shell. More recent gel-saline implants, from about 1979 onward, came with a valve, either *self-seal* or *leaflet* (Table 4–4). Note: *Double*-lumen Dow Corning implants are referred to in their literature as "gel-saline"; other manufacturers use the term "gel-saline" for this single-lumen type of implant, as we have adopted here.

Saline, Dextran, and Polyvinyl Pyrrolidone (PVP)-Filled Implants

Inflatable saline- and dextran-filled breast implants, with a silicone elastomer shell, have been available since the early 1960s. More recently, Bioplasty, Inc. manufactured PVP prefilled and inflatable implants. All these implants are in a single category because their appearance on MR images is

Table 4–4. Implant Valve Types

Valve type	*Description*
No valve	There was one early Heyer Schulte polyurethane-coated gel-saline implant that had no valve. Saline could be added to the silicone gel by placing a needle directly through the shell. Saline could later be added via the same route percutaneously.
Early valves	Some early breast implants inflated with saline or dextran had a tube that was intended to be folded and then ligated with a silicone rubber ring. Others had tube valve intended to be plugged with a Teflon stopper and then possibly inverted into the implant. Some early gel inflatable implants had a distinctive plug or valve.
Leaflet	Leaflet valves have been used in six types of breast implants: saline, gel-saline, "standard" double lumen, "reverse" double lumen, "reverse adjustable" double lumen, and triple lumen. The leaflet valve usually consists of two pieces of silicone elastomer with a hole at each end. A tube is placed through one hole into the central channel between the two pieces at the time of placement, and saline is added. All of the American breast implant manufacturers except Heyer Schulte used leaflet valves in at least some of their implants.
Double leaflet	One style of "reverse" double lumen breast implant used identical leaflet valves assemblies on both implant shells. The inner saline-filled lumen was intended to be filled through a tube first entering the implant through the outer leaflet valve, traversing the silicone gel–filled outer lumen, and then entering the inner leaflet valve. When the inner lumen was inflated, the tube was pulled out, and each leaflet valve rolled up like a window shade.
Diaphragm	This valve type is used commonly in saline-filled breast implants. A plug fits into the valve, attached to the shell by a strap on one or both sides.
Retention	This type of valve was used in some Heyer Schulte, Mentor, McGhan, and McGhan/3M breast implants. It consisted of a tube attached to a leaflet-like structure. It was largely discontinued by the early 1980s.
Self-seal	Surgitek was the only American breast implant manufacturer to use self-seal valves in their commercially available products. Dow Corning may also have used such a valve in a small number of early experimental saline inflatable implants in about 1969–70. This type of valve consisted of an ovoid lens-shaped structure about 27-mm diameter mounted on the outer implant shell, made of silicone elastomer (often Dacron reinforced), containing a small quantity of special silicone gel. This valve type was largely discontinued by the early 1980s.
Internal tube	Many "reverse" double lumen implants had a permanent tube to inflate the inner saline filled lumen, which was *not* removed along with the filler tube after inflation with saline.

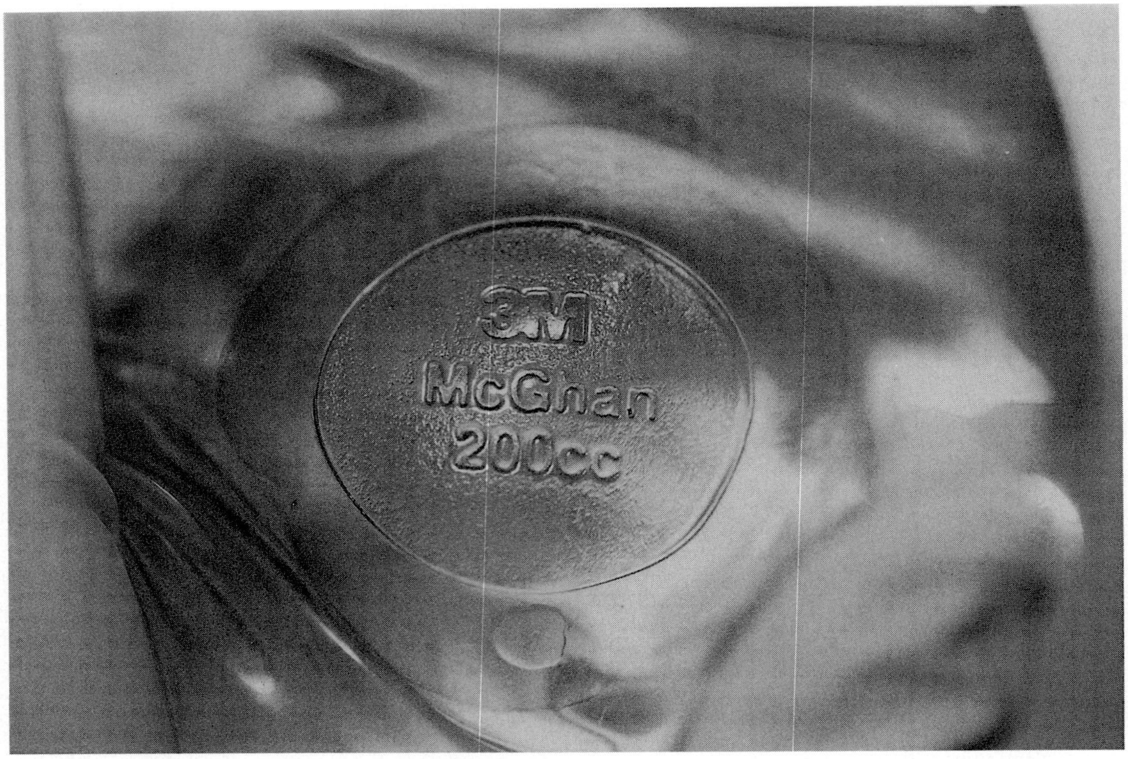

Figure 4–1. McGhan/3M smooth shell single-lumen silicone gel-filled breast implant, showing the name of the manufacturer and the implant size on the back patch.

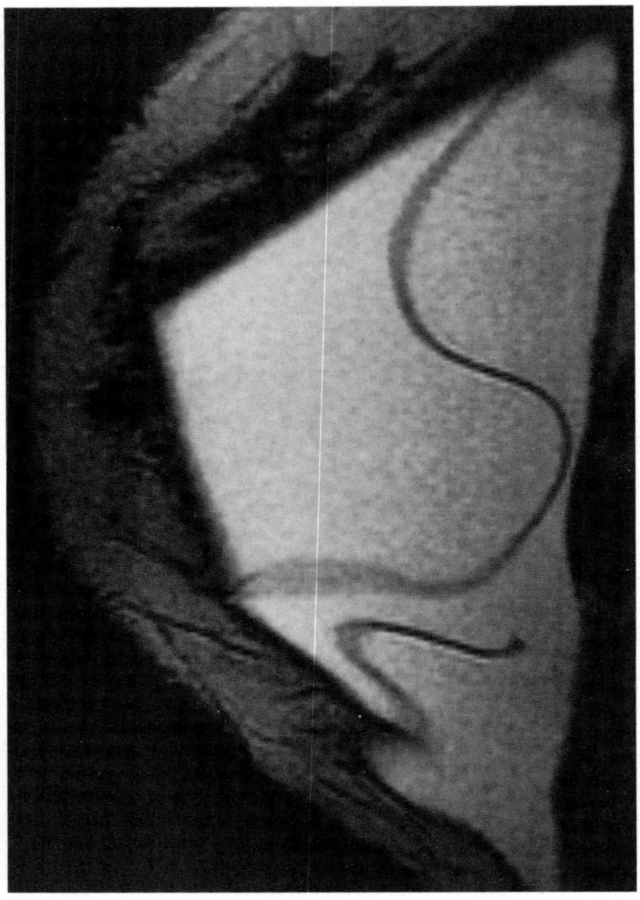

Figure 4–2. T2-weighted water-suppressed MR image of a smooth shell single-lumen silicone gel-filled breast implant, showing no evidence of rupture. Note that implant folds can be numerous and complex in appearance, and still be normal.

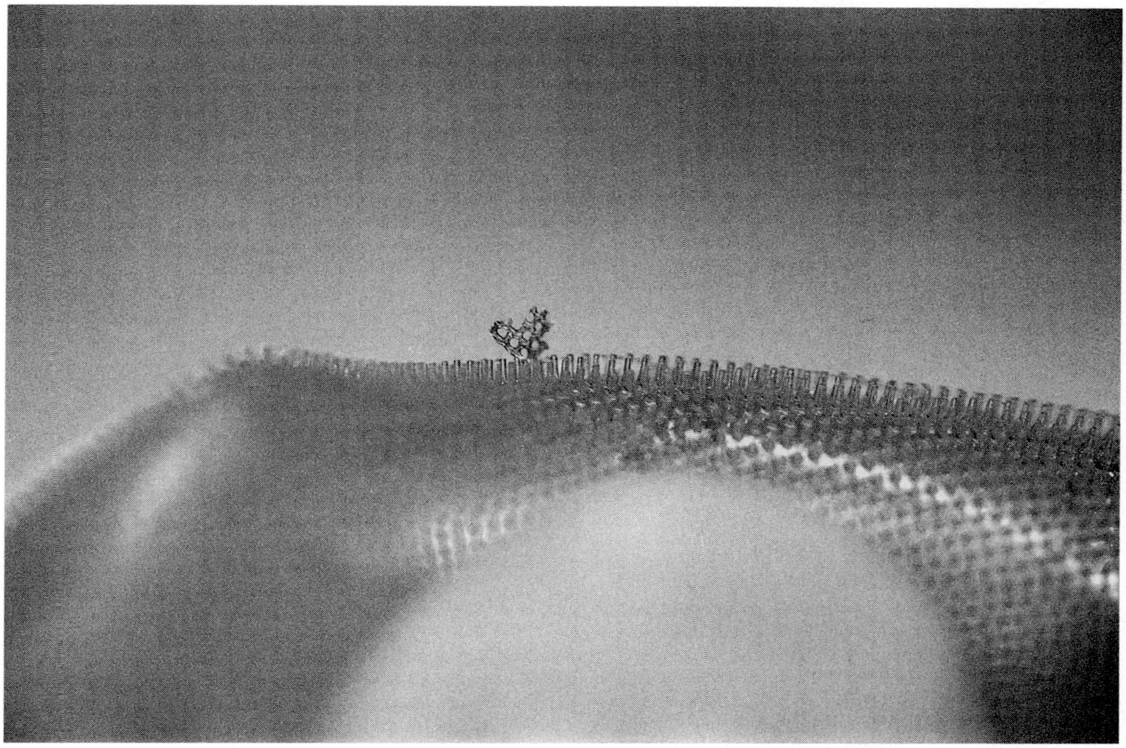

Figure 4–3. Textured surface (close-up) of a Dow Corning Silastic® II MSI single-lumen silicone gel-filled breast implant, which showed no evidence of rupture on MR or at surgery. Note small attached piece of adherant tissue, with holes corresponding to spacing of micropillar texturing of implant surface.

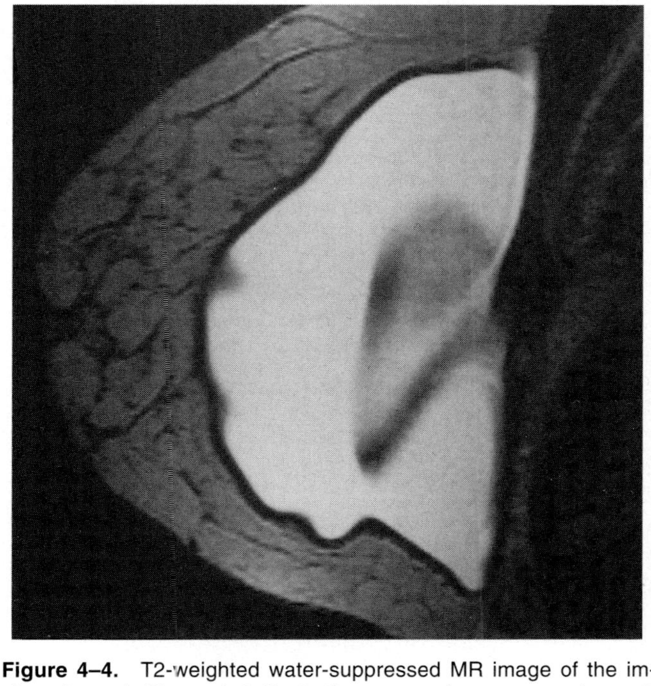

Figure 4–4. T2-weighted water-suppressed MR image of the implant shown in Figure 4–3, illustrating a normal appearance for such an implant. Note that the implant shell appears fairly thick, partly because of the presence of water-suppressed intracapsular water-like fluid surrounding the implant. Such intracapsular water-like fluid may have no significance, unless the amount is large.

identical. Early versions had self-seal or tube valves, and later versions had leaflet or diaphragm valves (Figs. 4–8 and 4–9).

"Standard" Double-Lumen Implants

About 15% of the silicone gel–filled breast implants we have imaged are "standard" double lumen, with saline in the outer and silicone gel in the inner lumen (Figs. 4–10 through 4–12). The outer lumen was provided to allow size adjustability at the time of placement. Double-lumen implants either had a *shared back patch* or a *bag-in-a-bag* configuration. In the former case, one complex back patch connected both shells (i.e., Heyer Schulte, McGhan, and McGhan/3M). In the latter case, each implant shell came complete with its own separate back patch (i.e., CUI, Dow Corning, Mentor, and Surgitek). The earliest standard double-lumen implants, which became available in about 1975, were of a design that had a relatively larger saline-to-gel ratio than later such implants.

(text continues on page 37)

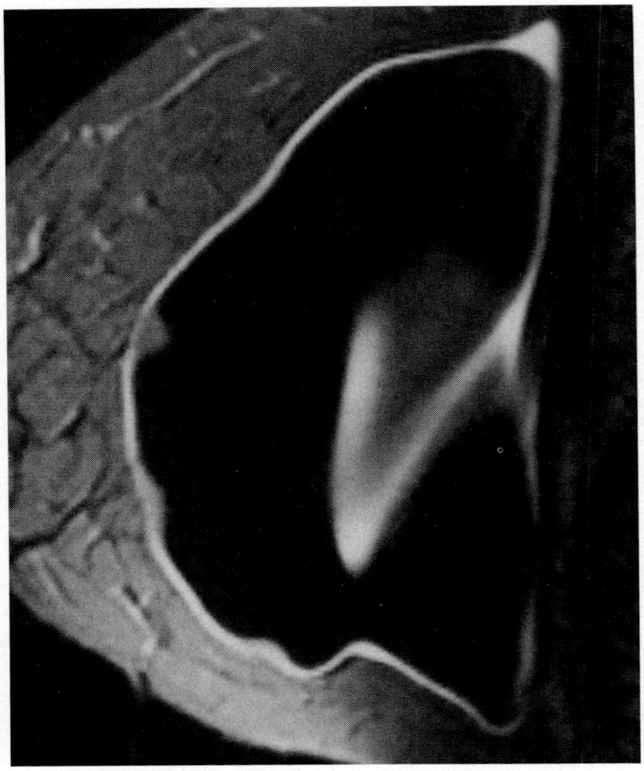

Figure 4–5. T2-weighted silicone-suppressed MR image of the implant shown in Figure 4–3, illustrating a normal appearance for this implant for this type of pulse sequence. The intracapsular water-like fluid images with bright signal, in contrast to the dark signal from the suppressed silicone gel inside the implant and the dark signal from the implant shell. The layer of fluid surrounding these implants is, as a rule, thicker than is seen surrounding other types of textured implant, perhaps because a "standoff layer" is created by the micropillars.

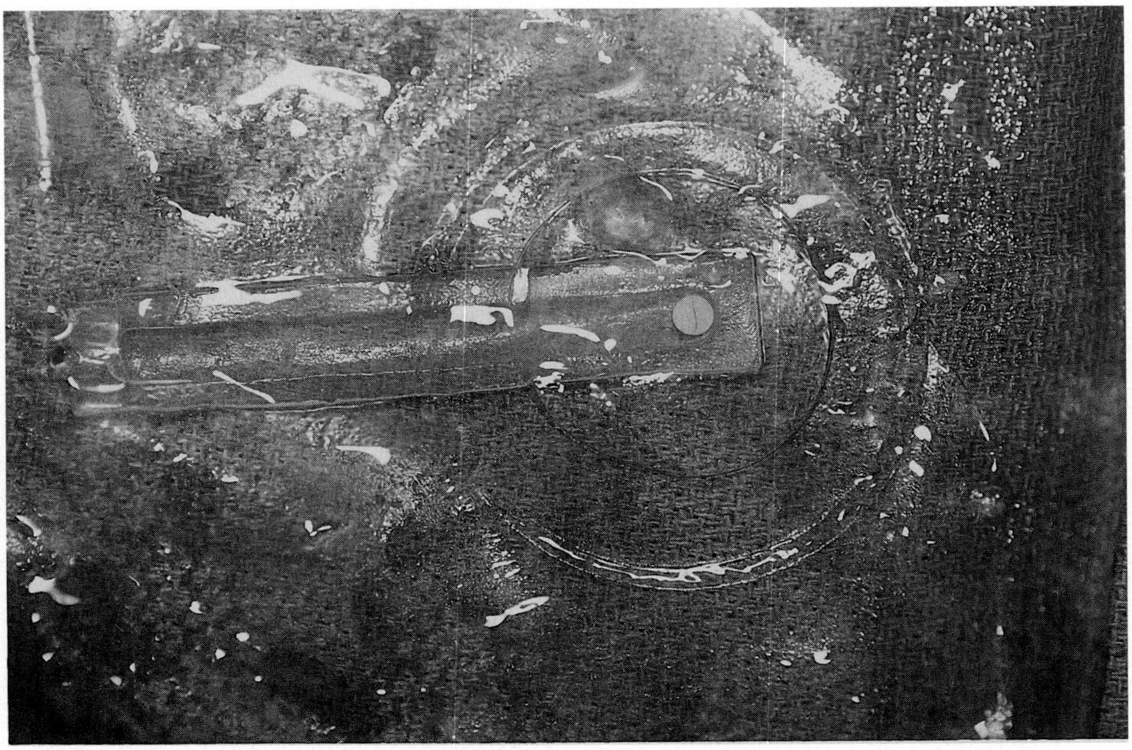

Figure 4–6. Surgitek single-lumen gel-saline breast implant, showing the leaflet valve (Quin-seal®) on the posterior surface. The beveled appearance of the back patch outside the implant shell, on which the valve is mounted, is characteristic for many Surgitek implants. The 3-mm white circle at the proximal end of the leaflet valve, with a slit in the middle, is also characteristic for these implants. As this is a gel-saline implant, a raised gel fill point is seen here peripherally on the back patch, next to the leaflet valve..

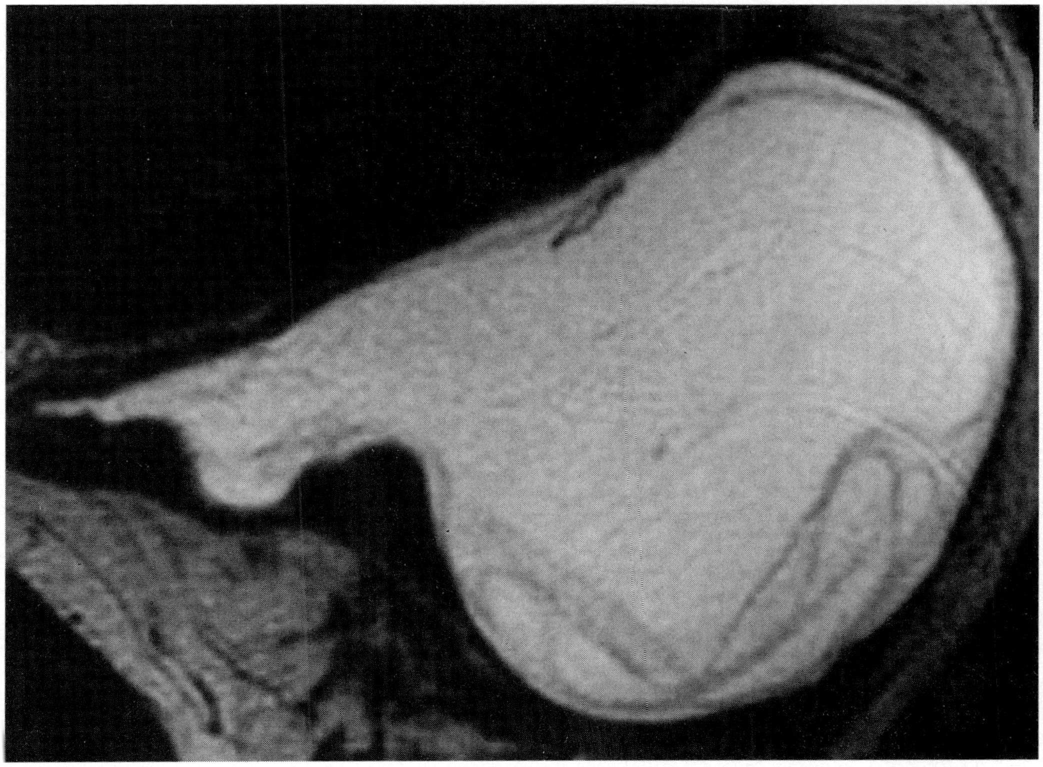

Figure 4–7. T2-weighted water-suppressed MR image of the implant shown in Figure 4–6. A cross section through the leaflet valve is seen within the silicone gel near the posterior surface of the implant.

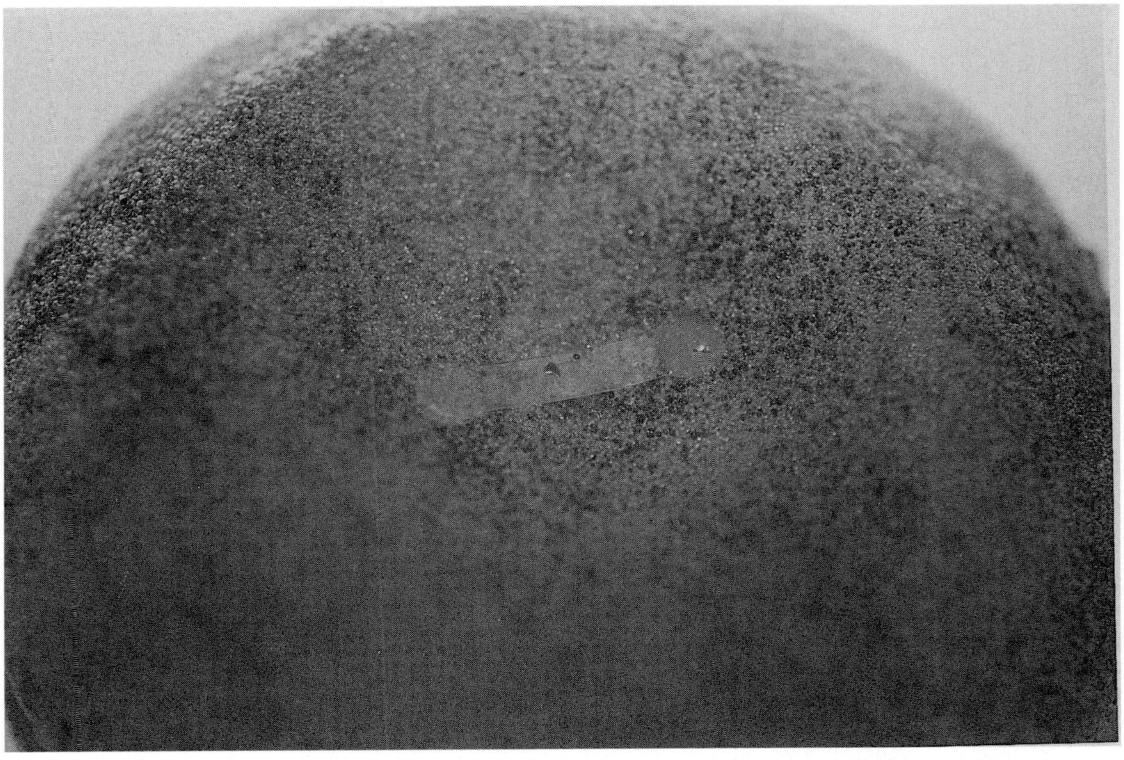

Figure 4–8. McGhan Style 168 textured saline-filled breast implant, anterior view, showing the diaphragm valve. A small plug fits into that valve which is attached to the implant shell by a strap, as shown in this figure.

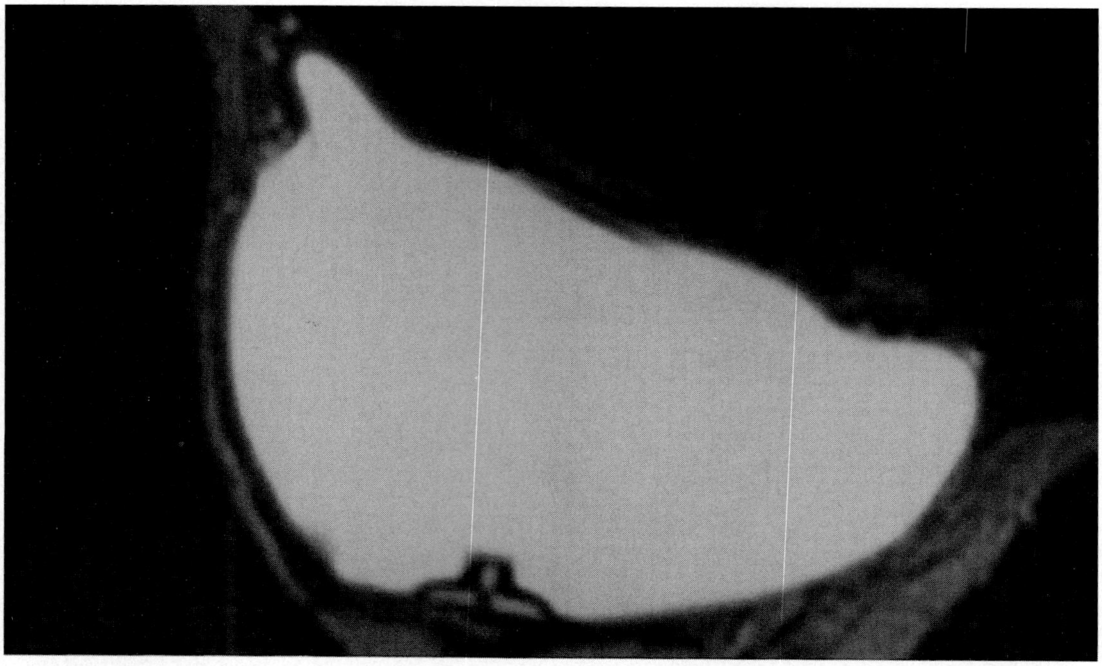

Figure 4–9. T2-weighted silicone-suppressed MR image of the saline-filled implant shown in Figure 4–8; shown in cross section is the diaphragm valve extending into the saline-filled lumen.

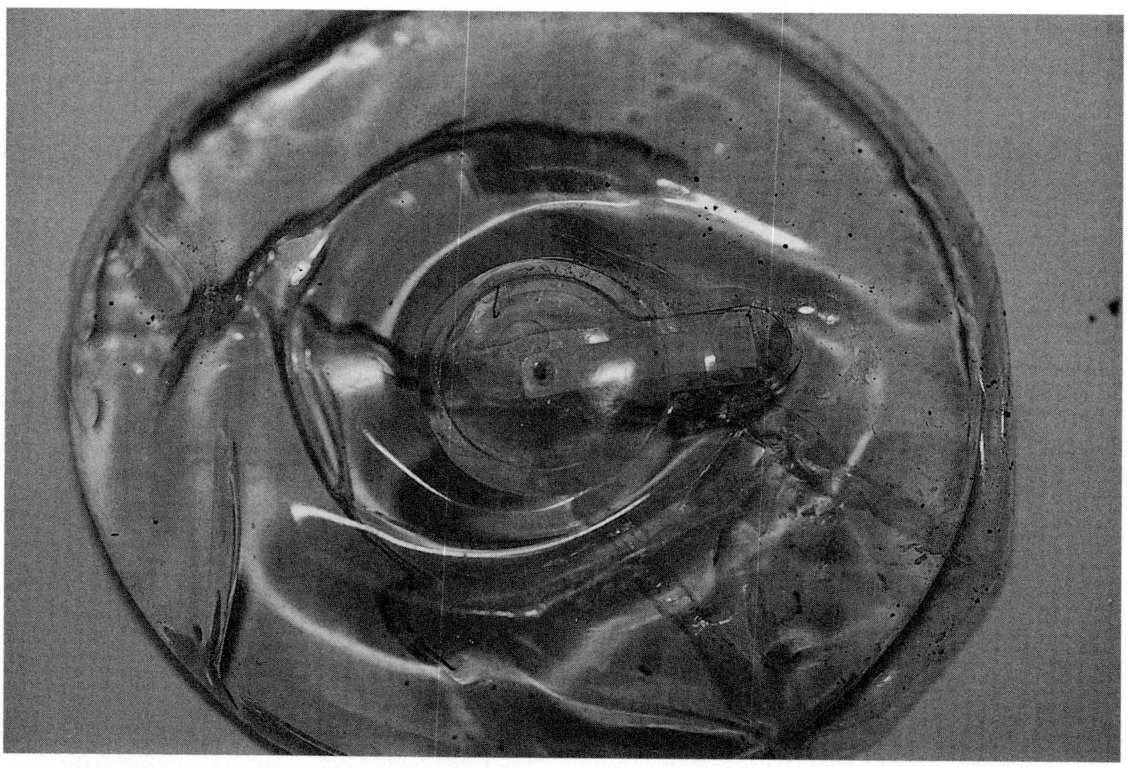

Figure 4–10. CUI "standard" double-lumen breast implant with a leaflet valve. The presence of the white strip within the valve, and the shape of the valve, are characteristic for some double-lumen implants from this manufacturer. The inner lumen has its own separate back patch (not shown).

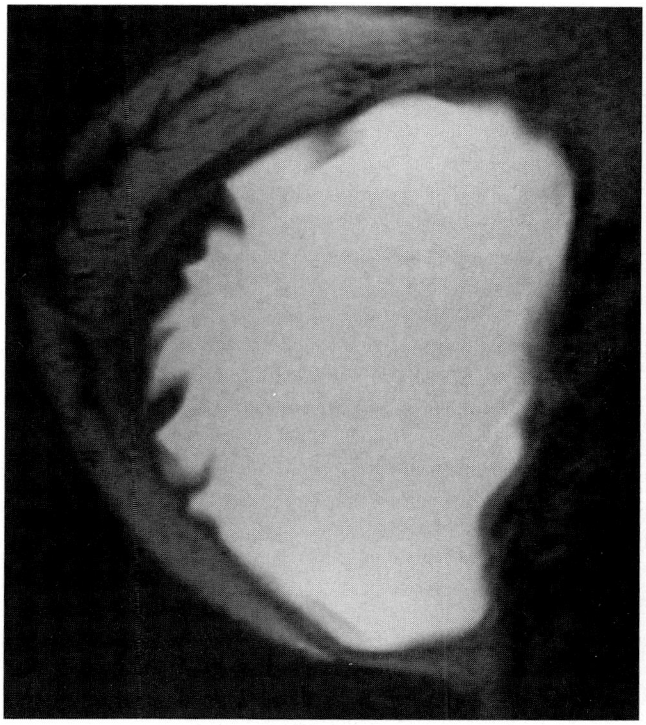

Figure 4–11. T2-weighted water-suppressed MR image of the double lumen implant shown in Figure 4–10, showing the inner lumen silicone gel as bright, and the outer lumen saline as dark.

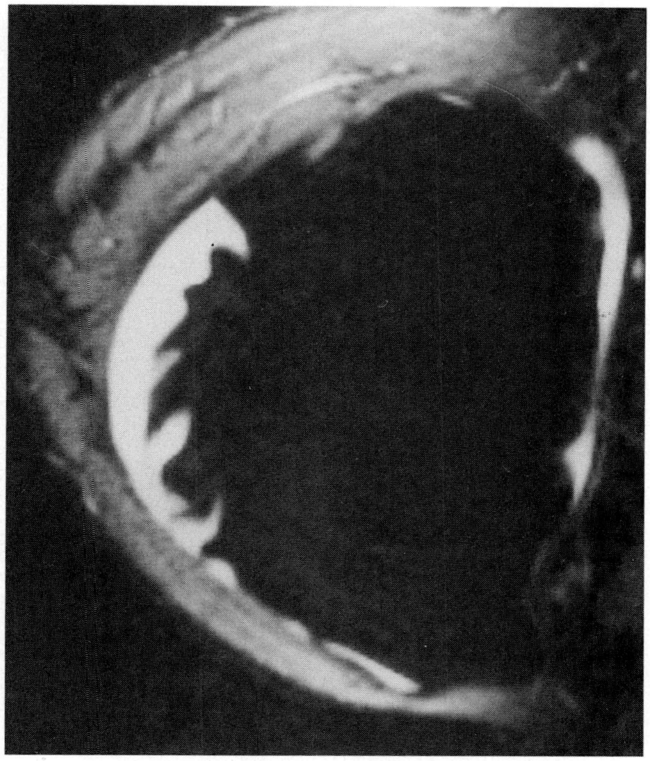

Figure 4–12. T2-weighted silicone-suppressed MR image of the double lumen implant shown in Figure 4–10, showing the inner lumen silicone gel as dark, and the outer lumen saline as bright.

"Reverse" Double-Lumen Implants

Less than 1% of the silicone gel–filled breast implants we have imaged have been "reverse" double lumen, with silicone gel in the outer and saline in the inner lumen (Figs. 4–13 through 4–15). This type of implant was mainly used in reconstructive surgery. Variable amounts of saline were added to the inner lumen through a valve or valves, which could be of the leaflet or internal tube types. To our knowledge, of the American manufacturers only CUI, McGhan, McGhan/3M, and Mentor produced this type of implant as commercial product.

"Reverse Adjustable" Double-Lumen Implants

Much fewer than 1% of the silicone gel–filled implants we have imaged are of the "reverse adjustable" double-lumen variety, with silicone gel in the inner *and* outer lumen (Figs. 4–16 and 4–17). Saline can be added to the inner silicone gel–filled lumen (only) to provide adjustability of size. Like the reverse double-lumen implants, these are used mostly in a reconstructive setting. To our knowledge, these were manufactured as a commercial product only by Surgitek.

"Gel-gel" Double-Lumen Implants

The McGhan style 153 textured implant has an inner, relatively overfilled, silicone gel–filled lumen, and an outer less-filled lumen also containing silicone gel (Fig. 4–18). Its shape was described as "anatomical," and there was no provision to add saline to the implant. Some McGhan/3M custom Birnbaum implants from the early 1980's were also gel-gel double lumen.

Triple-Lumen Implants

Fewer than 1% of the silicone gel–filled implants we have imaged are triple lumen (Figs. 4–19 and 4–20). In their most common form, the inner lumen is relatively overfilled with silicone gel, the middle lumen is relatively underfilled with silicone gel, and the outer lumen can be filled through a leaflet valve with saline at the time of implant placement. This type of implant was most often used in a reconstructive setting. CUI, McGhan/3M, and McGhan produced these implants as a commercial product.McGhan/3M also produced

(text continues on page 41)

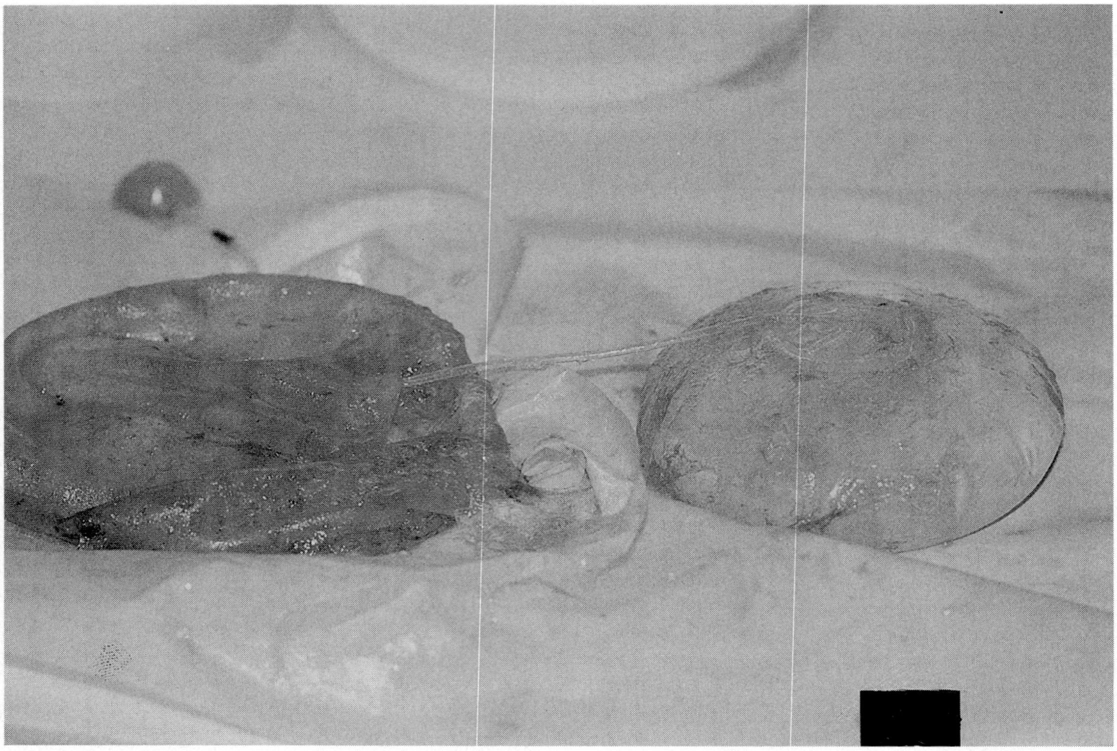

Figure 4–13. Mentor Becker "reverse" double-lumen breast implant (ruptured outer silicone gel-filled lumen), with a tube leading from the valve on the outermost implant shell, to the inner saline filled lumen (shown inflated here).

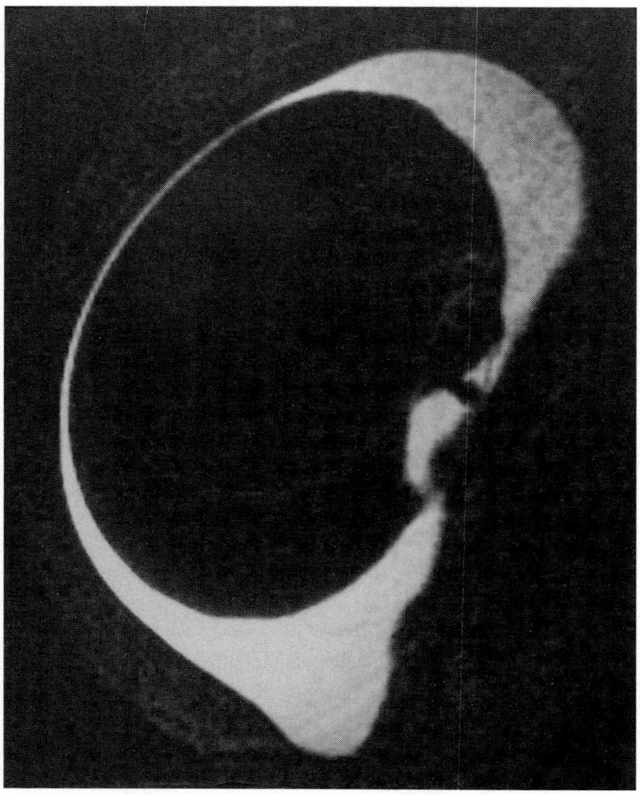

Figure 4–14. T2-weighted water-suppressed MR image of the reverse double lumen implant shown in Figure 4–13, showing the outer lumen silicone gel as bright and the inner lumen saline as dark. Note that the inner fill tube apparatus can be seen within the outer lumen silicone gel in the posterior part of the implant.

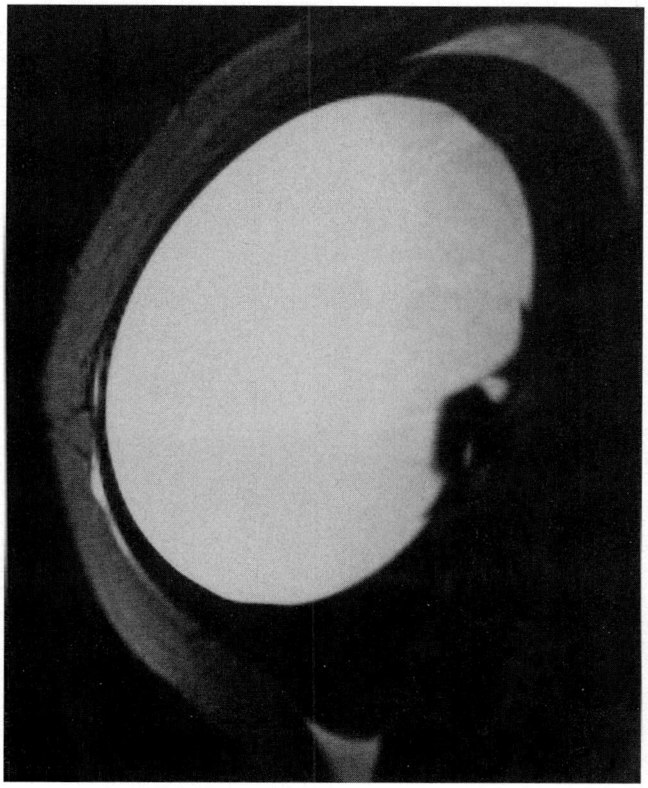

Figure 4–15. T2-weighted silicone-suppressed MR image of the reverse double lumen implant shown in Figure 4–13, showing the outer lumen silicone gel as dark, and the inner lumen saline as bright. A layer of water-like intracapsular fluid, outside the implant, is also seen here.

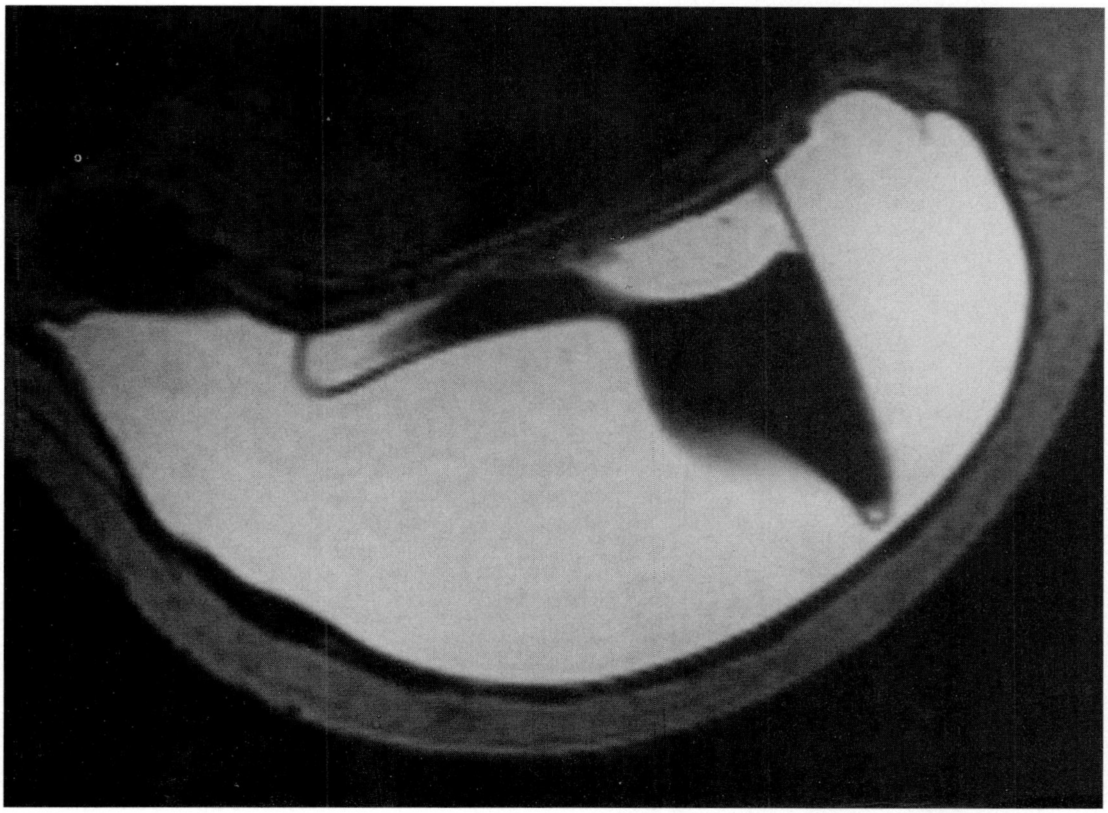

Figure 4–16. T2-weighted water-suppressed MR image of a Surgitek "reverse adjustable" double-lumen breast implant, showing the outer silicone gel as bright, the inner lumen silicone gel as bright, and the inner lumen saline mixed with that gel as dark. Leaflet valves were used to introduce saline into the inner gel filled lumen.

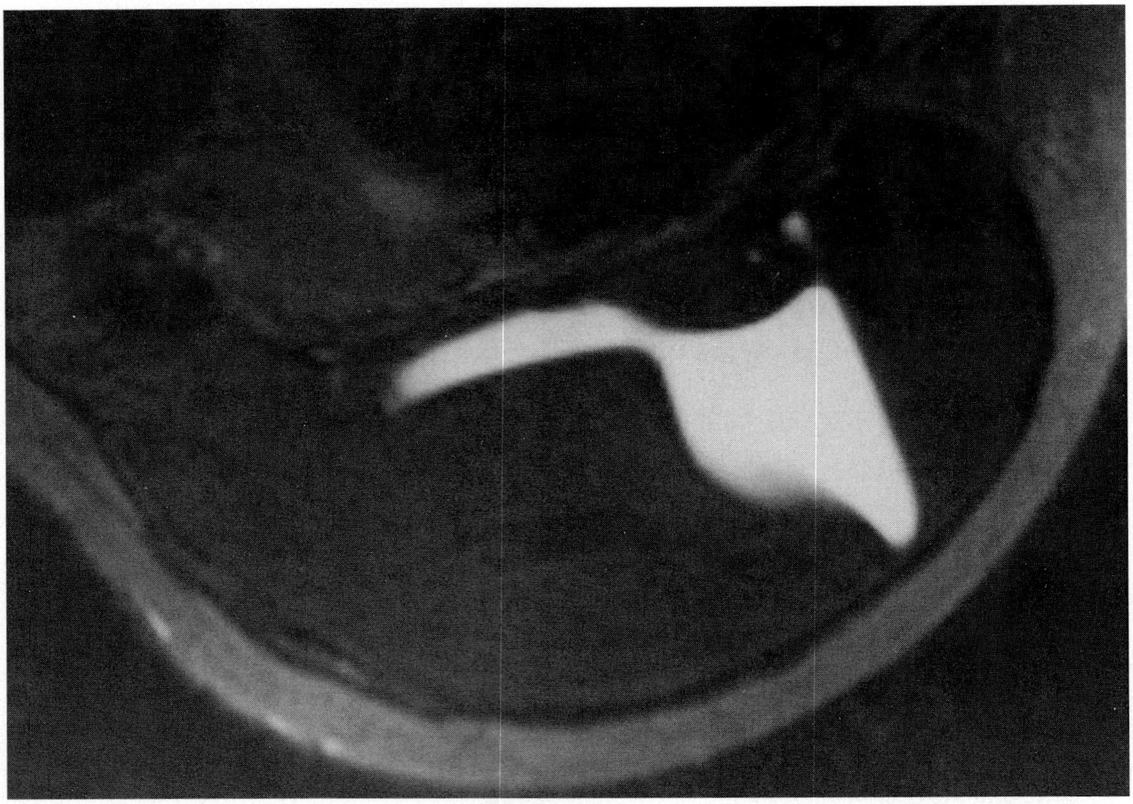

Figure 4–17. T2-weighted silicone-suppressed MR image of the Surgitek "reverse adjustable" double-lumen breast implant shown in Figure 4–16, showing the outer lumen silicone gel as dark, the inner lumen silicone gel as dark, and the inner lumen saline mixed with that gel as bright.

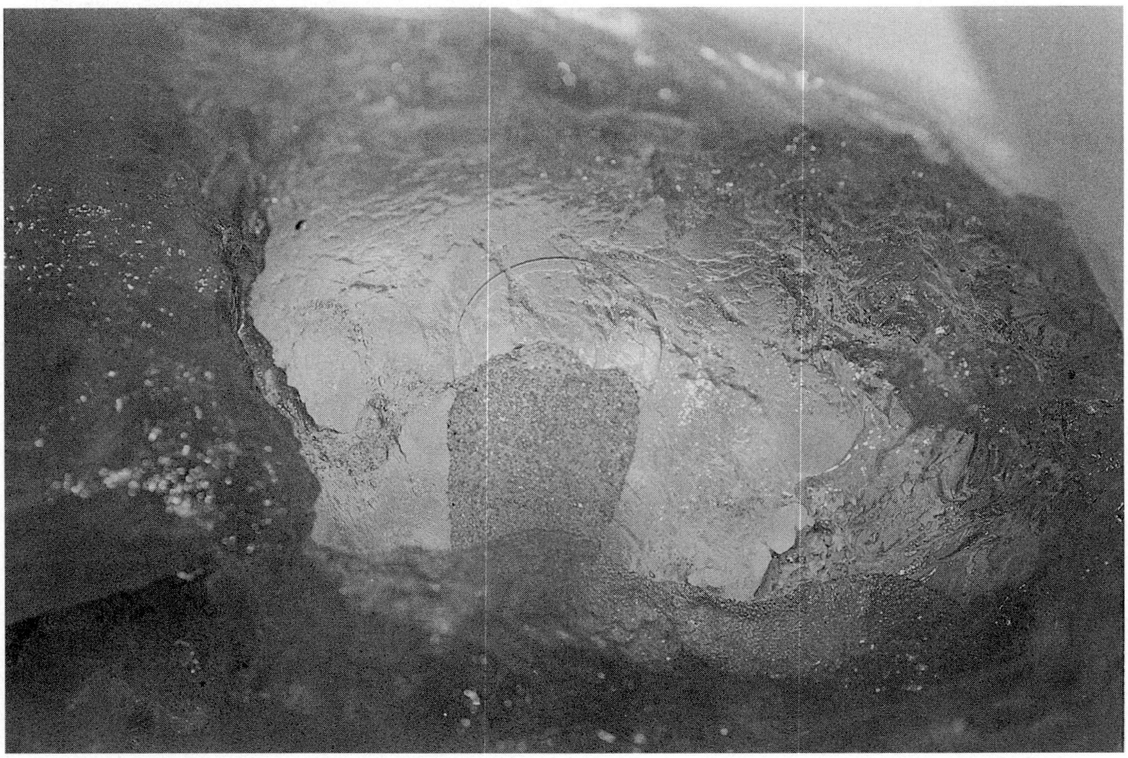

Figure 4–18. McGhan Style 153 "gel-gel" double-lumen implant (outer lumen ruptured), showing the inner lumen and its back patch, a portion of the textured outer lumen shell, and some of the outer lumen gel pushed aside.

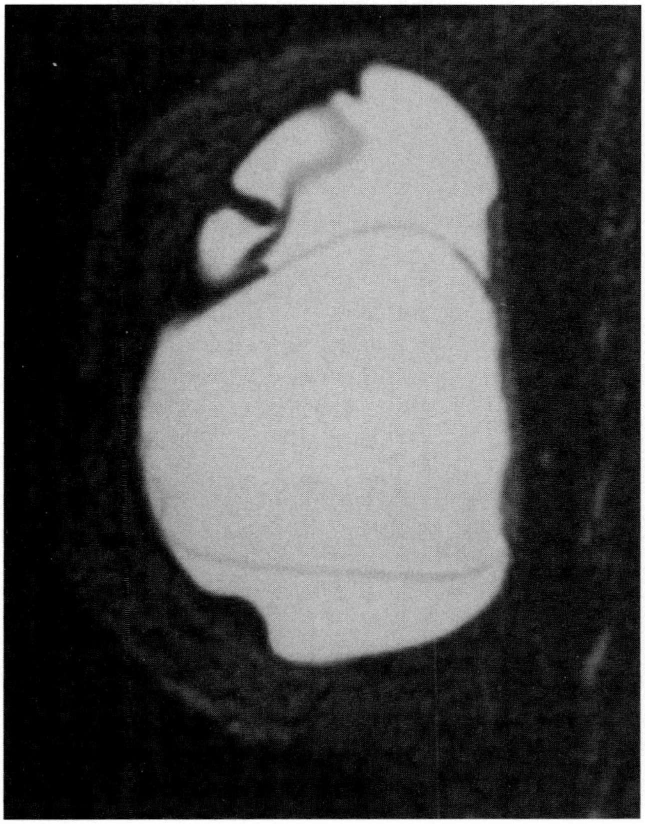

Figure 4–19. T2-weighted water-suppressed MR image of a McGhan triple-lumen breast implant, showing the inner and middle lumen silicone gel as bright, and the outer saline-filled lumen as dark. A leaflet valve is used to introduce saline into the outer lumen.

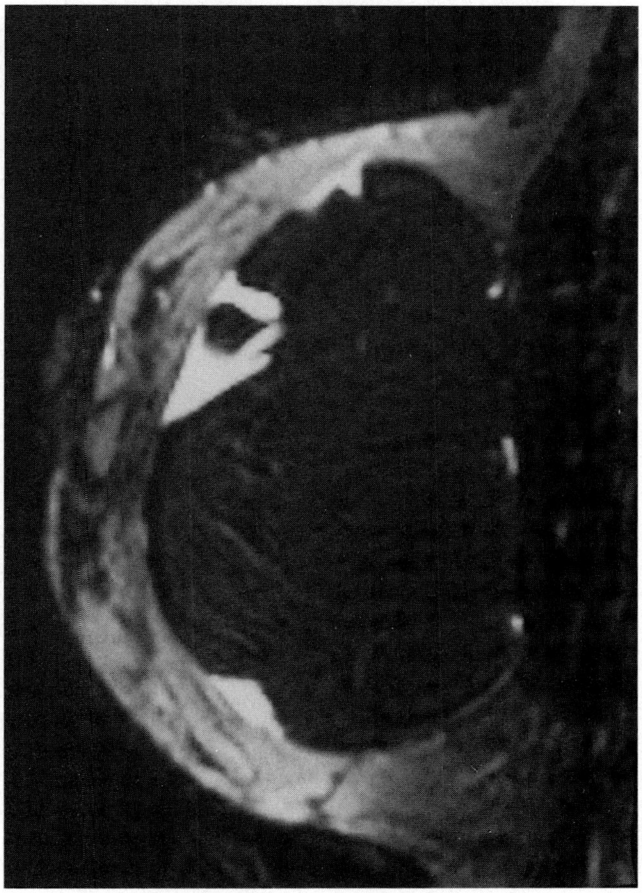

Figure 4–20. T2-weighted silicone-suppressed MR image of the McGhan triple-lumen implant shown in Figure 4–19, showing the inner and middle lumen silicone gel as dark, the outer lumen saline as bright.

custom tri-lumen Birhbaum implants, with a more underfilled inner silicone gel-filled lumen.

Cavon "Cast Gel" Implants

Dr. Joseph F. Cavon designed a breast implant with no shell and very cohesive gel (Fig. 4–21), which was available from Cox Uphoff, and then Aesthetech, from about 1980 to 1985. Very few were ever placed.

Custom Implants

Custom implants individualized to a patient's needs could be ordered by prescription. These were usually used to correct acquired or congenital breast deformity (Fig. 4–22).

Pectus Implants

Pectus implants are solid implants used to correct acquired or congenital pectoralis muscle absence (Fig. 4–23). They were usually constructed of solid silicone elastomer, and image dark on all MR pulse sequences.

Solid Sponge

Solid sponge implants were being used for breast augmentation in the 1950s (Figs. 4–24 and 4–25). With the introduction of silicone gel–filled breast implants in 1962, their use was essentially discontinued. They were made from Etheron (polyurethane) and Ivalon.

Sponge Adjustable

Early hollow polyurethane sponge implants were available in the 1950s and could be inflated with dextran or saline. In the early 1970s, polyurethane sponges contained within a silicone elastomer shell were manufactured by Polyplastics, Inc. Those implants consisted of a silicone elastomer shell

(text continues on page 44)

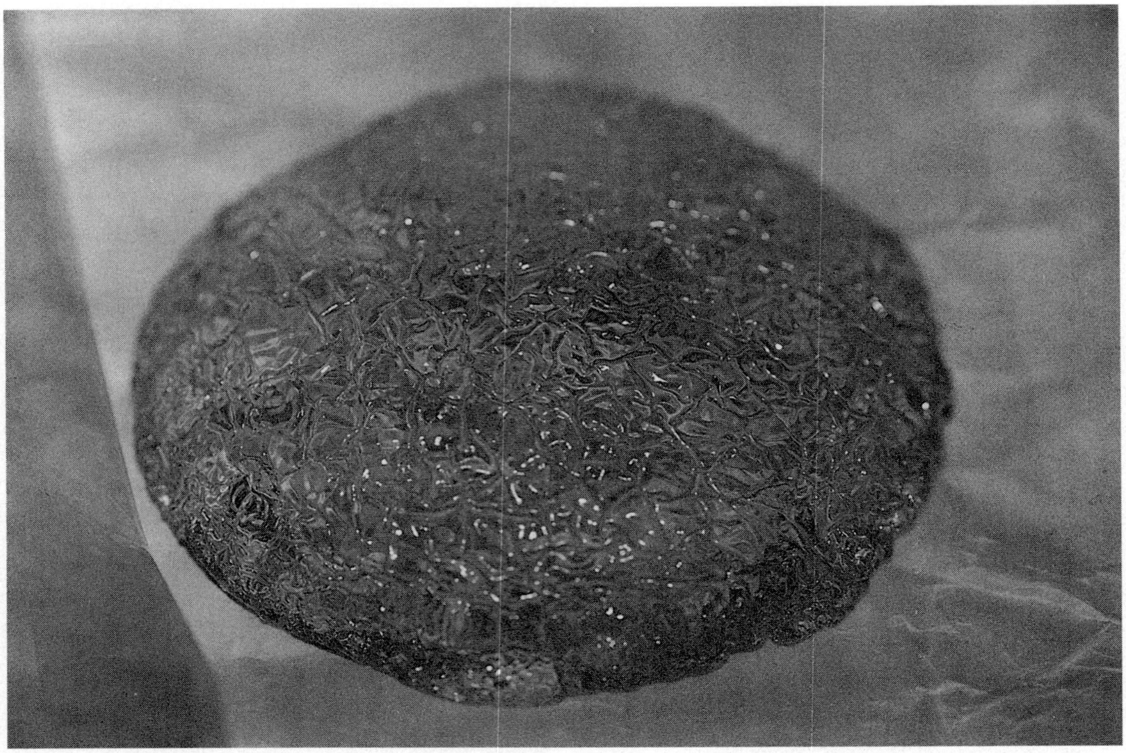

Figure 4–21. Cavon implant, showing the distinctive "elephant-skin" appearance of these implants at time of removal. This implant had no shell, and hence no back patch. The gel was of increased cohesiveness compared to most other implants.

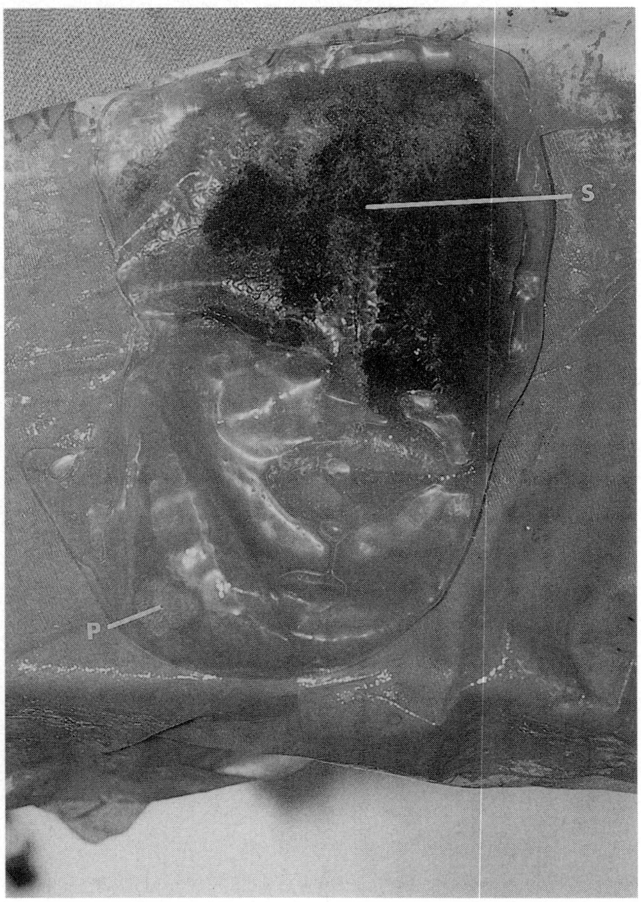

Figure 4–22. Heyer Schulte custom silicone gel-filled single-lumen breast implant with Dacron-reinforced elastomer back patches (P), Dacron rectangular "Velcro-style" fixation patches (on posterior implant surface, not shown here), and an internal polyurethane sponge (S) within the silicone gel. This implant was used to correct a congenital deformity from Poland syndrome.

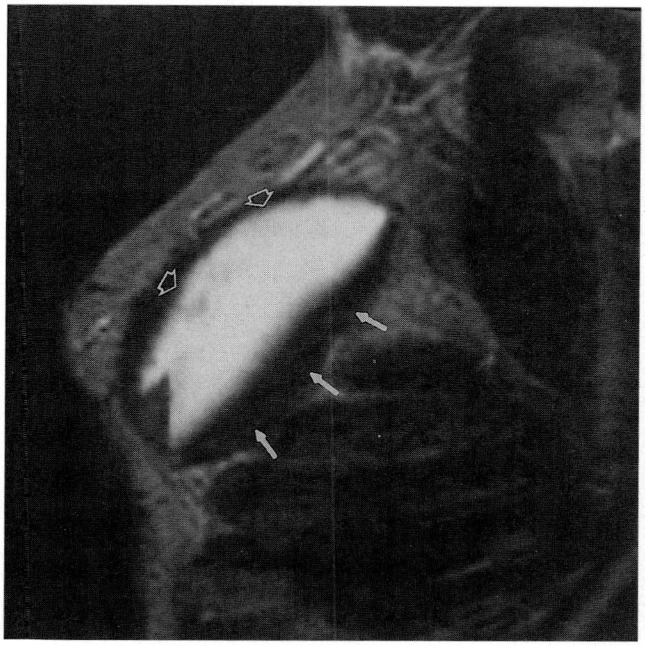

Figure 4–23. T2-weighted MR image (without suppression) of a soft pectus implant (solid arrows), placed in this male to correct absence of pectoralis major due to Poland syndrome. Since the implant is solid, it images as dark on all sequences. In the case shown here, this patient suffered trauma to the upper chest with hematoma formation, seen here as increased T2 signal (open arrows) anterior to the dark pectus implant.

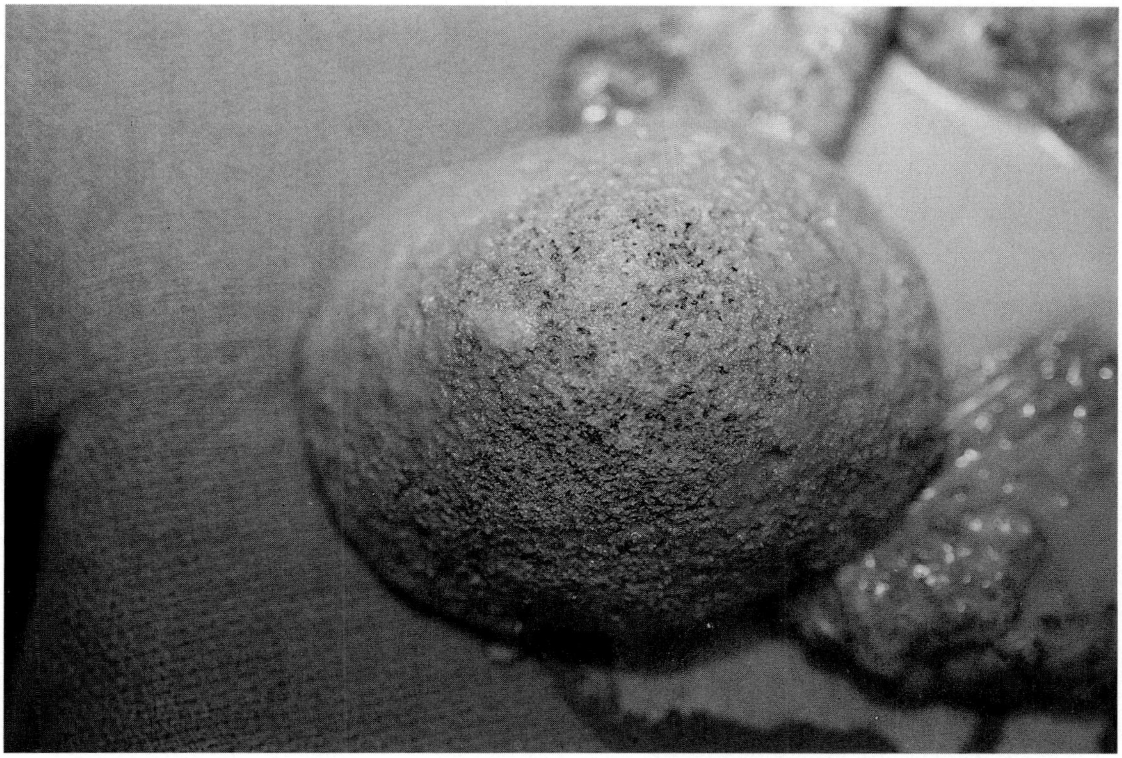

Figure 4–24. Solid sponge breast implant placed in 1956, shown here at time of removal 38 years later. Note the abundant fluid around the implant containing particulate sponge material, still pooled in the fibrous capsule behind the implant.

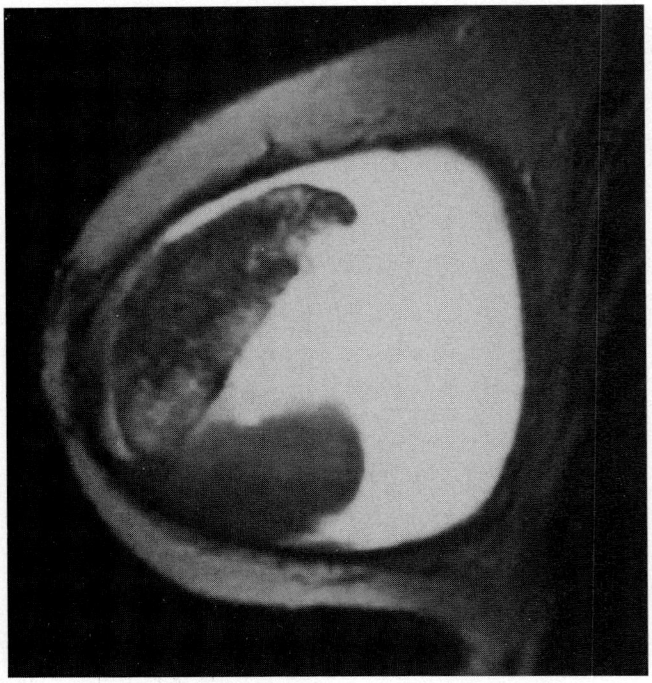

Figure 4–25. T2-weighted silicone-suppressed MR image of the solid sponge breast implant shown in Figure 4–24. The dome-shaped sponge is seen centrally, surrounded by a large intracapsular water-like fluid collection, that upon removal was seen to contain abundant dissolved particulate sponge material. The more inferior homogeneous material next to the implant represents the settled particulate sponge material within the fluid collection.

coated on its outer surface with polyurethane, contained a polyurethane sponge, and were inflatable with dextran or saline.

Other

Experimental implants now being developed include some with silicone elastomer shells, filled with soybean oil. T1-weighted MR pulse sequences may be useful to image these implants.

■ SUMMARY

The breast implant classification scheme described in this chapter will help facilitate a better understanding of normal and abnormal appearances of common and unusual implants, as well as allowing stratification of future research data.

■ ACKNOWLEDGEMENTS

I am grateful for monetary support in the form of unrestricted gifts either to the San Diego Radiology Research and Education Foundation, or to the Regents, University of California, from Dow Corning as well as plaintiff attorneys, one defense attorney, physicians, and patients, as well as for the loan of equipment or the donation of materials from General Electric, Medical Advances, 3M, Acuson, and Konica. We also have been funded by a University of California Academic Senate grant. The condition, appearance, or manufacturer of the implants chosen to be shown in this chapter are not intended to imply anything about the rupture rate of those products, or possible local or systemic effects caused by those products.

REFERENCES

1. Braley SA. The use of silicones in plastic surgery. *Plast Reconstr Surg.* 1973;51:280–288.
2. Gerow FJ. In: Georgiade NG, ed. *Reconstructive Breast Surgery.* St. Louis: Mosby; 1976.
3. Gerow FJ. A pictorial inventory of breast implants. In: Owsley JQ, Peterson RA, eds. *Symposium on Aesthetic Surgery of the Breast.* St. Louis: Mosby; 1978.
4. Berg WA, Caskey CI, Hamper UM, et al. Diagnosing breast implant rupture with MR imaging, US, and mammography. *Radiographics.* 1993;13:1323–1336.
5. Steinbach BG, Hardy NS, Abbitt PL, Lanier L, Caffee HH. Breast implants, common complications, and concurrent breast disease. *Radiographics.* 1993;13:95–118.
6. Middleton MS, McNamara MP. Breast implant classification and identification—a pictorial review. Oral abstract presentation and poster, 1995 RSNA Annual Meeting.
7. Middleton MS, McNamara MP. Mammary implant product list—1962 to 1996. In: *Breast Implant Imaging.* Lippincott-Raven Press; in preparation.

5

Mammographic Evaluation of the Augmented Breast

G. W. EKLUND AND GILDA CARDENOSA

In the United States, 2 million women have undergone augmentation mammoplasty, and over 150,000 undergo this procedure annually. Women with implants face the same risk of developing breast cancer as women who do not have implants. Although many issues and controversies surround the practice of breast augmentation and the local and systemic effects of implants, it is imperative that all women over 40 have annual mammograms. Early detection of breast cancer is the most important factor affecting breast cancer mortality.

With standard mammographic techniques, subglandular and subpectoral implants obscure significant amounts of breast tissue while absorbing the effects of compression, leaving visualized tissue around the implant inadequately compressed.[1–4] The modified compression technique (implant displacement view) described by Eklund et al[1,2] increases the amount of visualized tissue and allows adequate compression without risk to the implant (Figs. 5–1 through 5–5). When screening women with augmentation implants, four views are obtained of each breast.[1,2]

Standard craniocaudal (CC) and mediolateral oblique (MLO) views include the implants and remain important in the mammographic evaluation of women with augmented breasts.[1,2] Maximal upward mobilization of the breast is undertaken for the standard CC views and maximal medial mobilization of the breast is undertaken for the standard MLO views.[5] Because the implant is the limiting factor to compression with standard views, only enough compression to immobilize the breast is required. The minimal compression required for immobilization of the breast imposes no risk for damage to the implant. We must recognize that on standard views compression and optimal tissue visualization are significantly limited. Standard views are always obtained before displacement views are attempted, so as to establish a baseline for the implants. Standard views are also needed to evaluate the implants, posterior tissue surrounding the implant, and the lower axillary area[6,7] (Figs. 5–1 and 5–5A,B). The implant contour and pericapsular regions are evaluated for signs of implant herniation or disruption.

Implant displacement views are done by pulling breast tissue forward, away from the implant, at the same time the implant is displaced posteriorly against the chest wall[1,2] (Figs. 5–2 and 5–3). Compression is then applied to the tissue in front of the implant (Fig. 5–3). No direct compression is applied to the implant during implant displacement views, thereby eliminating the risk of damage to the implant by compression. Firm fibrous encapsulation, the most common complication of breast implant augmentation, is suspected when the implant demonstrates a spherical shape on the standard MLO view.[8,9] Encapsulated implants feel hard, are immobile, and cannot be flattened against the chest wall. In many women with firm implant encapsulation, it is still possible to pull breast tissue over and in front of the implant. When imaging women with firmly encapsulated implants, we add a 90°lateral view to the standard CC and MLO views[1,2] (Fig. 5–6). The rationale for this fifth image is to include some posterior tissue above and below the implant, not otherwise included on the CC and MLO views.

In spite of efforts to maximize the amount of tissue imaged free of the implant, optimal tissue visualization is com-

(text continues on page 51)

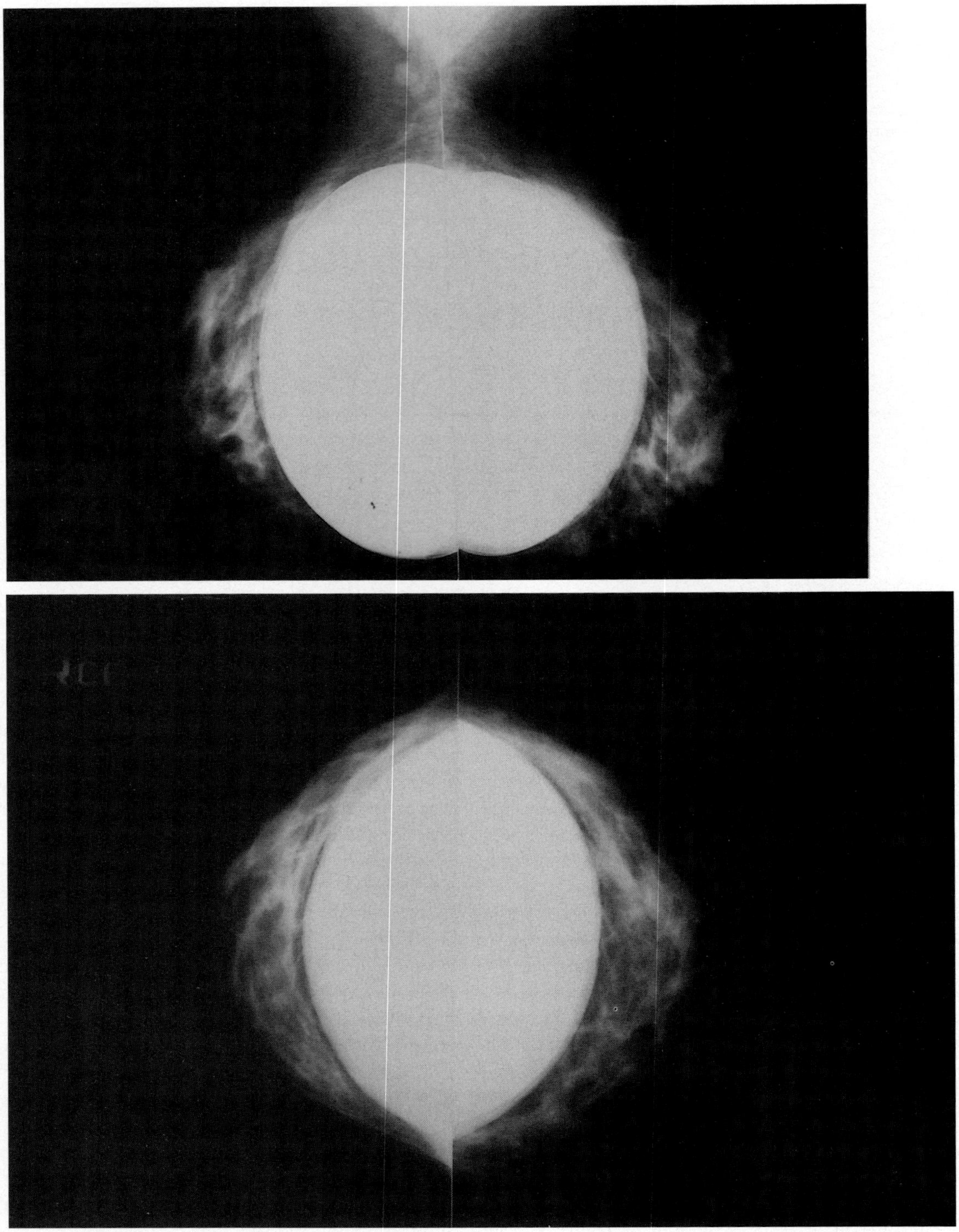

A

B

Figure 5–1. (**A,B**) Standard MLO and CC views of both breasts, show augmentation with double-lumen, subpectoral implants. Most of the implant is included in the field. Only the most posterior portion of the implant is not visualized. (See Figure 5–11 for imaging technique to visualize the posterior implant wall.) Standard views are important to visualize the implant and the posterior tissue surrounding the implant. The standard MLO view also provides the best visualization of the lower axillary area. Compression is required only to immobilize the breast. Because the implant limits compression, the visualized tissue will remain uncompressed.

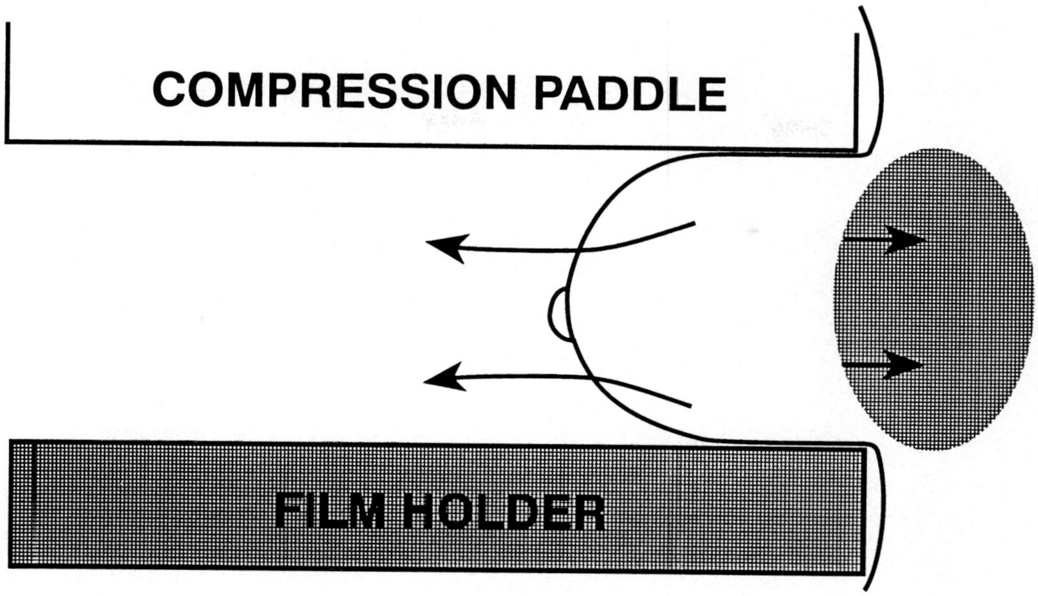

Figure 5–2. Implant displacement view is obtained by pulling breast tissue over and in front of the implant while pushing the implant posteriorly against the chest wall (arrows). With the implant out of the field, proper compression of the visualized breast tissue is possible as shown in Figure 5–3.

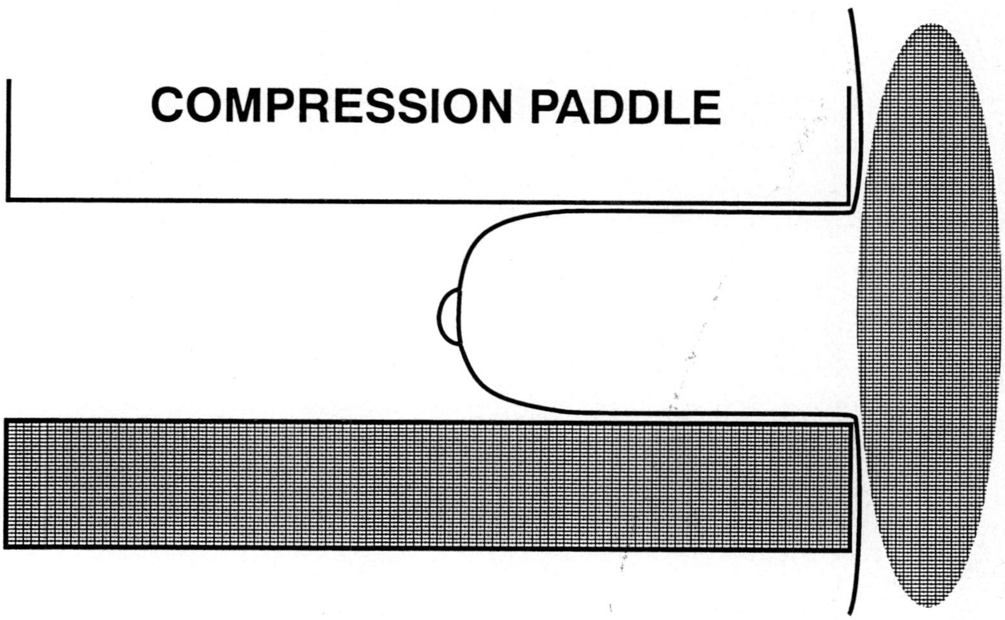

Figure 5–3. Full compression of breast tissue is possible with the implant displaced and flattened against the chest wall. The extent to which the implant can be flattened depends on the degree of fibrous encapsulation.

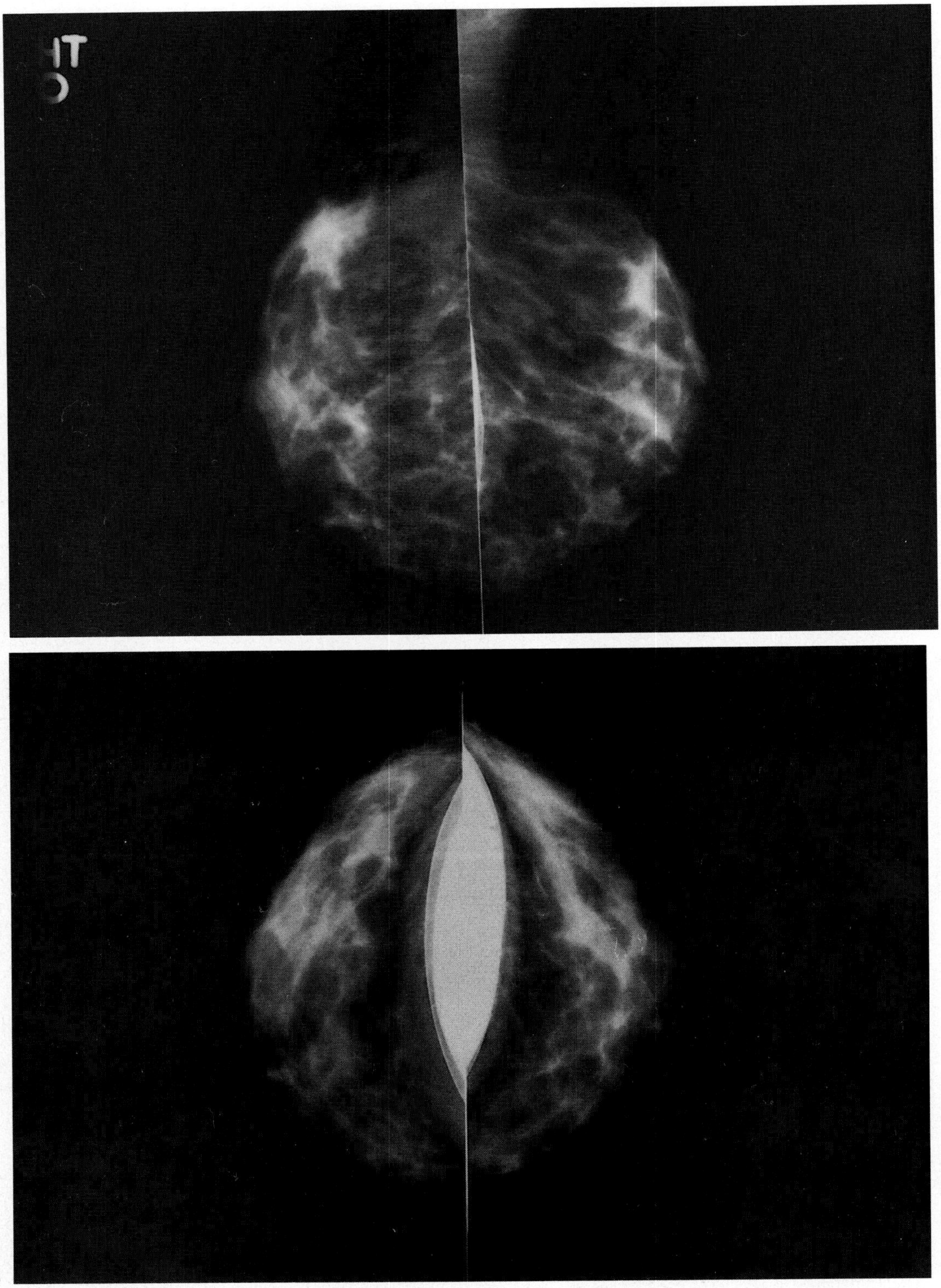

Figure 5–4. (**A,B**) MLO and CC implant displacement views of the same breast shown with standard views in Figure 5–1. Significantly better compression of breast tissue is possible with the implant displaced posteriorly.

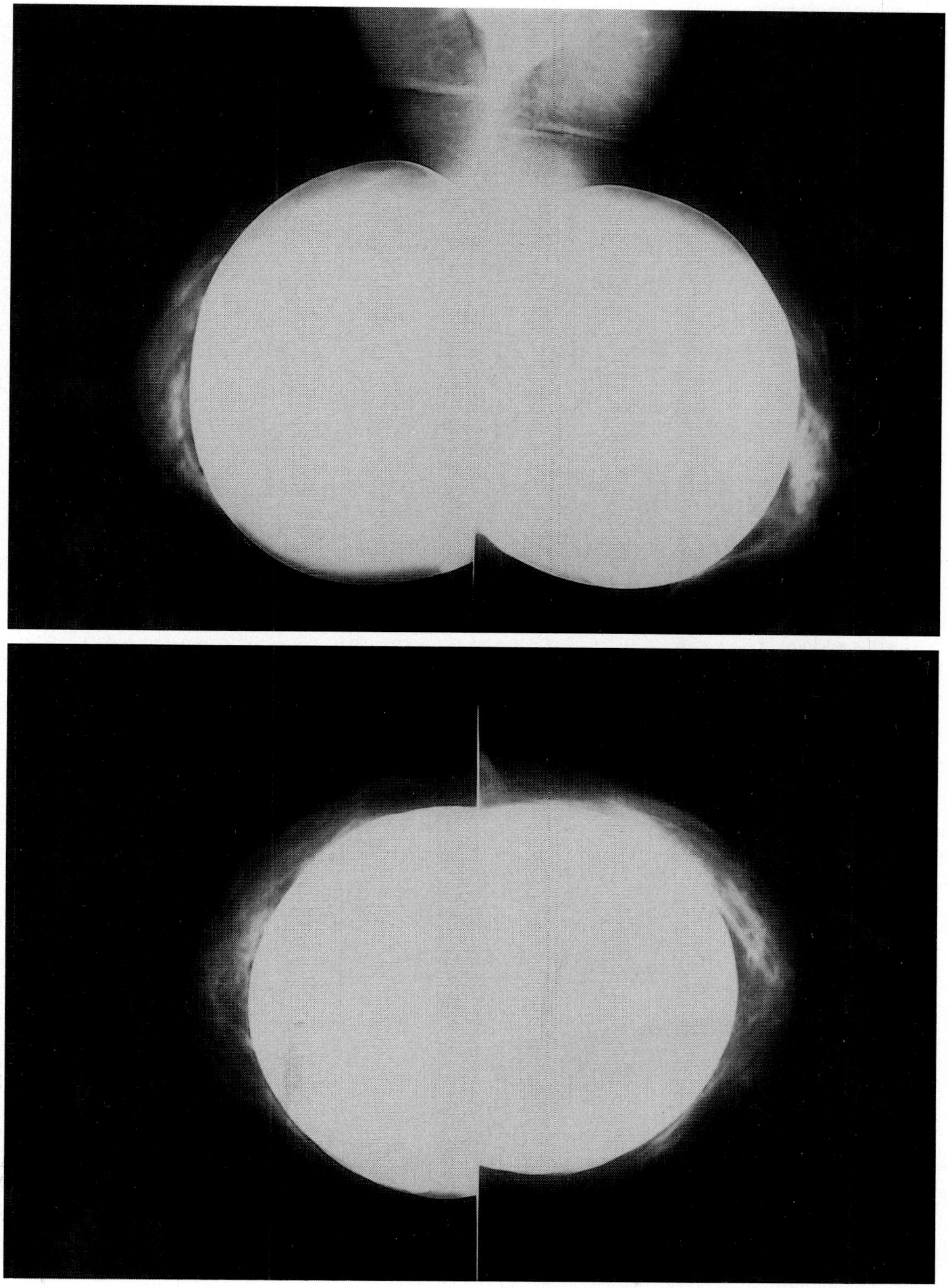

A

B

Figure 5–5. (**A,B**) Standard MLO and CC view of both breasts, show augmentation with subglandular, saline implants. Again, it is important to note that the visualized tissue is uncompressed when the implants are included in the field.

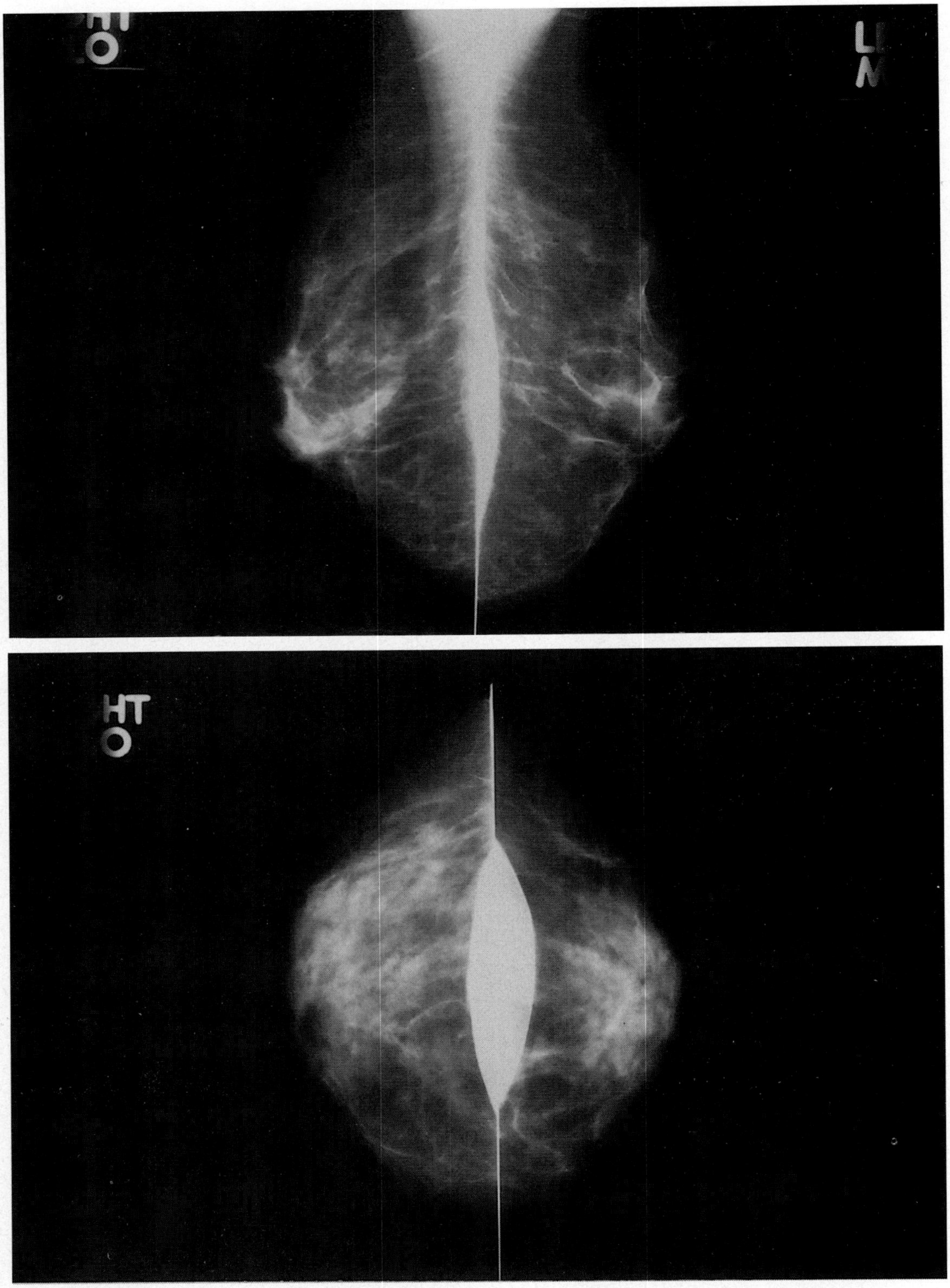

C

D

5–5. (***Continued***) (**C,D**) Implant displacement MLO and CC views provide better visualization of more breast tissue.

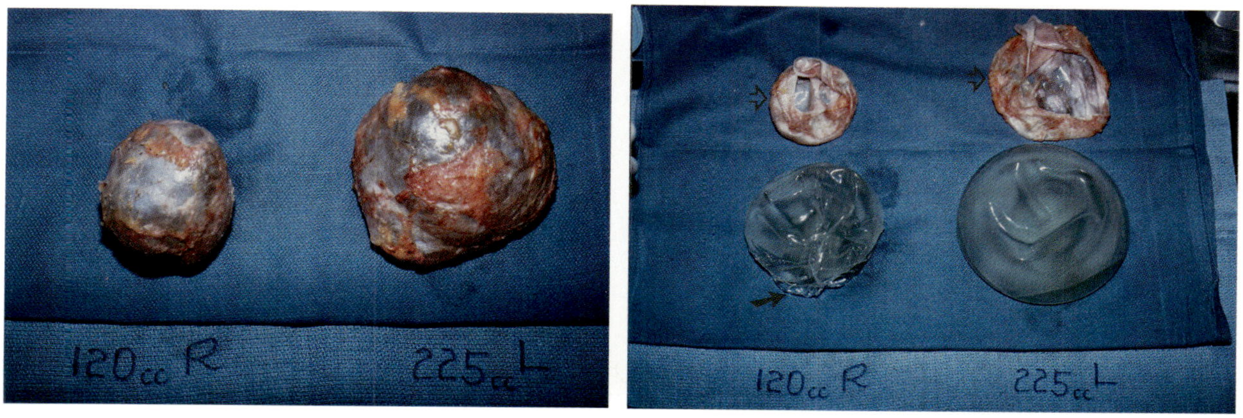

A B

Plate I. Ruptured and intact silicone gel–filled implant from the same patient. (**A**) Periprosthetic fibrous capsules surrounding the ruptured right implant and the intact left implant. (**B**) The periprosthetic capsules have been removed from the silicone implants (open arrows). The ruptured right implant has free silicone outside the implant shell (arrow). This patient had different size implants in her breasts; a 120-cc implant had been placed in her right breast and a 225-cc implant had been placed in her left breast.

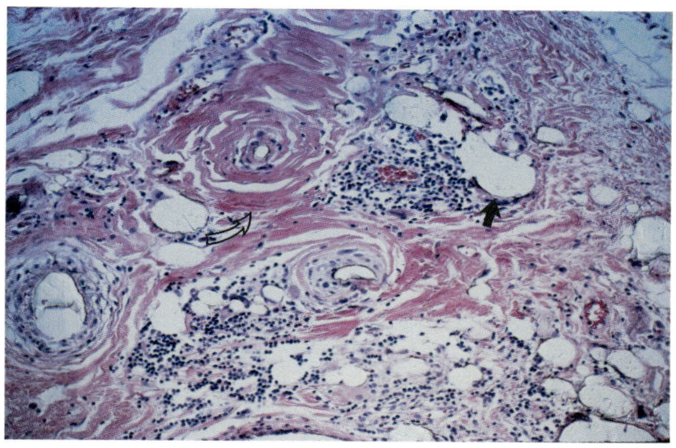

Plate II. Microscopic histology of periprosthetic capsule showing silicone granuloma (arrow) and dense irregular collagen fibrils (open arrow).

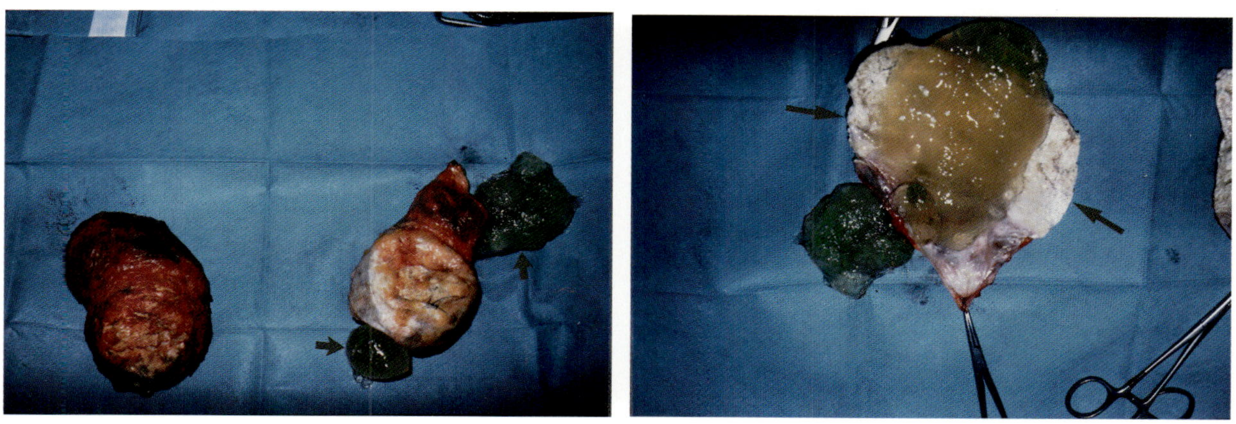

A B

Plate III. Ruptured and intact gel-filled silicone implant. (**A**) The ruptured left implant demonstrates extruded free silicone (arrows) extending from the calcific periprosthetic capsule. The right implant was intact. (**B**) Close-up photograph of the ruptured left implant with a partially calcified periprosthetic capsule (arrows).

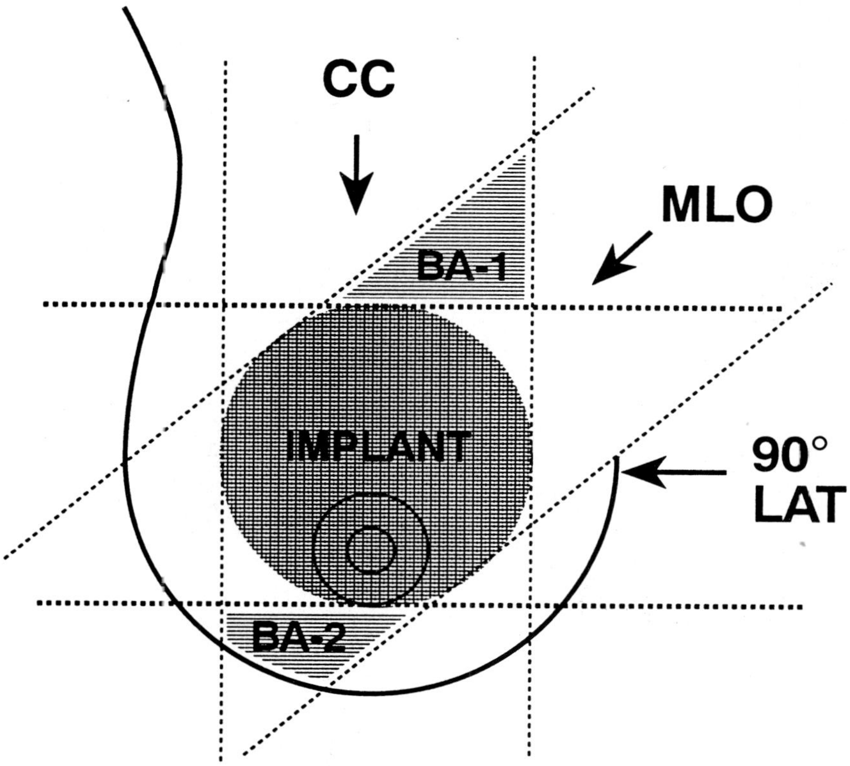

Figure 5–6. Illustration of the right breast illustrates a spherical, firmly encapsulated implant and areas that are "blind" (BA-1 and BA-2) on either the MLO or CC projections. Lesions in these areas will be obscured by the implant in either an MLO or CC view. By including a 90° lateral (standard view) these areas will be visualized.

promised in most women. In women with little native tissue or who have had a subcutaneous mastectomy, implant displacement views are limited to the extent that breast tissue, especially tissue in areas of focal concern, can be pulled forward and compressed free of the implant. Patients who have had a subcutaneous mastectomy with preservation of the nipple areolar complex and reconstruction with implants have variable amounts of breast tissue remaining in the subareolar region.[8] Tissue must be left in the subareolar region to preserve the blood supply and viability of the nipple-areolar complex. Using spot compression and the implant displacement procedure described above, subareolar tissue can be imaged well in most women who have had subcutaneous mastectomies. Tailored spot compression views, using the implant displacement technique, should be obtained to optimize visualization of any focal area of radiographic or palpable concern that is incompletely or inadequately seen with routine CC and MLO displacement views (Fig. 5–7).

Two common questions pertaining to breast cancer detection arise in women with implant breast augmentation: (1) Can we quantify the amount of breast tissue imaged in the augmented breast? (2) Is it possible to screen the augmented breast as well as the nonaugmented breast?

Currently, there is no accurate method available to quantify the amount of breast tissue imaged. Several recent publications have dealt with the limitations imposed by augmentation implants on screening mammography.[10] These studies have tried to compare the amount of tissue obscured in standard views to that seen with implant displacement views. All of these articles are flawed by measuring "area" rather than "volume" of visualized tissue. To properly quantify "amount" of tissue imaged, the thickness of imaged tissue must be included in the calculations. In other words, because we are dealing with a compressible, three-dimensional structure, "amount" is a volumetric, not a "surface," measurement. This concept is easier to understand if one considers what happens to the area of an image of a shot pellet BB viewed from above, before and after flattening with a hammer (Fig. 5–8). It may appear as an area about 2 mm in diameter before flattening, but 4 mm in diameter after flattening. We are not seeing more BB when it is flattened, but the same amount of BB spread over a larger surface area. The measurement techniques described in these publications are further flawed by a failure to recognize how the tissue is distributed over the surface of the implant. If breast tissue is spread evenly over the surface of the implant (rarely the case), a proportionately larger amount of tissue will be obscured by the implant. If most of the breast tissue in a moderate-sized breast lies anterior to the implant (not an uncommon occurrence), there may be minimal masking with implant displacement views. In women with very little native tissue, thinly stretched and mostly obscured by the implant, a 75% increase in the amount of visualized tissue may be negligible. If 90% of the breast tissue is masked because

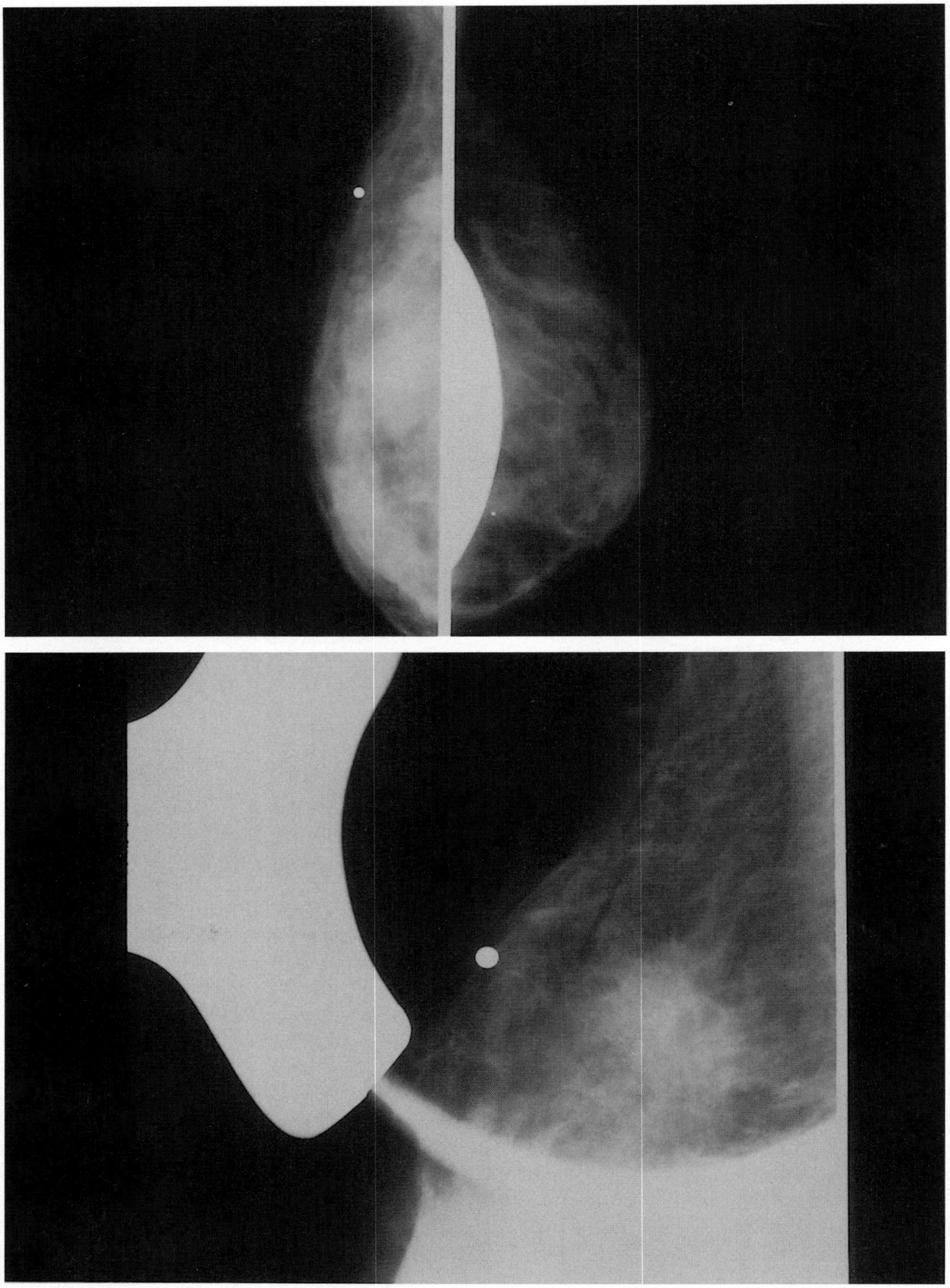

A

B

Figure 5–7. (**A**) Patient presented with a palpable "fullness" in the upper outer aspect of the right breast. Images are implant displacement MLO and CC views of the right breast (positioned back to back). A lead BB was placed over the area of palpable concern. The BB is excluded on the CC view and seen only on the MLO view. Prominence of glandular tissue deep to the marker on the MLO view is insufficiently visualized to characterize as a mass. Further workup is indicated. (**B**) A tailored spot film over the area of concern with implant displacement technique, and an exaggerated CC view would be helpful. At this time, it is especially helpful for the radiologist to examine the patient and prescribe the tailored images needed to optimize visualization of the palpable finding. This spot film is taken with implant displacement technique in a modified MLO projection to direct the x-ray beam tangentially to the overlying skin. The image reveals a 2-cm spiculated mass, highly suspicious for malignancy.

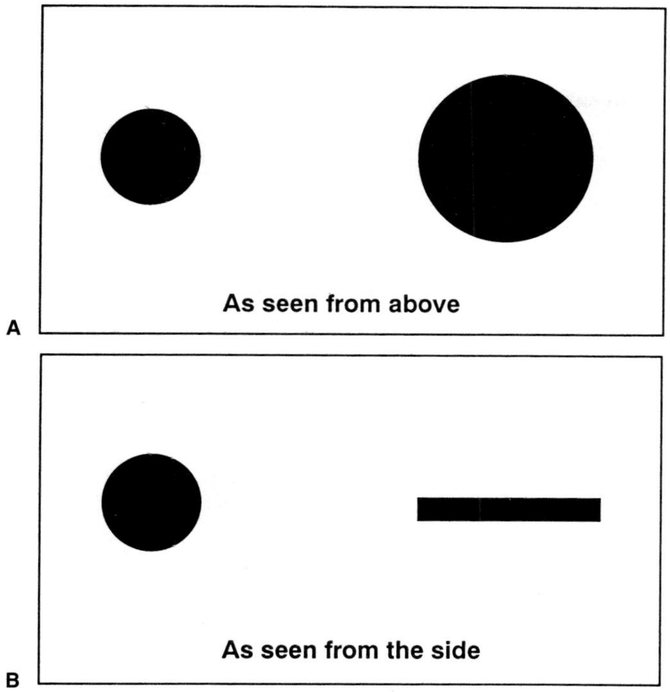

Figure 5–8. (**A**) The images of two BBs as seen from above. No accurate assumptions regarding the size of these BBs can be made without knowledge of the respective thickness of each BB. (**B**) The BB on the right has been flattened. Although the image of the right "BB" seen in **A** is considerably larger than that of the left BB, their respective volumes are identical, and the "amount" of BB seen is the same for each.

it is spread thinly over the entire surface of the implant, and implant displacement views triple the amount of visualized tissue (from 10% to 30%), however, 70% of the tissue remains obscured.

Although not accurately quantifiable, two important advantages are provided by the implant displacement views: (1) more breast tissue is seen in most patients, and (2) better compression of the tissue, possible only when the implant is out of the field, means better image quality. Reasonable estimates of additional tissue imaged with the implant displacement views are best made with attention to specific landmarks within the breast, such as the relationship of anatomic landmarks to the margin of the implant. Using this subjective estimation technique in women with soft compressible implants, significantly more breast tissue is imaged with the implant displacement technique than with the standard images. With firm implant encapsulation and/or a small amount of native tissue, the amount of additional tissue imaged using implant displacement techniques is limited. With native tissue stretched thinly over the implant, additional tissue imaged using implant displacement techniques may be negligible. The degree of limitation remains a subjective estimate. Significant tissue masking by implants occurs in some mammographic studies. Very little (and occasionally no) masking occurs in other mammographic studies.

Areas of clinical concern should be marked with lead BBs to provide assurance that the area is included adequately on the mammographic images. When significant masking potential is apparent, the examination should be "tailored" or focused to optimize tissue visualization. If glandular tissue predominates laterally, an appropriately tailored CC implant displacement view can maximize lateral tissue visualization (Fig. 5–9). Similarly, if glandular tissue is found predominantly in the upper portion of the breast, the implant displacement MLO can be tailored to maximize visualization (Fig. 5–10).

In our experience, breast physical examination is not compromised by the presence of implants. Some would argue that the presence of an implant, with its smooth anterior surface, against which the examiner can palpate, facilitates physical examination. Thinning of native tissue over the surface of the implant increases the sensitivity of palpation. The most important observation for women doing breast self-examination (BSE) is "interval change." Once the woman becomes familiar with the contour and surface of her implant, she becomes very astute in detecting subtle changes. BSE is also aided by the thinning effect of breast tissue over the surface of the implant. Tailored mammographic views are often needed to properly image areas of palpable concern. The

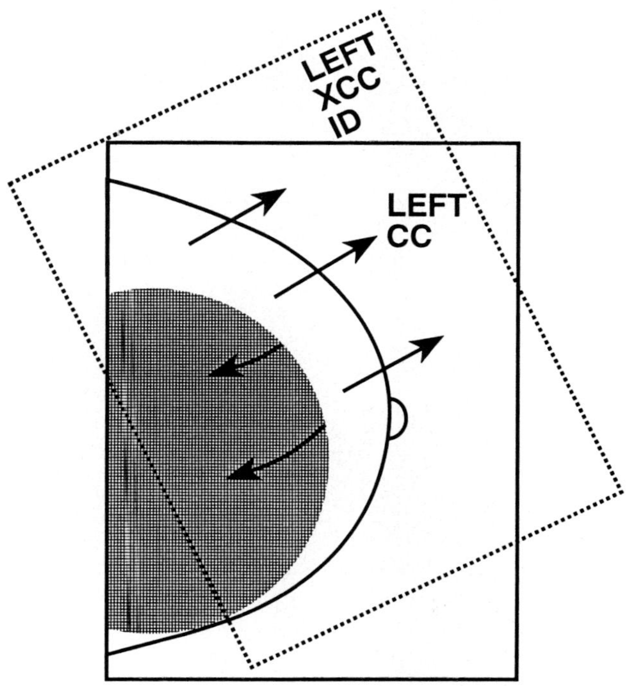

Figure 5–9. A standard left CC image illustrates a somewhat medial position of the implant, with dominance of the breast tissue more laterally. To optimize visualization of breast tissue, the implant displacement view (dotted outline) will be exaggerated to include more lateral breast tissue.

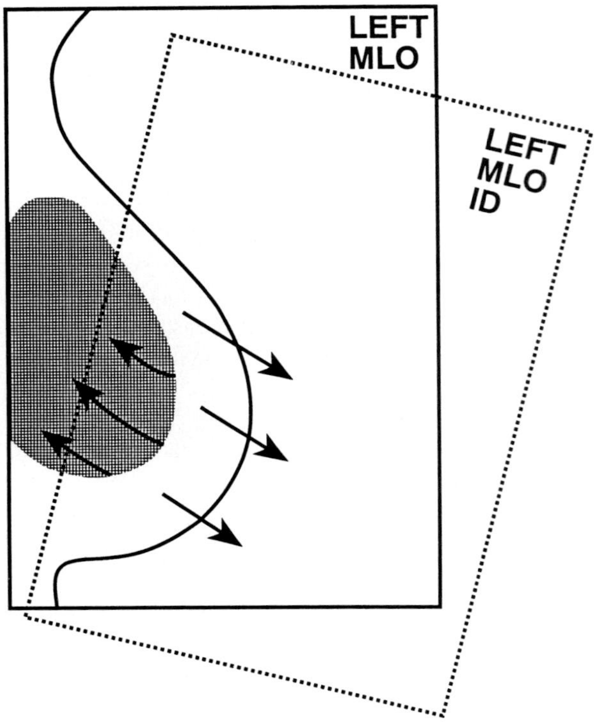

Figure 5–10. If the standard MLO image shows dominance of glandular tissue anteriorly and inferiorly, the implant displacement view (dotted outline) can be tailored to optimize tissue visualization.

tangential spot film, combined with implant displacement technique, is useful for optimal visualization of the area in question.

Without special chest wall techniques, the posterior wall of the implant and the retroimplant area remains obscured on both standard and implant displacement views. High kilovolt peak (kVp) and use of an aluminum, rather than molybdenum filter, allow techniques ideally suited for excellent images of the chest wall and posterior wall of the implant (Fig. 5–11). We have not found routine use of this view helpful. Although we have not identified a rupture that was not apparent clinically or with routine implant imaging, we use the chest wall view selectively to better visualize the upper posterior extension of silicone from implant rupture or herniation.

There is growing interest in the ability of breast imaging procedures to assess the integrity of breast implants. Although highly specific mammographic findings may be seen with disruption of the implant envelope, intracapsular rupture of silicone implants has no specific mammographic or clinical signs. Magnetic resonance imaging (MRI) is the most sensitive and specific modality for detection of extraluminal silicone.[13–16] Sonography, although less sensitive or specific, is less costly and often a valuable tool for detecting intracapsular rupture and the presence of extracapsular accumulations of silicone.[3,9]

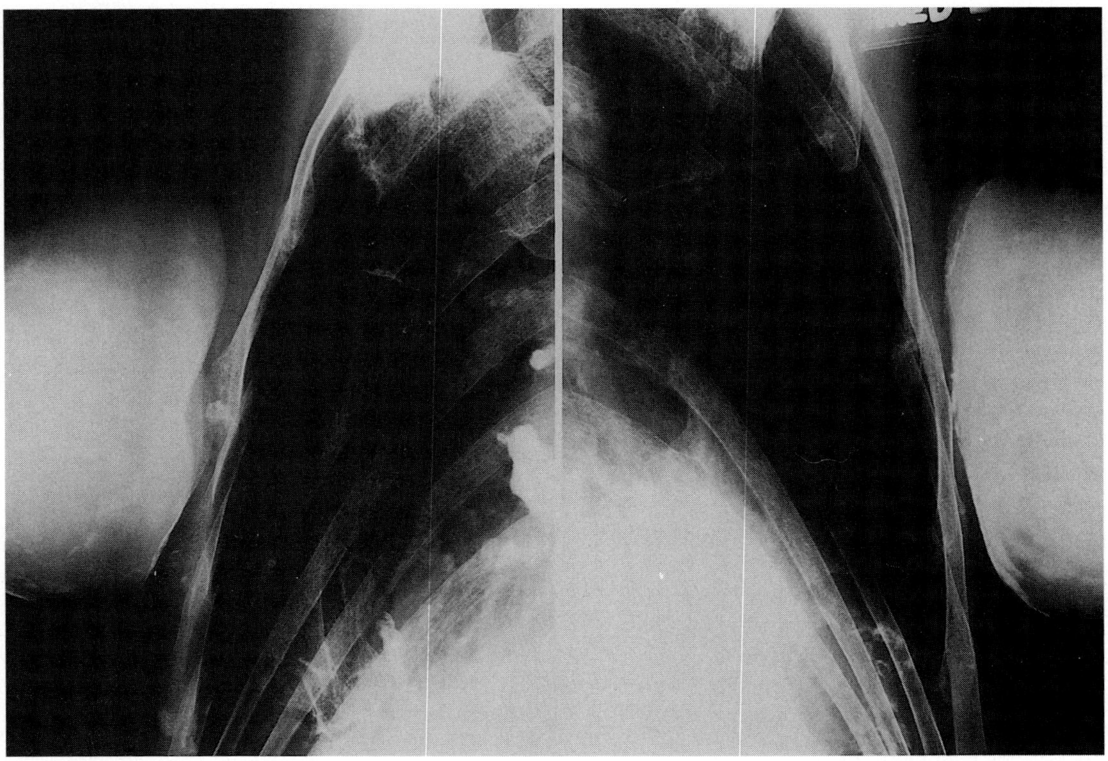

Figure 5–11. Chest wall view is obtained using high kVp (38 to 40), aluminum in place of the molybdenum filter, and no compression. The patient stands in front of the Bucky and rotated so that the x-ray beam is directed tangentially to the chest wall and between the chest wall and posterior wall of the implant. Although this view provides an exquisite look at the posterior wall of the implant, it has not proven to be of sufficient benefit to be included in routine imaging of the augmented breast.

Detectability of breast cancer in patients with augmentation implants is primarily dependent on the following: (1) appropriate patient selection for augmentation surgery, (2) appropriate selection of implant size relative to the amount of native breast tissue, (3) vigilance in obtaining annual physical examination by an experienced examiner, (4) proper instruction in doing monthly BSE, (5) immediate attention to clinical concerns, (6) properly done mammographic studies at appropriate intervals with on-site supervision of an experienced radiologist. Imaging the augmented breast frequently requires tailored supplemental implant displacement views or ancillary studies such as ultrasonography, to achieve optimal visualization of breast tissue (especially areas of clinical concern). For this reason, we regard imaging of the augmented breast as a diagnostic mammogram. Patients are allocated more time for the study and are scheduled when the radiologist is present to participate as needed.

To date, there is no scientific proof that the presence of implants delays detection of breast cancer when the above protocol has been followed.[17,18] In addition, published research from epidemiology studies shows that there is no increase in breast cancer incidence in women with breast implants.[17,18]

REFERENCES

1. Eklund GW. Busby RC, Miller SH, Job JS. Improved imaging of the augmented breast. *AJR.* 1988;151:469–473.
2. Eklund GW. Mammographic imaging of the augmented breast. *Admin Radiol.* 1988;12:42–43.
3. Leibman AJ, Kruse B. Breast cancer: mammographic and sonographic findings after augmentation mammoplasty. *Radiology.* 1990;174:195–198.
4. Clark CP, Peters GN, O'Brien KM. Cancer in the augmented breast: diagnosis and prognosis. *Cancer.* 1993;72:2170–2174.
5. Eklund GW, Cardenosa G. The art of mammographic positioning. *Radiol Clin North Am.* 1992;30:21–53.
6. Cardenosa G, Eklund GW. Imaging the altered breast. In: Taveras JM, Ferrucci JT, eds. *Radiology: Diagnosis—Imaging—Intervention.* Philadelphia: J.B. Lippincott;1994:1–32.
7. Destouet JM, Monsees BS, Oser RF, et al. Screening mammography in 350 women with breast implants: prevalence and findings of implant complications. *AJR.* 1992;159:973–978.
8. Noone RB. *Plastic and Reconstructive Surgery of the Breast.* St. Louis: CV Mosby–Year Book; 1991.
9. Ganott MA, Harris KM, Ilkhanipour ZS, Costa-Greco MA. Augmentation mammoplasty: normal and abnormal findings with mammography and US. *Radiographics.* 1992;12:281–295.
10. Handel N, Silverstein MJ, Gamagami P, et al. Factors affecting mammographic visualization of the breast after augmentation mammoplasty. *JAMA.* 1992;268:1913–1917.
11. Argenta LC. Migration of silicone gel into breast parenchyma following mammary prosthesis rupture. *Ann Plast Surg.* 1983;7:253–254.
12. Capozzi A, Dubou R, Pennisi VR. Distant migration of silicone gel from a ruptured breast implant. *Plast Reconstr Surg.* 1976;62:302.
13. Gorczyca DP, Sinha S, Ahn CY, et al. Silicone breast implants in vivo: MR imaging. *Radiology.* 1992;185:407–410.
14. Gorczyca DP, Debruhl ND, Mund DF, Bassett LW. Linguine sign at MR imaging: does it represent the collapsed silicone implant shell? *Radiology.* 1994;191:576.
15. DeAngelis GA, de Lange EE, Miller LR, Morgan RF. MR imaging of breast implants. *Radiographics.* 1994;14:783–794.
16. Mund DF, Farria DM, Gorczyca DP, et al. MR imaging of the breast in patients with silicone-gel implants: spectrum of findings. *AJR.* 1993;161:773–778.
17. Deapen DM, Brody GS. Augmentation mammoplasty and breast cancer: a 5-year update of the Los Angeles study. *Plast Reconstr Surg.* 1992;89:660–665.
18. Deapen DM, Pike MC, Casagrande JT, Brody GS. The relationship between breast cancer and augmentation mammoplasty: an epidemiologic study. *Plast Reconstr Surg.* 1986;77:361–367.

6

Mammographic Evaluation of the Failing Implant

DEBRA L. MONTICCIOLO

Most patients undergo mammography to evaluate or rule out parenchymal breast disease. Evaluation of the implant has traditionally been of secondary concern. The routine use of implant displacement views (Chapter X) has been tremendously helpful in the radiographic evaluation of the augmented patient. These views are specially designed to visualize more breast tissue and, consequently, less of the implant. Still, much information is present on both the routine and displacement views regarding the implant and its status. Over time the variety of implants has grown as have the known radiographic manifestations of the complications associated with them. Mammography has, therefore, found a special role in evaluating these women. Patients are often as interested in the radiographic information gained about their implant as they are in the findings regarding their breast tissue. The Food and Drug Administration (FDA) warnings and moratorium of 1992 no doubt have played a significant role in this. Prior to this debate, findings related to the implant were reported almost incidentally. In the current climate, much more demand has been placed on as complete a mammographic description as possible. A thorough knowledge of implant types and their expected radiographic manifestations has become not only useful but essential.

■ IMPLANT TYPES

Silicone Gel–Filled, Single Lumen

Simple single-lumen silicone implants were the first silicone prostheses introduced and have been available since the early 1960s. The single-lumen variety consists of an envelope, made of silicone elastomer, that contains a variable amount of silicone polymer (polydimethylsiloxane) in the form of a gel. Modifications over time have primarily involved the outer envelope. The first envelopes were clear in vitro and smooth in texture. In the absence of other complications, they appear smooth mammographically (Fig. 6–1). Their high incidence of contracture[1] led to attempts to alter the envelope in the hope of decreasing the body's fibrous reaction. Textured, single-lumen implants are now widely used and have been found to have lower contracture rates.[2] The textured surface has an opaque appearance in vitro. It is usually smooth mammographically as well, although it can sometimes be noted as a corrugated edge, especially on magnified views.

A special case of envelope modification is the polyurethane-coated variety. These implants have a coating of polyurethane foam, which is yellow-colored in vitro, adherent to the silicone envelope. Their appearance mammographically is usually indistinguishable from smooth single-lumen implants. More than one polyurethane-coated implant can be placed in a single implant cavity in a "stacked" configuration (Fig. 6–2). The two implants are placed adjacent to each other in the coronal plane with the smaller of the two anterior. The polyurethane coating prevents slippage. The polyurethane coat also retards the formation of fibrous capsule contracture,[3,4] but other complications have occurred, such as fluid collections, separation of the coating from the envelope, and difficulty in removal.[5–7] These implants were removed from the market after reports suggested that patients with polyurethane-coated prostheses may be ex-

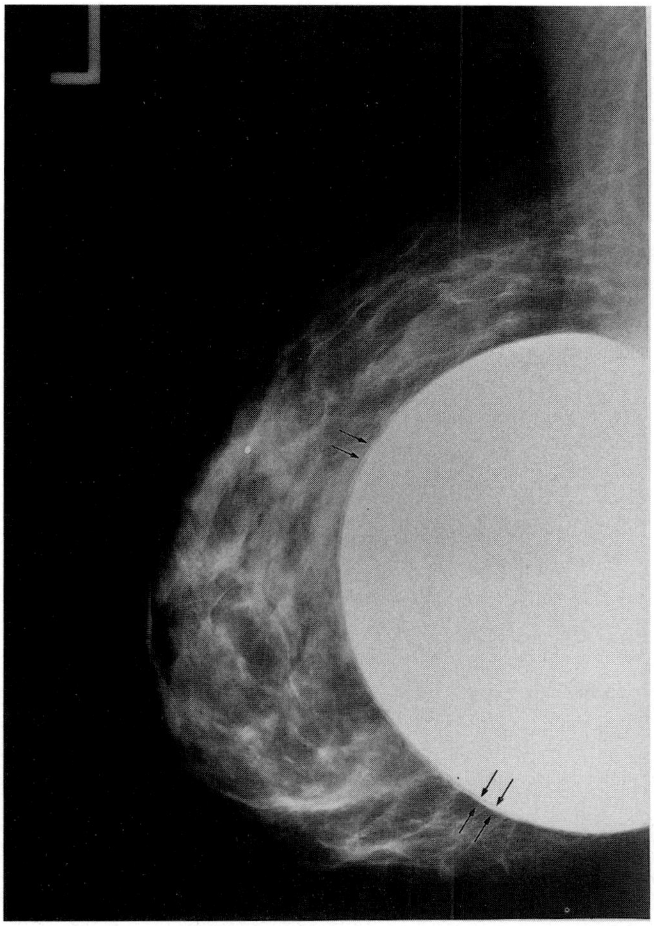

Figure 6–1. Single-lumen silicone implant placed anterior to the pectoralis major muscle. The anterior surface is smooth. There is minimal visible capsule formation (arrows).

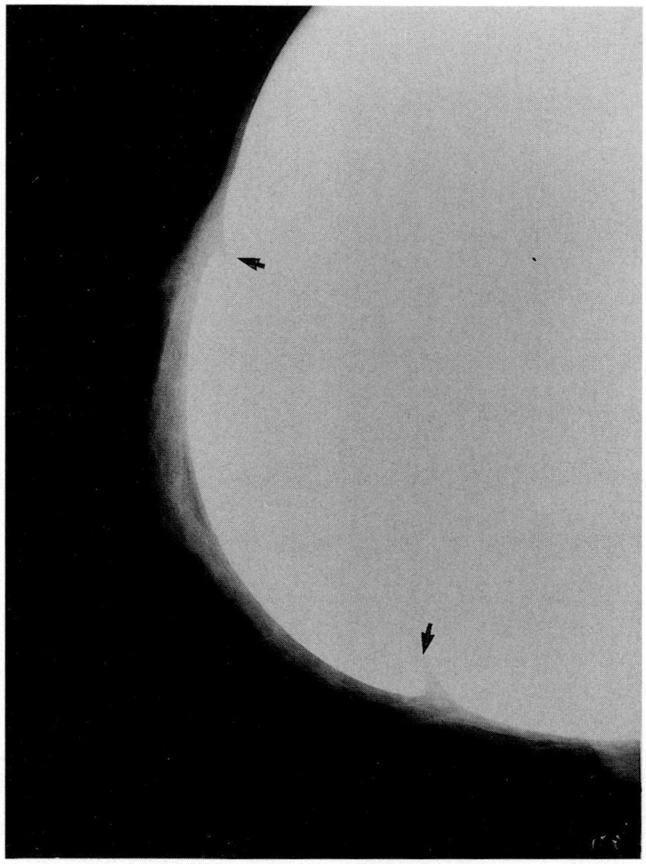

Figure 6–2. Stacked polyurethane implants. Two implants have been placed anterior to one another in the retromammary position. The edge of the space between the two implants is visible mammographically (arrows). The polyurethane coating prevents slippage.

posed to a metabolite of polyurethane, 2,4-toluenediamine (TDA), which has caused tumors in animals.[8] Patients are not currently advised to have their polyurethane implants removed.[9]

Saline-Filled, Single Lumen

Saline-filled implants all have a silicone outer shell (envelope). The saline fill renders this implant less radiopaque than their silicone counterparts, although visualization of the tissue obscured by the implant is still not sufficient for diagnosis. Often the fill valves of these implants and/or the circular placement disks are visible mammographically (Figs. 6–3 through 6–6). Folds are often more obvious because of the relative radiolucency of the enclosed saline (Figs. 6–5 through 6–7). These implants have a less natural feel in vivo than silicone but have the advantage, if ruptured, of releasing a harmless, fully absorbable substance.

Double Lumen

Double-lumen implants have a sphere-within-a-sphere configuration. The earliest of these implants has an inner lumen filled with silicone and an outer lumen filled with saline. This offers protection against silicone leakage after rupture. If the inner lumen ruptures, the silicone would still be contained by the saline-filled shell. An outer lumen rupture will simply result in the release of saline into the surrounding tissue. Of course, the protective mechanism will then be gone.

The normal mammographic appearance of a double-lumen implant with a saline-filled outer envelope reveals the less radiopaque saline lumen just outside the silicone inner lumen (Fig. 6–8). The saline is often forced to those regions of least resistance; with the breast compressed, the saline lumen may be visible only posteriorly at the edges of the film. Leakage of saline from the outer shell is diagnosed mammographically by the absence of the saline lumen where one was previously known to be present. This radiographic ap-

(text continues on page 60)

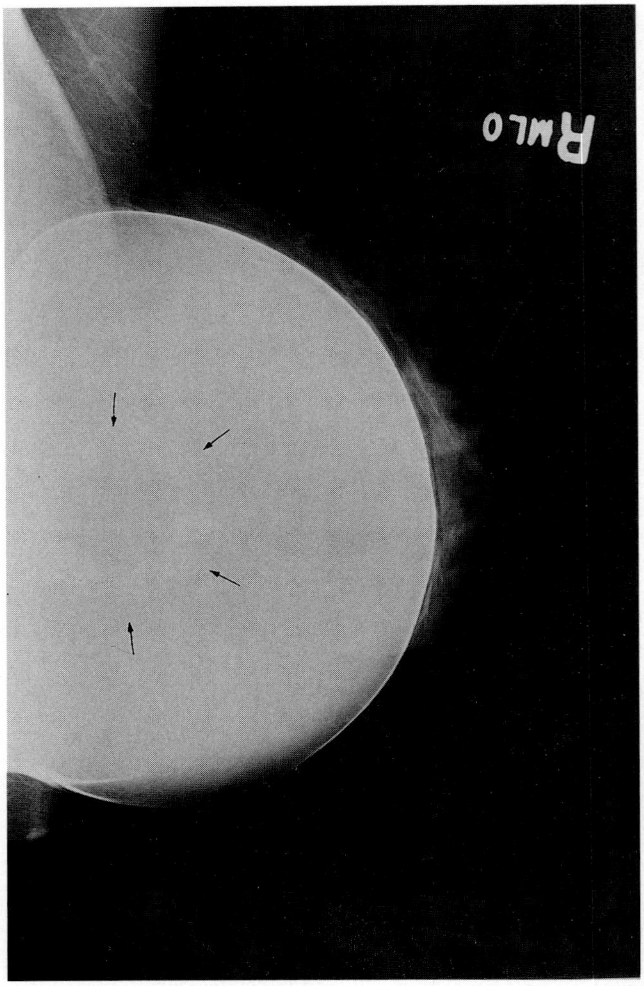

Figure 6–3. Circular placement disk (arrows) is faintly visible through this single-lumen saline implant.

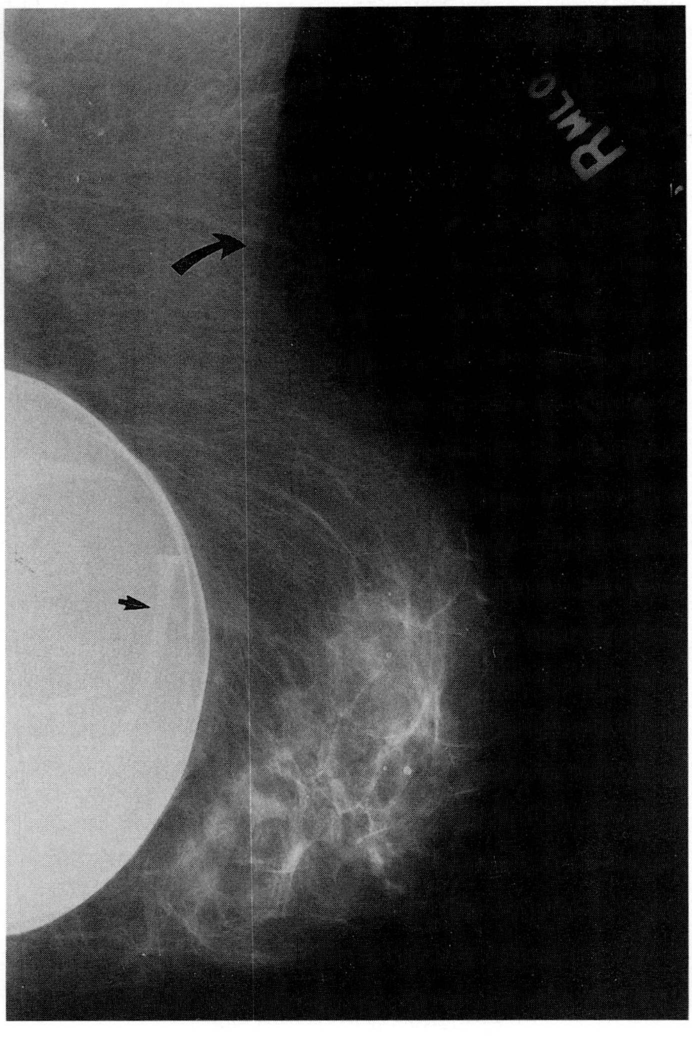

Figure 6–4. Saline implant with visible fill valve and tube (arrow). Pectoralis muscle overlying implant (curved arrow).

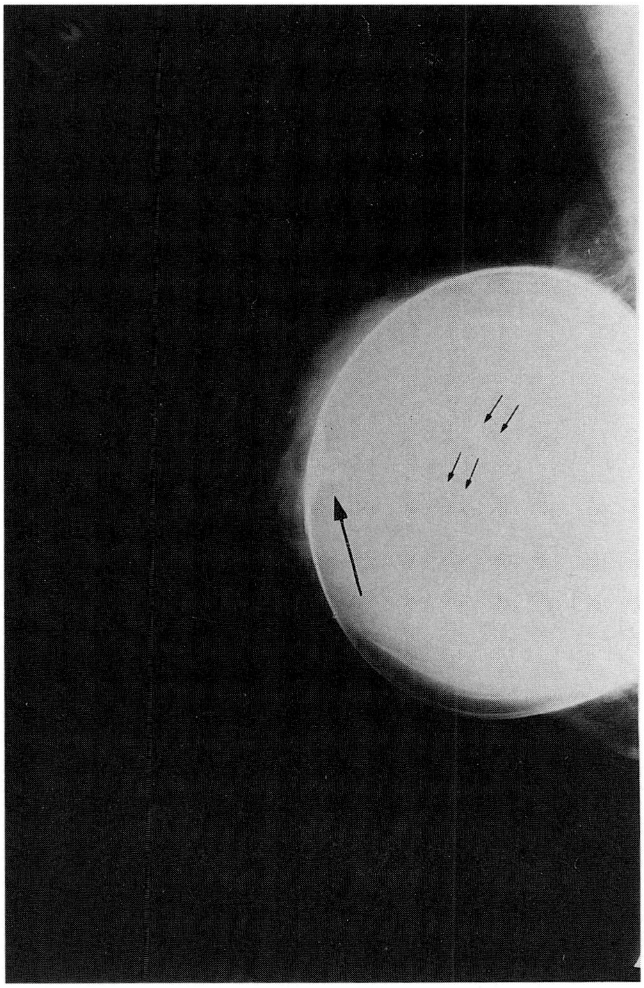

Figure 6–5. Single-lumen saline implant. Fill valve (long arrow) and folds (short arrows) are visible.

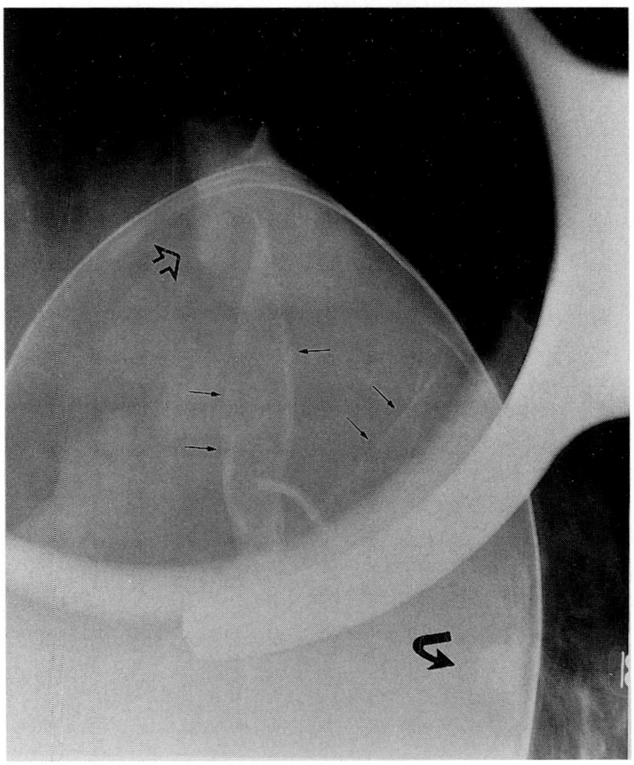

Figure 6–6. Spot-compression, magnification image obtained to evaluate masses of free silicone (open arrow). The patient now has a saline implant; folds (arrows) and valve (curved arrow) are visible.

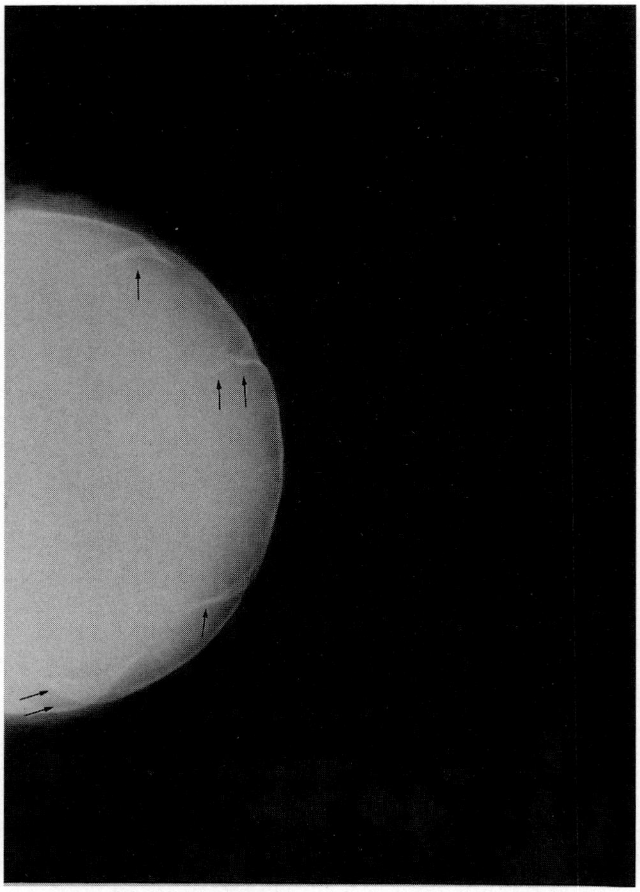

Figure 6–7. Normal folds (arrows) visible in a saline implant.

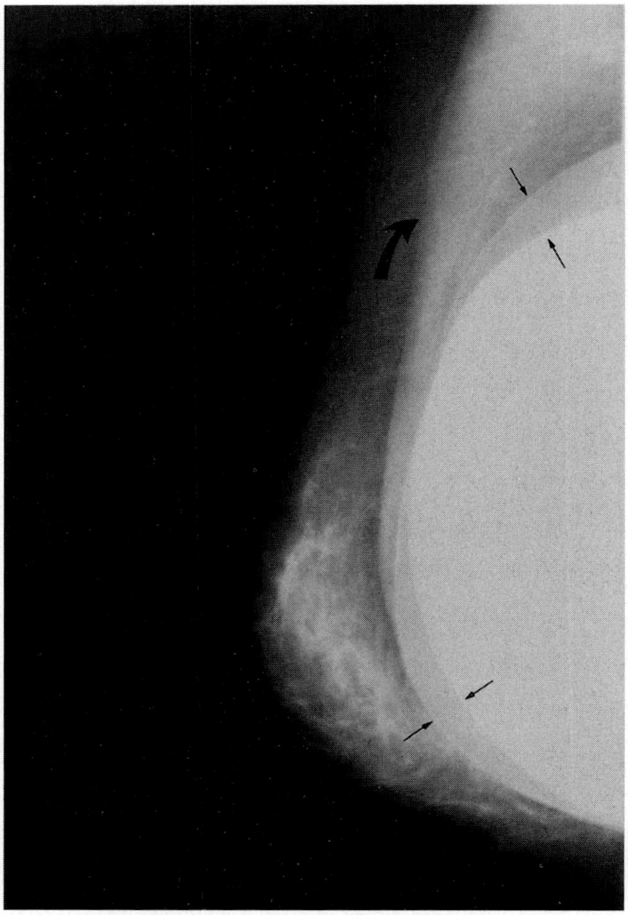

Figure 6–8. Normal double-lumen implant with a saline outer lumen (arrows). Pectoralis muscle (curved arrow).

pearance is indistinguishable from a single-lumen, silicone gel–filled implant without the proper history or prior films. The presence of a visible, double lumen in the contralateral breast is a good indication that the same implant was once present on the side of concern, but this is not always necessarily so.

Rupture of the inner silicone lumen into the surrounding, saline-filled outer shell results in admixture of the two compartments, which can be seen mammographically (Figs. 6–9 and 6–10). There is loss of the normal acute angle between the silicone and saline compartments (Fig. 6–11). As the mixing of the two substances is more complete, the distinction between them becomes less obvious and the appearance may be similar to a single-lumen silicone implant. This depends on the relative amounts of saline and silicone and on the size and location of the rupture. Some partially mixed ruptures remain stable for years. If enough saline is present, the rupture may still be evidenced by the presence of two distinct substances mammographically, regardless of the extent of admixture (Fig. 6–12). If the amount of saline is small relative to the amount of silicone, rupture of the inner silicone lumen will be indistinguishable in mammographic

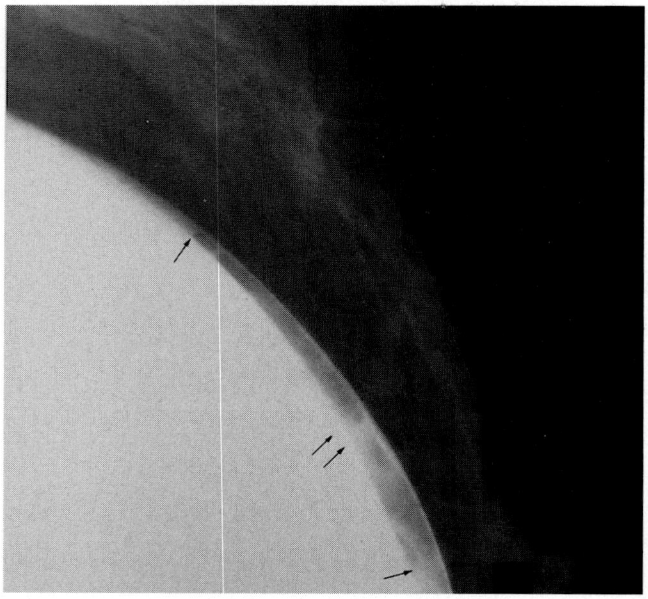

Figure 6–9. Double-lumen rupture. Early admixture (arrows) seen as a result of rupture of the inner silicone lumen.

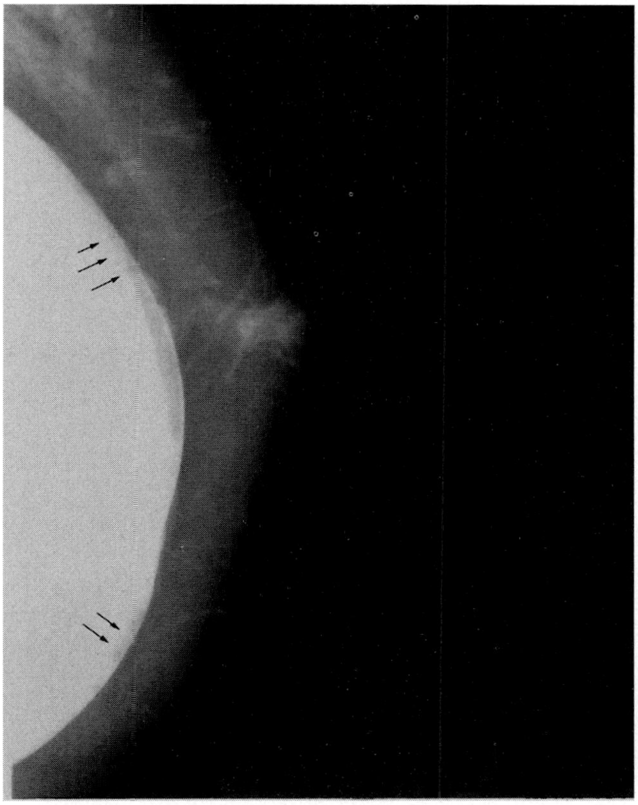

Figure 6–10. Double-lumen rupture. More complete admixture with silicone inner lumen rupture.

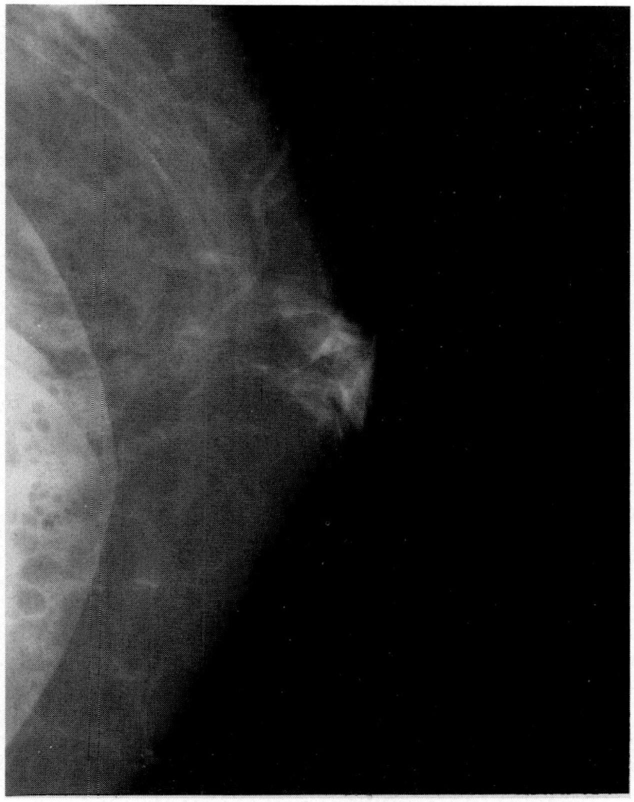

Figure 6–12. Long-standing double-lumen implant rupture. Presence of two distinct substances is still evidenced by saline within silicone even though the inner lumen rupture is remote (4 years).

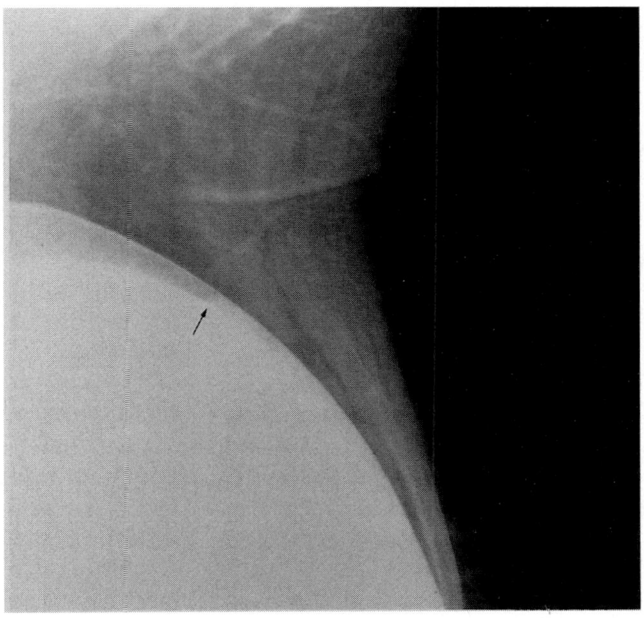

Figure 6–11. Double-lumen rupture. Rupture of inner silicone lumen. The normal acute angle between the two compartments is blunted (arrow).

appearance from either a single-lumen silicone or a double lumen with leakage of the saline outer shell. That is, in a double-lumen rupture with complete admixture it may be impossible to determine which lumen has been compromised unless interim films are available that show the materials gradually mixing. If the only films available show only the prerupture intact implant and, later, the completely mixed postrupture state, one clue is to assess the implant size. Rupture of only the outer saline shell results in a single-lumen appearance that has the size of the original silicone component alone. The ruptured double-lumen implant should, therefore, be smaller than the original and its mammographically visible silicone compartment should be the same size as prior to rupture. Double-lumen rupture involving the inner silicone lumen results in expansion of the available silicone into a larger volume space. Therefore, the visible silicone compartment postrupture will appear larger than the intact silicone inner lumen before admixture (Fig. 6–13).

Another type of double-lumen implant is the expander, which is a later innovation. These implants have a saline inner lumen, which can be filled incrementally, and a thin outer lumen of silicone gel fill. They do not offer the leakage protection of the reverse configuration but have a more nat-

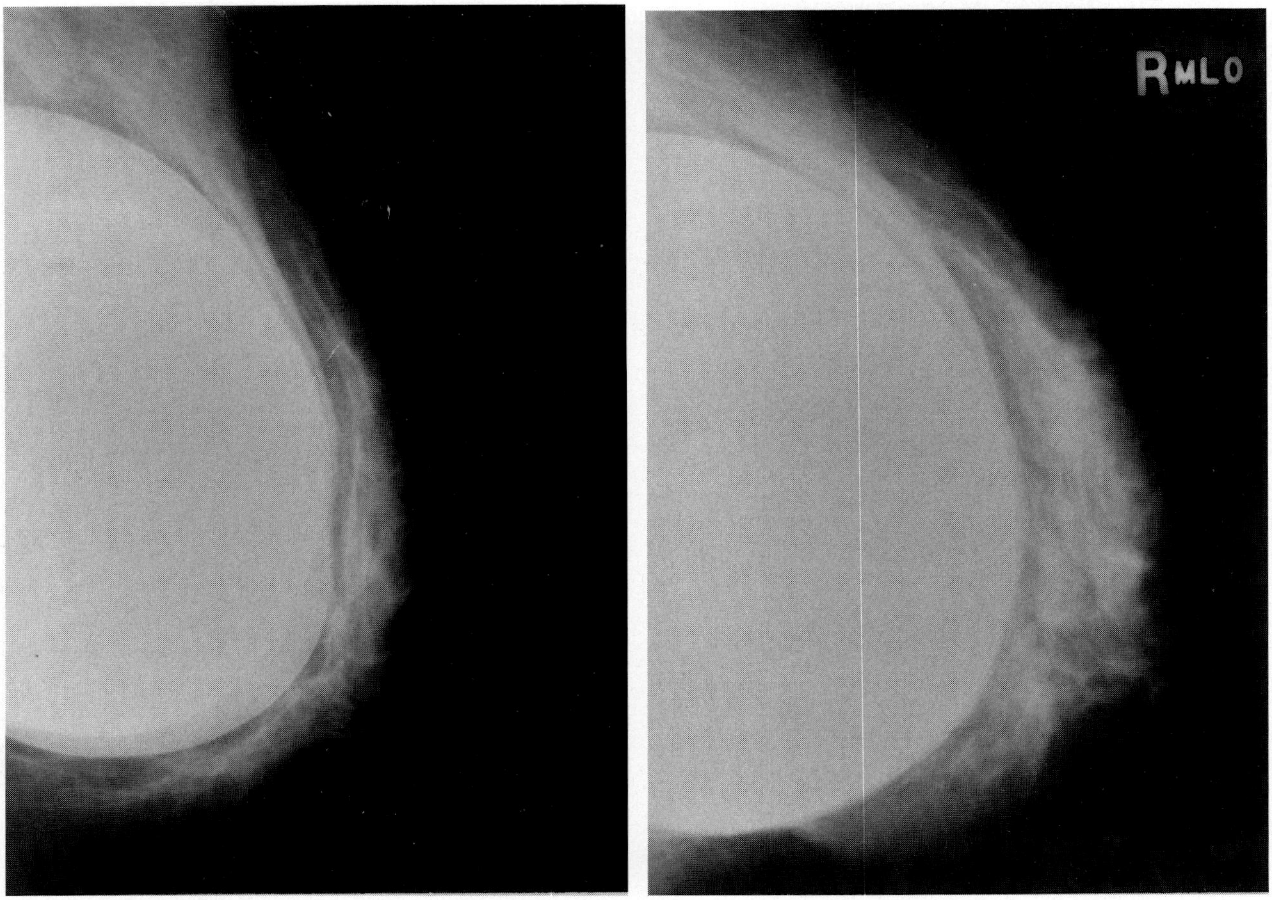

A B

Figure 6–13. (**A**) Subpectoral intact double-lumen implant. (**B**) Seven years later the saline lumen is no longer apparent. Size of silicone compartment suggests the inner lumen has ruptured and expanded into the space formerly held by the outermost shell.

ural feel and can be slowly expanded to stretch the surrounding tissues to an appropriate degree. Mammographically, the expander looks like a silicone single-lumen implant except that the former is slightly more radiolucent (Figs. 6–14 and 6–15).

■ IMPLANT PLACEMENT

Implants can be placed anterior or posterior to the pectoralis muscle. When anterior, they are termed retroglandular, subglandular, or retromammary. The posterior placement is known as submuscular, subpectoral, or retropectoral. The pectoralis muscle should be radiographically visible in front of the implant's anterior surface if the placement is subpectoral (Figs. 6–4 and 6–8). This is sometimes a difficult distinction because the muscle layer can be quite thin. Conversely, a thickened capsule can be confused with overlying pectoralis muscle. Therefore, although placement anterior or posterior to the muscle is usually obvious, caution should be used in making this distinction and designation.

■ MAMMOGRAPHY OF IMPLANT COMPLICATIONS

Implant Failure

The most obvious and definite radiographic sign of implant rupture is free silicone in the surrounding tissues. Silicone granulomas (Fig. 6–16) have an intermediate density relative to dense fibroglandular tissue and calcifying masses. Silicone can also be detected in lymph nodes (Fig. 6–17). This is not always indicative of rupture; the silicone envelope is a semipermeable membrane and silicone can bleed through it. Silicone can be found in surrounding tissue and concentrated by the lymph system.

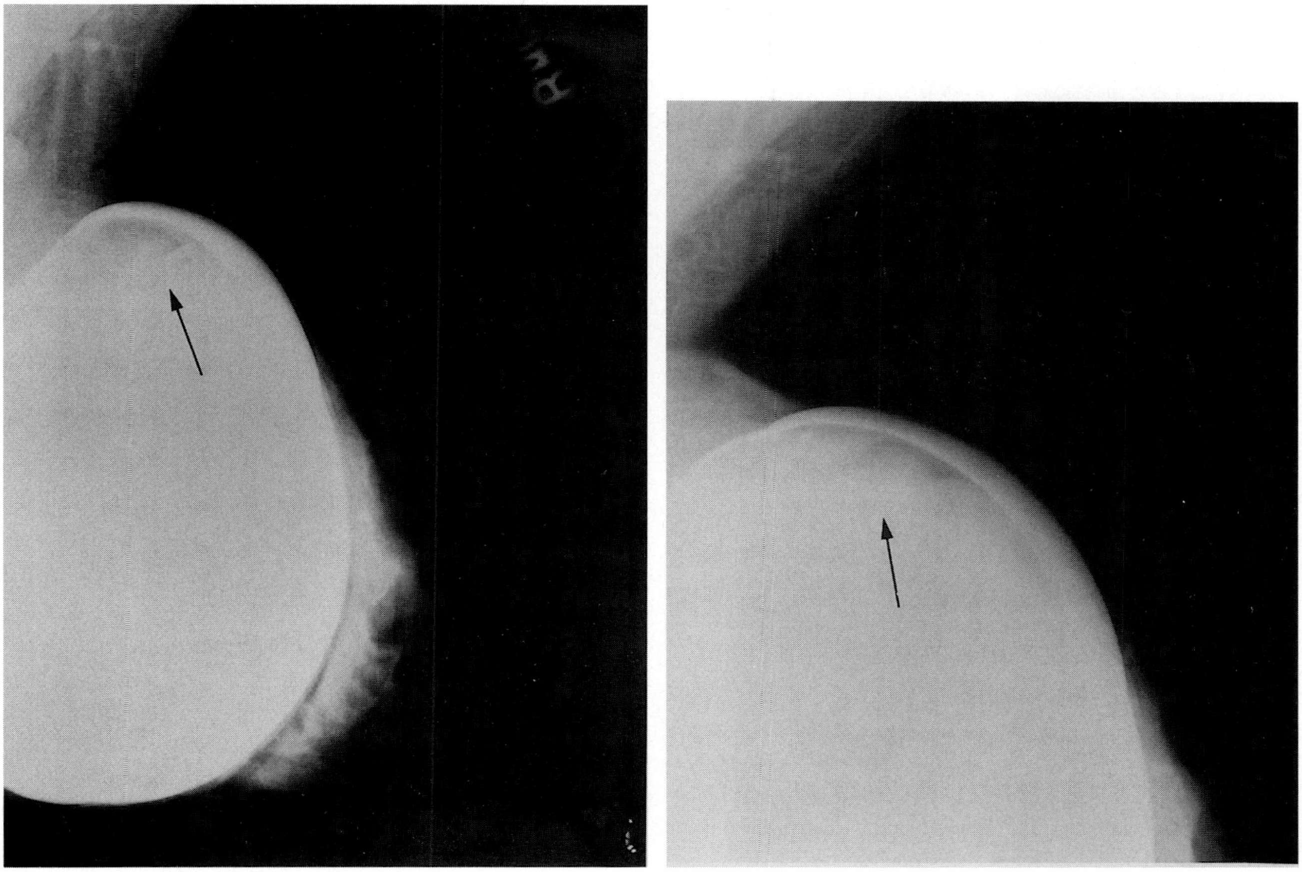

A B

Figure 6–14. Double-lumen expander with silicone in the outer lumen. (**A**) Presence of the inner saline lumen is apparent superiorly (arrow). (**B**) Closeup of **A**.

If silicone has escaped the envelope but is still limited by a well-developed fibrous capsule, it may be visualized close to the implant surface (Fig. 6–18). Encapsulated rupture may be seen better on the implant displacement views (Fig. 6–19).

Another mammographic sign of prosthesis rupture is change in the apparent implant size or shape. Often these ruptures are walled-off or partially contained by a well-developed fibrous capsule. The leaking silicone will seek the point of least resistance, usually the axilla. A peaked appearance directed toward the posterior-superior aspect of the implant cavity, therefore, often indicates rupture (Fig. 6–20). If the extension is large and/or the leaking silicone separates from the main body of the implant, the underlying rupture is obvious (Figs. 6–21 and 6–22). Smaller leaks can produce more limited radiographic changes. The differential then includes simple herniation, which may be impossible to exclude based on mammography alone (Figs. 6–22 and 6–23). Large leaks may eventually disburse so that the free globules of silicone in the tissues are more apparent (Fig. 6–21).

Other Implant Complications

Implants can produce a spectrum of minor complications, some of which have radiographic sequelae. The most common complication is fibrous capsule formation, which may or may not cause clinical capsular contracture. Although there are radiographic signs to suggest the condition, implant contracture is strictly a clinical diagnosis. The Baker classification is commonly used to describe the degree of contracture and has four grades[10]:

- Grade I — Soft with natural appearance
- Grade II — Implant can be palpated, less soft; natural appearance
- Grade III — Firm with visible distortion
- Grade IV — Breast is hard, obvious spherical distortion.

Contracture may not be apparent radiographically. The formation of a fibrous capsule occurs with all implants and is usually a millimeter or so thick.[11–13] Once the capsule be-

(text continues on page 67)

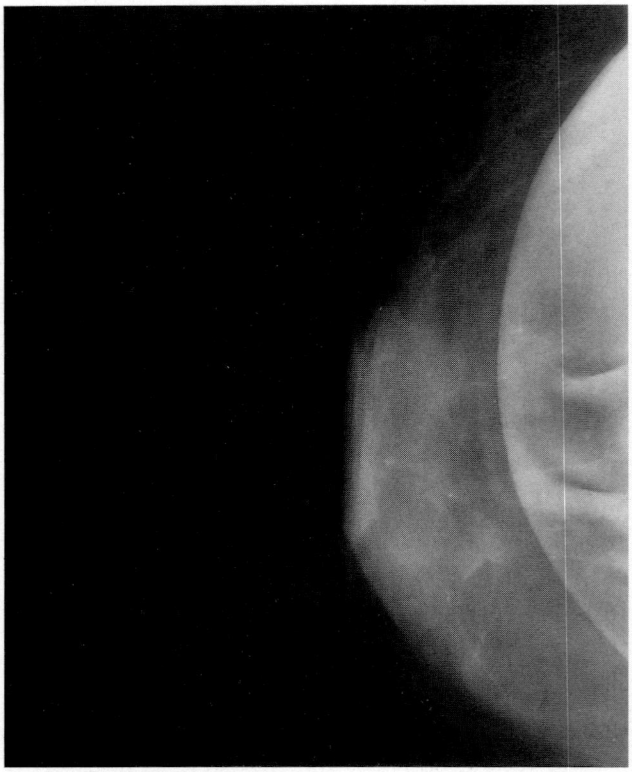

Figure 6–15. Expander, double-lumen implant with saline interior appears more radiolucent than a normal single-lumen silicone implant on this push-back view.

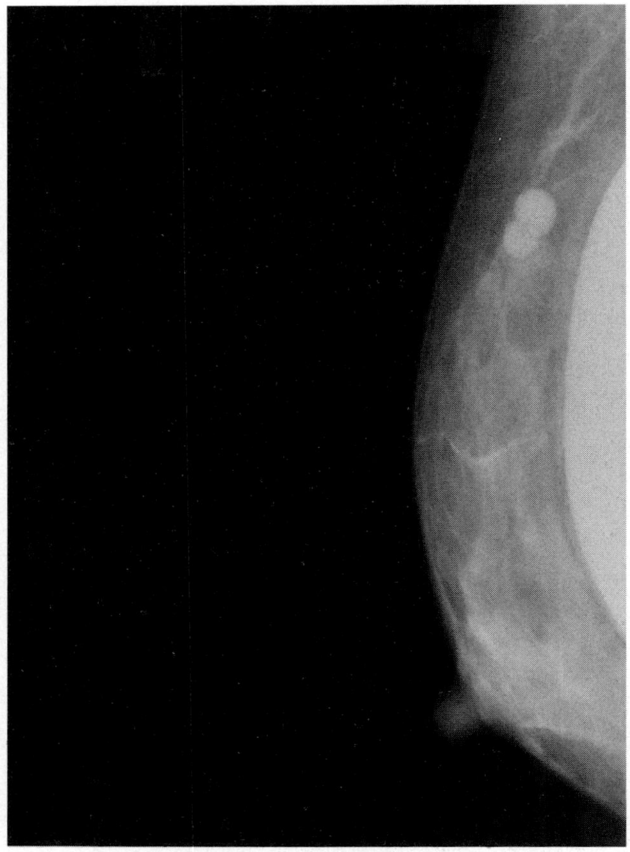

Figure 6–16. Silicone rupture. Silicone granulomas in tissue indicate implant rupture.

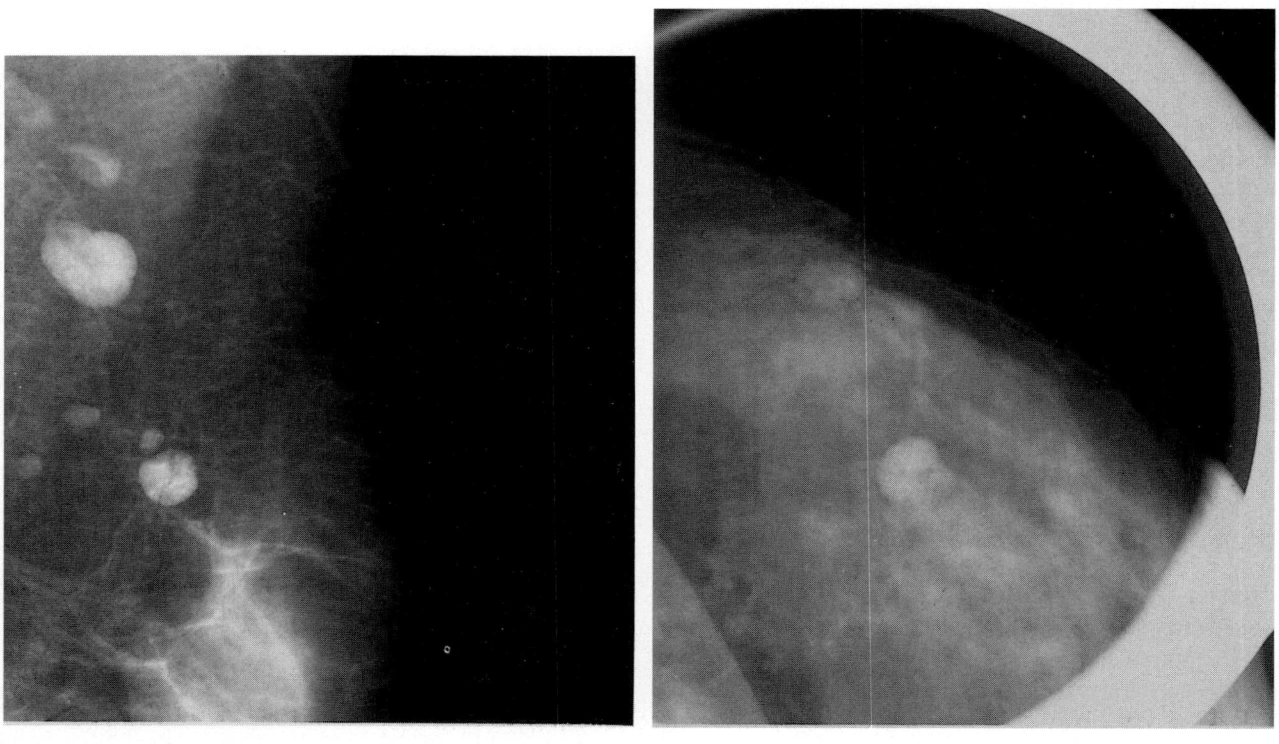

A B

Figure 6–17. (**A,B**) Silicone within lymph nodes causes increased density similar to that seen in silicone granulomas (Fig. 6–16).

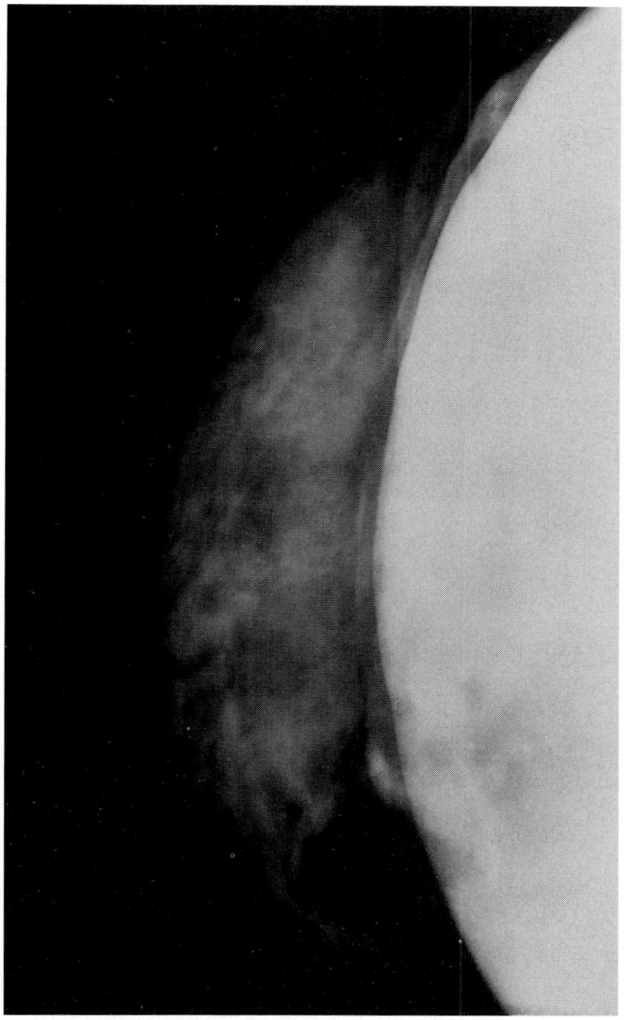

Figure 6–18. Ruptured implant with silicone contained close to implant by fibrous capsule.

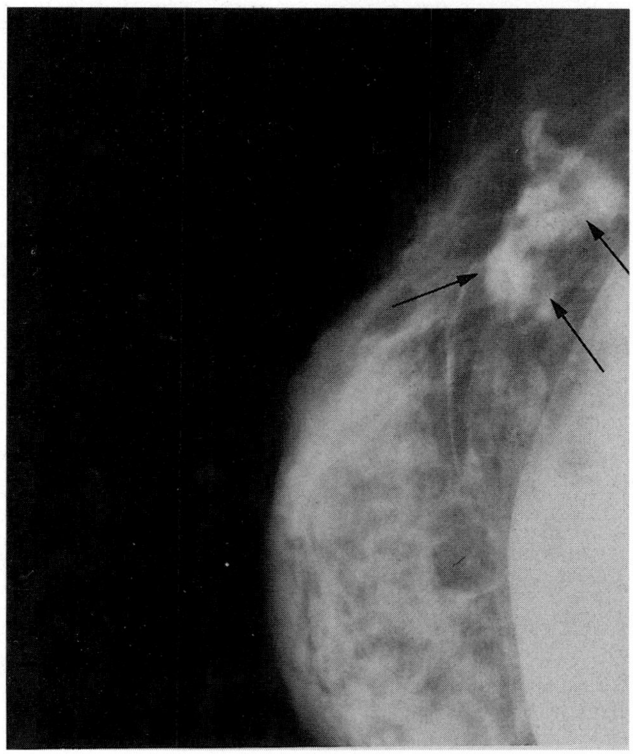

Figure 6–19. Push-back view of same patient as in Figure 6–18. Escaped but encapsulated silicone is more apparent (arrows).

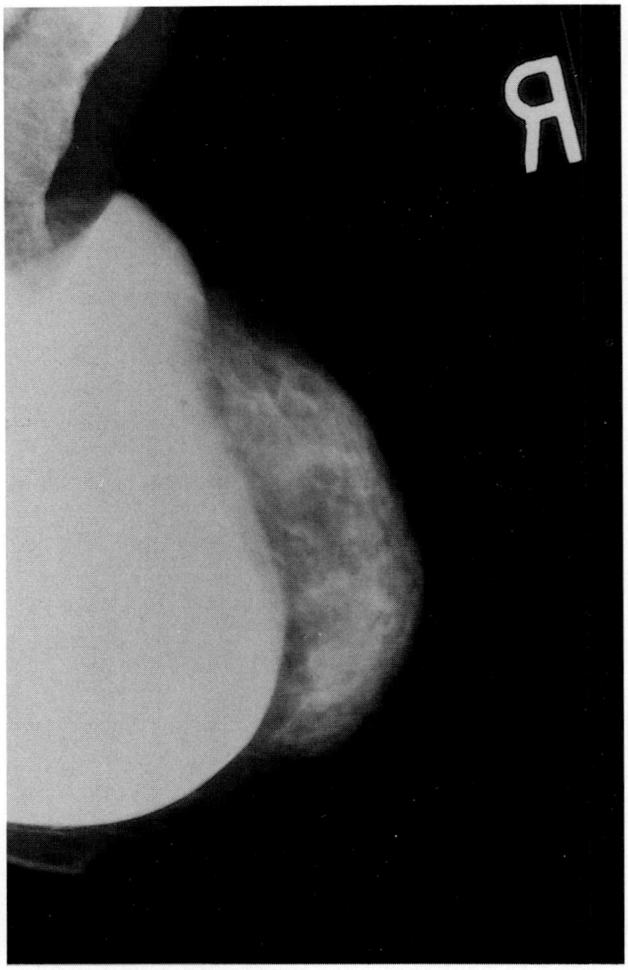

Figure 6–20. Right mediolateral oblique shows single lumen implant with superior "peak." This implant is ruptured and the silicone, still encapsulated, is taking the path of least resistance—toward the axilla.

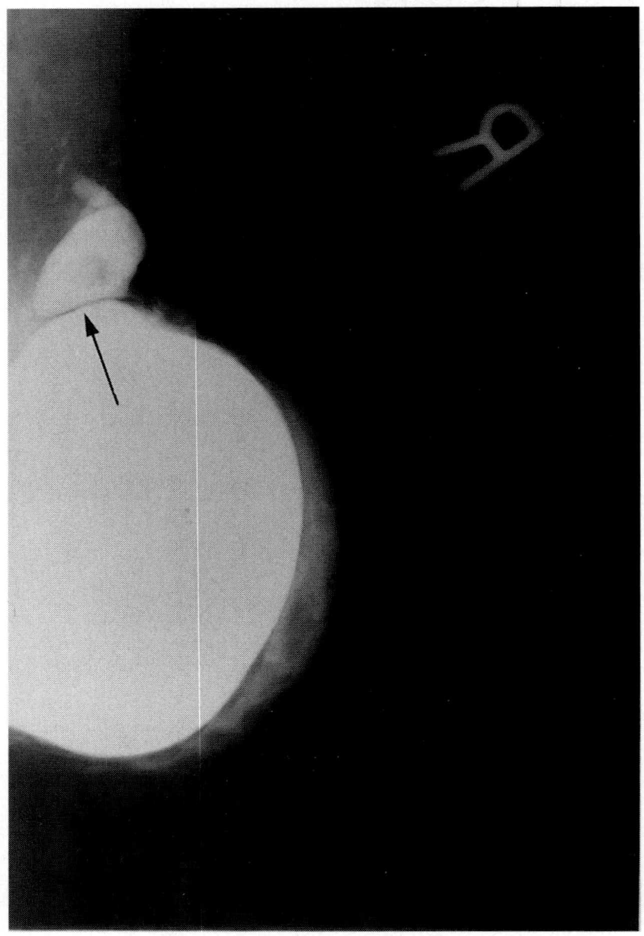

Figure 6–21. Superior leak of ruptured single-lumen implant. Silicone extends into the axilla and has separated (arrow) from the main body of silicone, indicating a free leak.

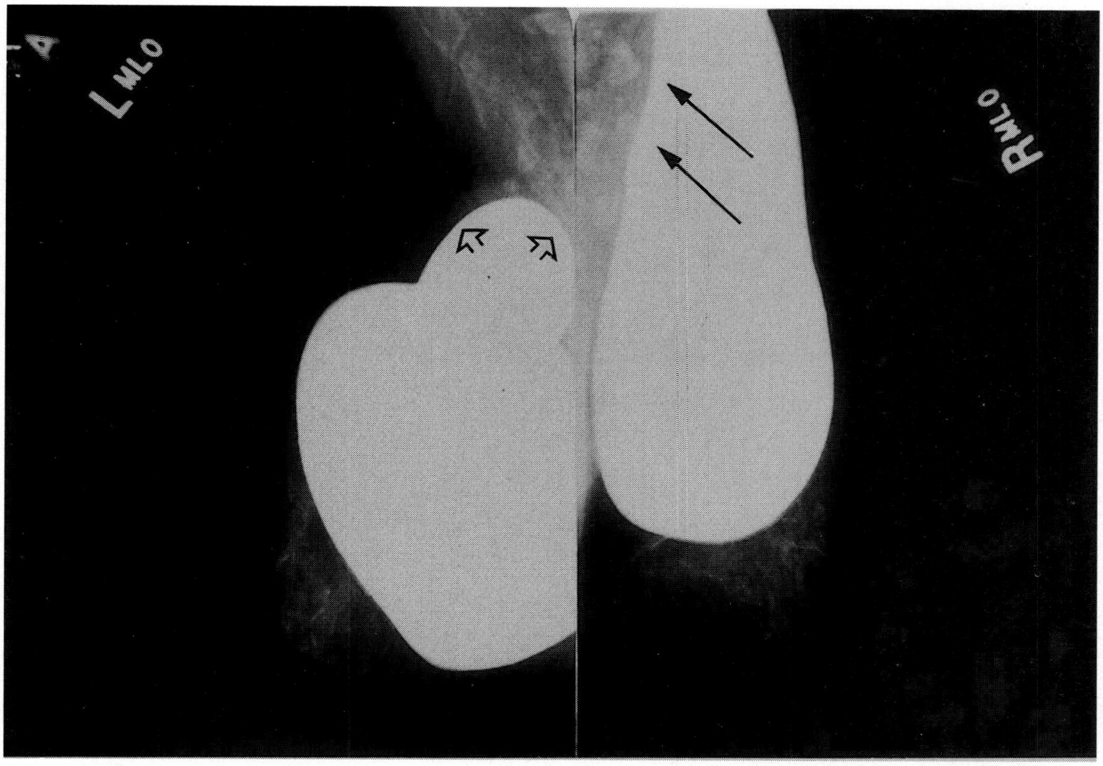

Figure 6–22. Bilateral mediolateral oblique views show large axillary extension on the right (solid arrows), which represents rupture with an axillary extension. Posterior bulge on the left (open arrows) also is due to implant rupture; the differential here includes a (large) herniation.

gins to contract, the implant becomes more spherical. This may be detected mammographically, especially if there are precontracture films available for comparison (Fig. 6–24). With increased pressure, minor focal bulges may appear (Fig. 6–25) and the visible circumference may take on an undulated appearance. Sometimes a thickened fibrous capsule can be identified (Figs. 6–26 and 6–27). Typically, with clinically significant contracture, the technologist is the first to know; obtaining the push-back views on such a patient is difficult. The films that result verify the lack of mobility of the overlying tissues (Fig. 6–28).

Capsular calcifications are another minor complication of implant placement. They typically take years to form and are seen in approximately 20 to 30% of cases.[12,13] Calcification present in the fibrous capsule does not have a definite clinical correlate; the radiographic finding is usually incidental. Capsular calcifications are easier to detect with saline implants and are often more obvious on the push-back views (Figs. 6–26 and 6–29 through 6–32).

■ LIMITS OF MAMMOGRAPHY FOR FAILED IMPLANTS

Silicone gel–filled implants have been available since the early 1960s. Many of these original prostheses are still in place and are now being routinely imaged as these patients reach middle age and enter mammography screening programs. Implants continue to be designed to resist compression and other stresses that could lead to rupture. Earlier models had thinner envelopes that were more prone to rupture and had more gel fill. The incidence of implant failure increases with the time in vivo (especially after a decade in place) and increases with chest wall or breast trauma (such as seat-belt injury). The overall expected rate of rupture is, however, not known with certainty.[14,15] Data evaluating the use of mammography specifically for diagnosing implant failure are scant. Many ruptures are clinically silent, and ex-

(text continues on page 73)

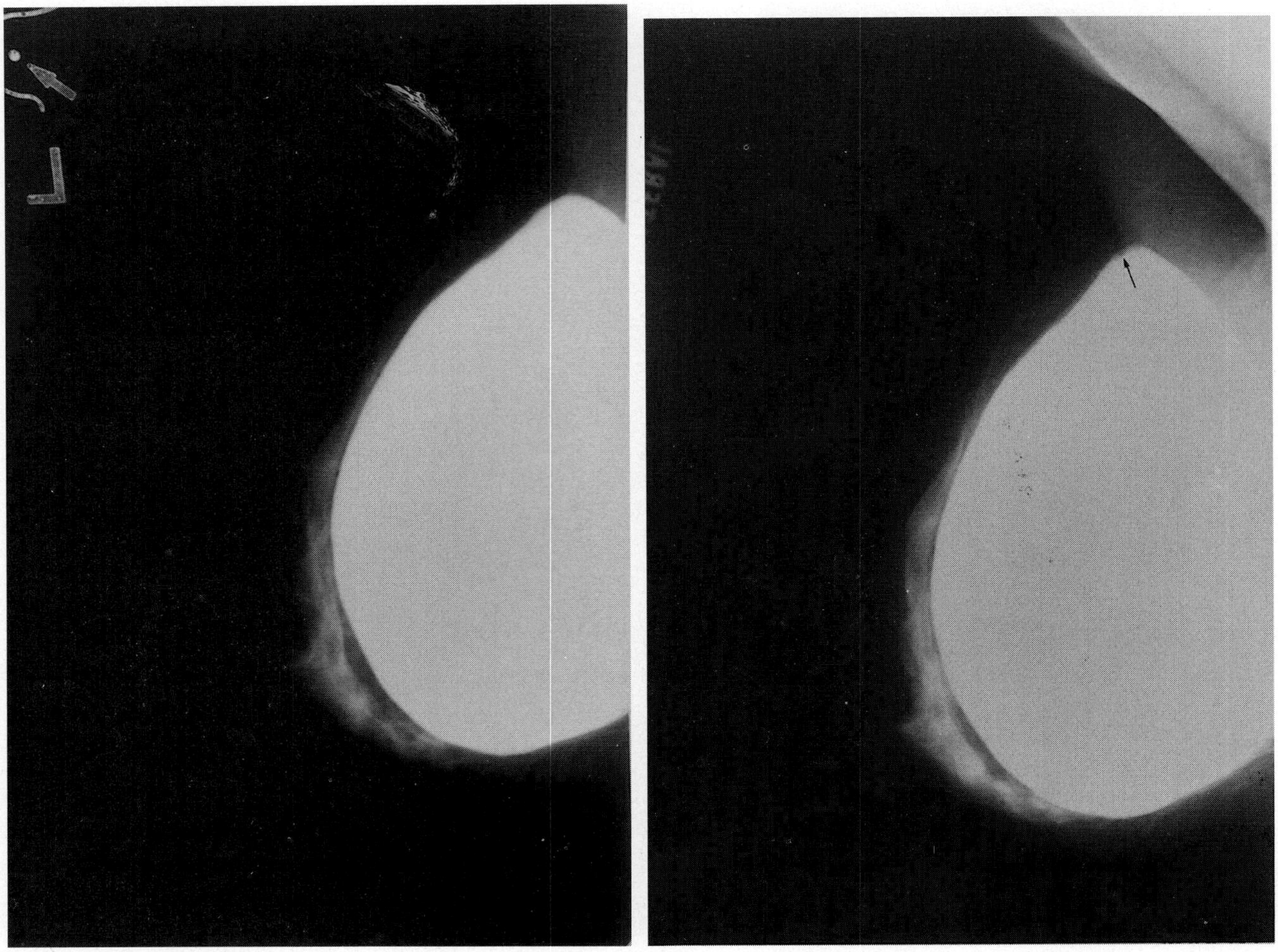

A B

Figure 6–23. (**A**) Left mediolateral oblique shows superior "peaking," assumed at the time of interpretation to represent herniation. (**B**) One year later a tiny bubble seen superiorly (arrow) indicates underlying rupture.

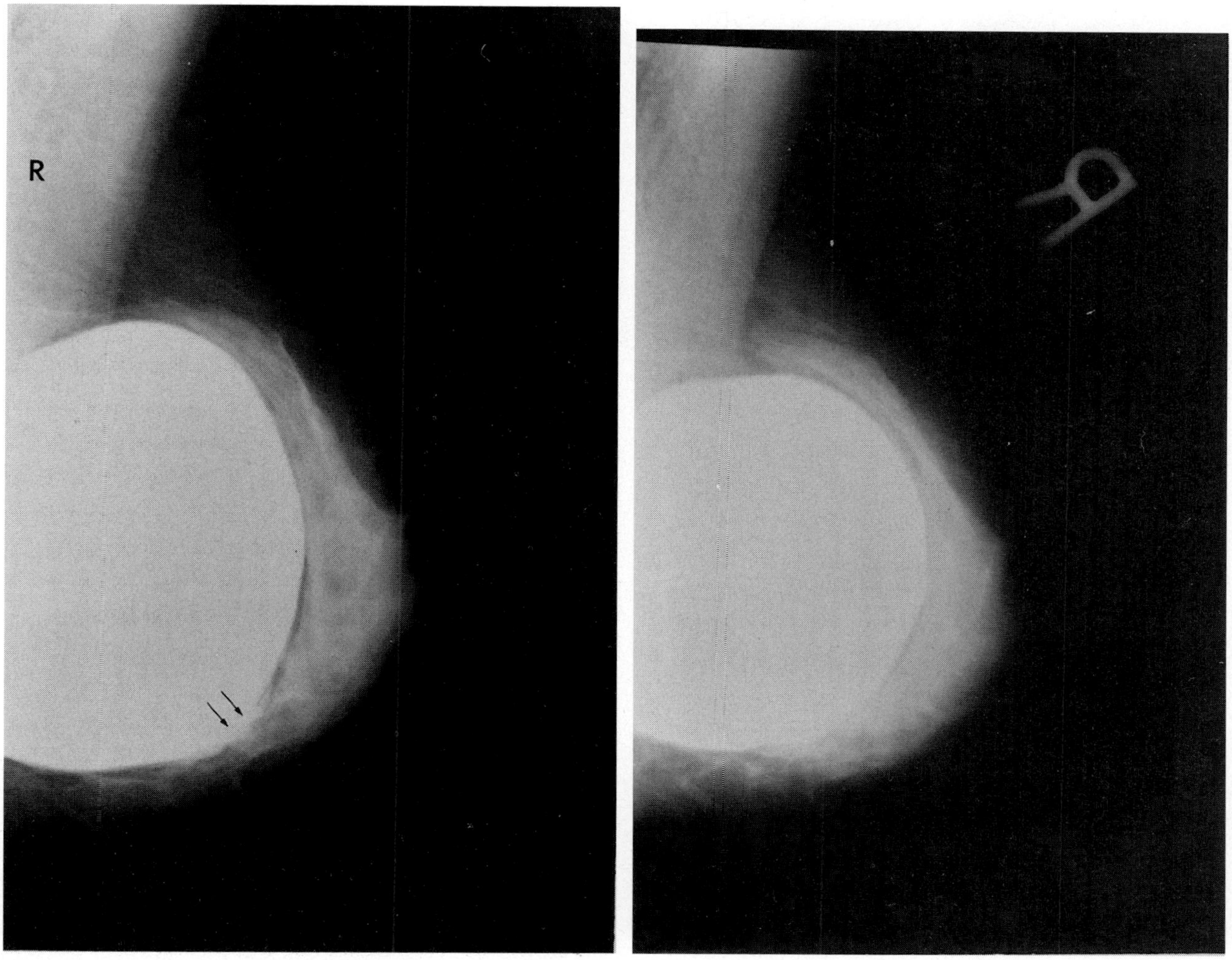

A B

Figure 6–24. Contracture. (**A**) Right mediolateral oblique shows single-lumen implant. There is evidence of encapsulated leak (arrows). Clinically, however, the implant was satisfactory and no revision was done. (**B**) Four years later there is significant clinical contracture. Mammographically the only clue is the more spherical appearance of the implant compared to the prior image.

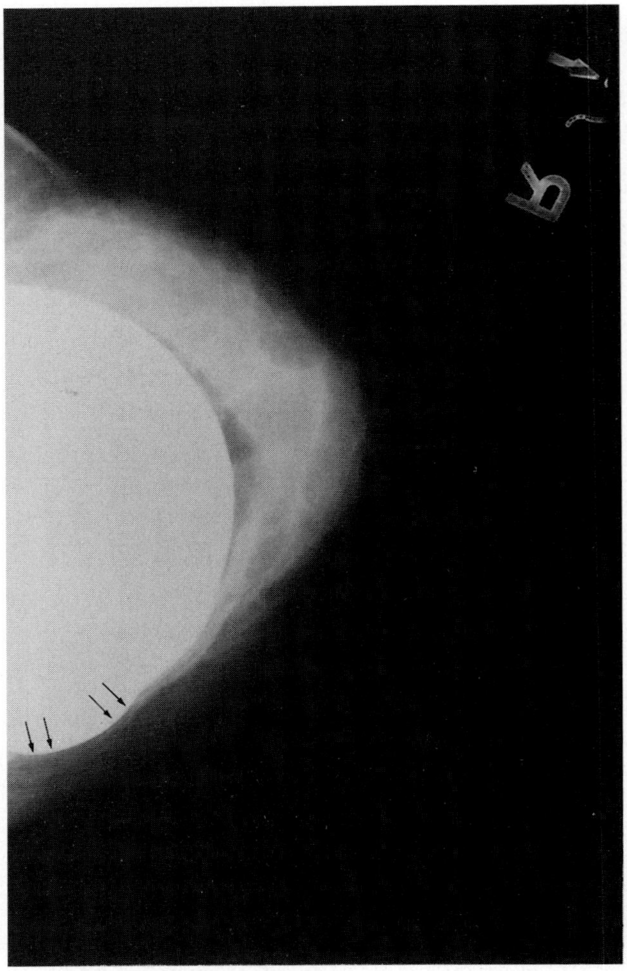

Figure 6–25. Focal bulge (arrows), seen on this craniocaudal projection, developed as contracture did clinically.

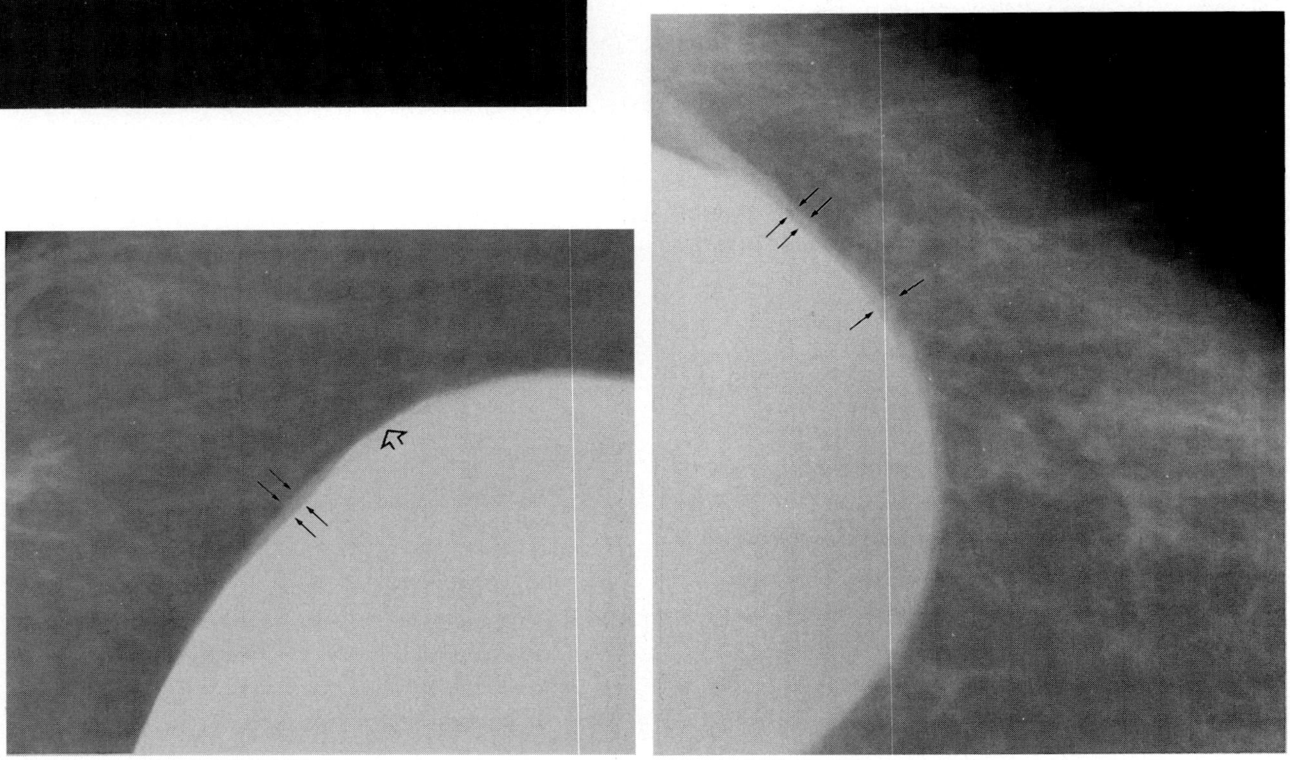

A

B

Figure 6–26. Thickened capsule. (**A**) Patient with retromammary implant shows capsule measuring 1 to 2 mm (arrows) and capsular calcifications (open arrow). (**B**) Same patient, 3 years later, now with clinical contracture. Mammogram shows increase in fibrous capsule (arrows).

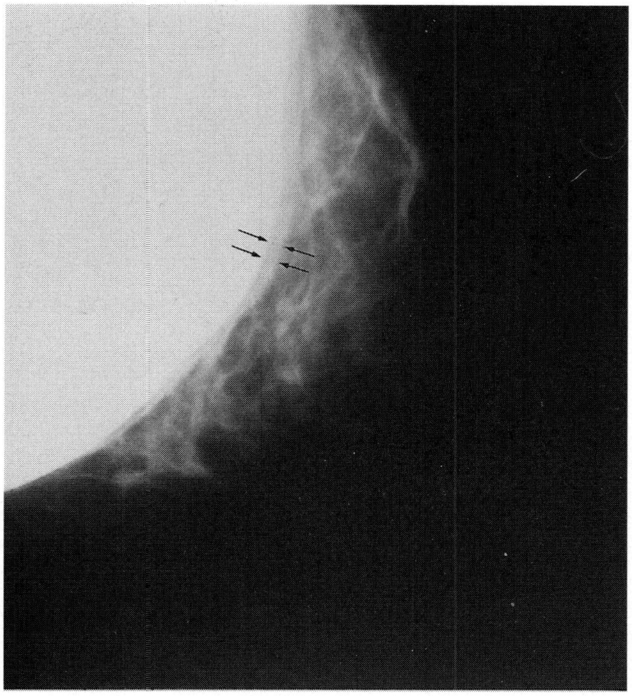

Figure 6–27. Thickened capsule. Retromammary implant with visible thick capsule (arrows). Implant was soft.

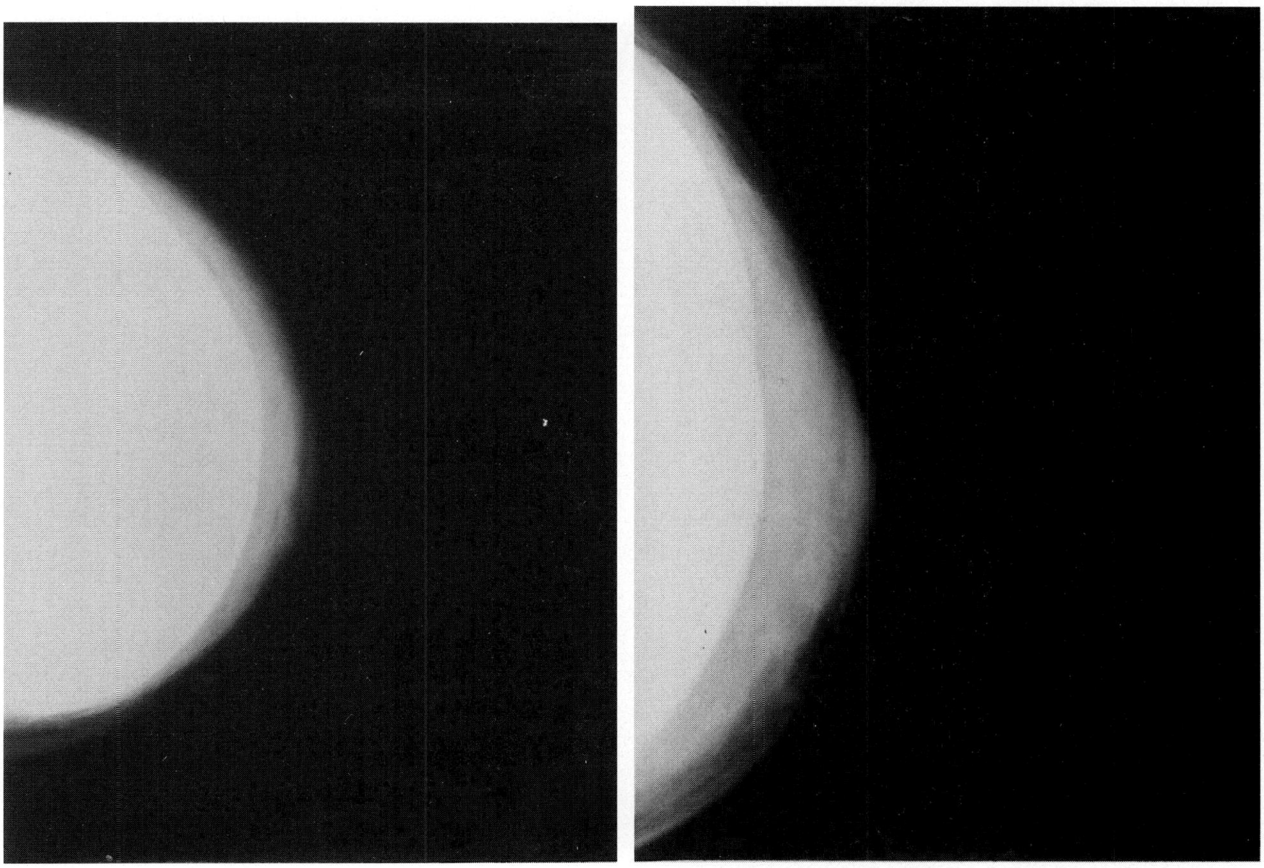

A B

Figure 6–28. Poor implant displacement views with contracture. (**A**) Standard CC image shows implant and dense tissue. (**B**) Eklund view shows little improvement in visualizing anterior tissue. Patient has significant clinical contracture, which limits mobility for this image.

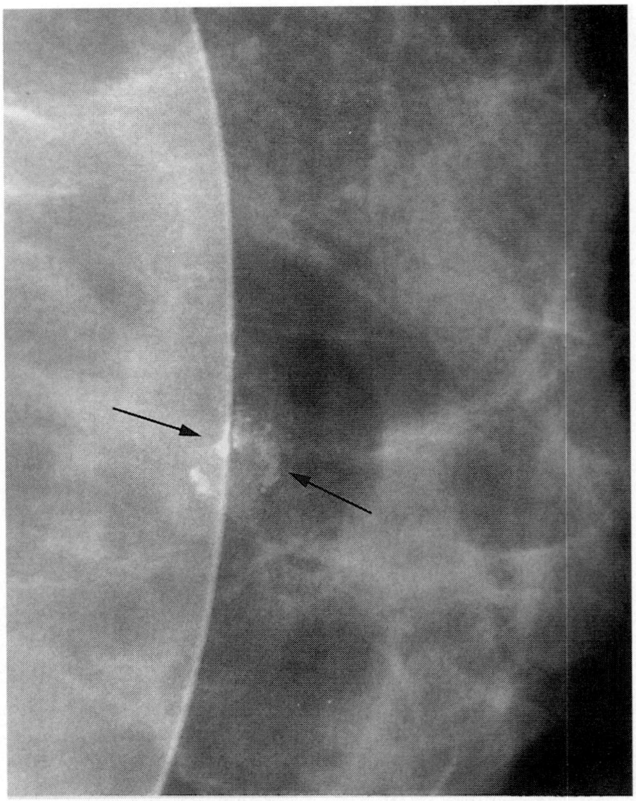

Figure 6–29. Closeup of push-back view showing capsular Ca^{2+} (arrows) in this patient with a saline implant.

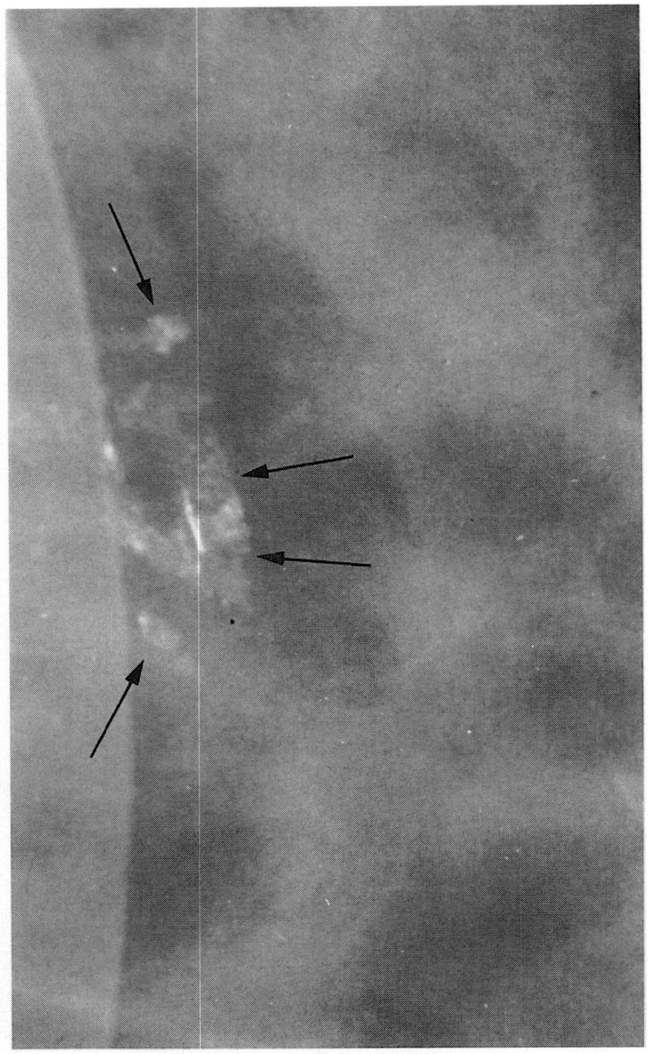

Figure 6–30. Capsular calcifications (arrows).

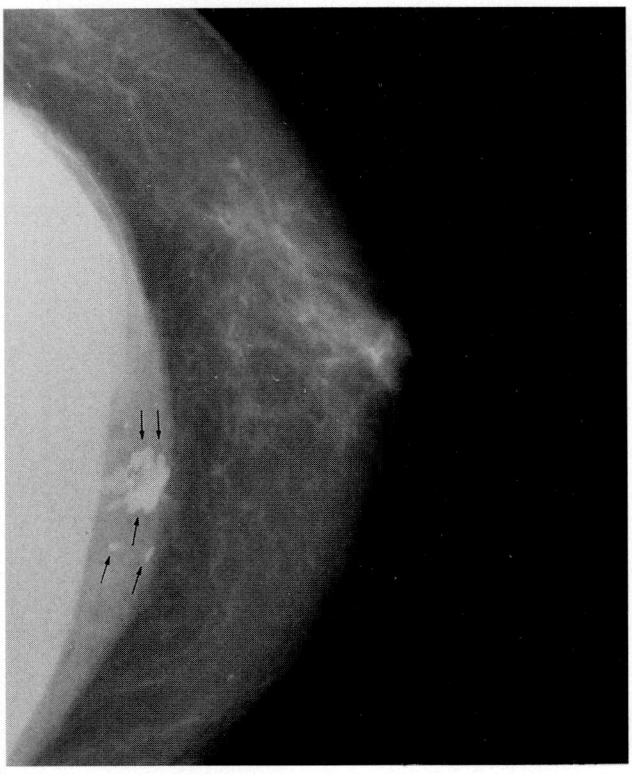

Figure 6–31. Capsular calcifications (arrows) in a patient with a subpectoral, double-lumen implant.

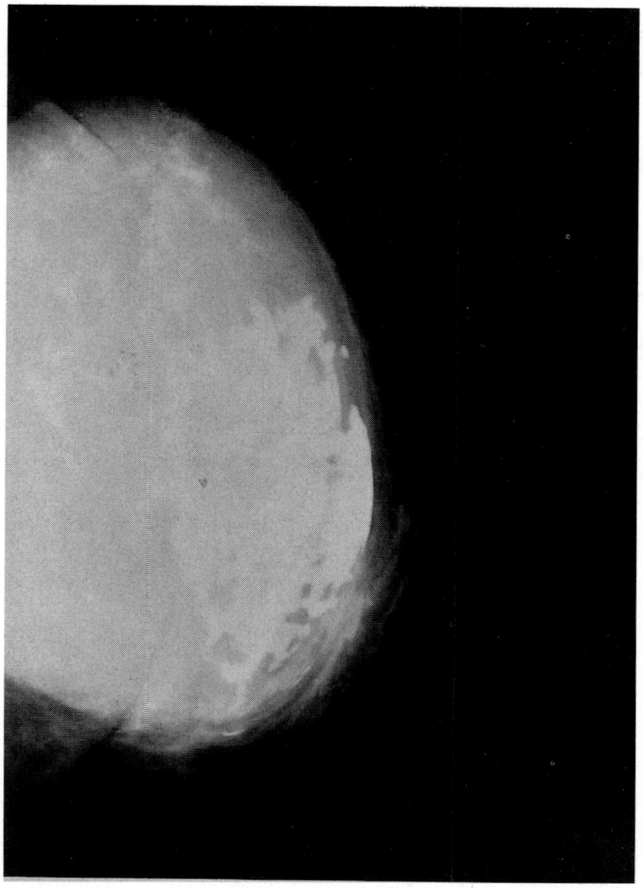

Figure 6–32. Extensive capsular calcification in a patient with a nonsilicone implant placed prior to 1960.

plantation, which provides surgical proof of any imaging modality's findings, was until just recently reserved for significant clinical dysfunction. It is expected that mammography would be much more useful in detecting extracapsular leakage than one contained within the fibrous capsule. Intracapsular rupture may be mammographically inapparent and will be a significant source of false-negatives for rupture using this imaging method. In animal models mammography has been shown to be much less accurate than magnetic resonance imaging (MRI) or computed tomography (CT) (although no implant displacement views were used, which are routine in human patients).[16] In vivo studies of human subjects show the sensitivity of mammography for rupture varies widely (11–81%). Studies that include a high percentage of encapsulated leaks find sensitivity to be low[17]; when more extracapsular ruptures are represented, sensitivity for mammography improves.[18] Specificity for mammography has been good (89–100%).

Mammography is clearly limited in evaluating the posterior wall of the implant. Anterior herniations, bulges, and capsule thickenings and calcifications are readily apparent. Leaks anteriorly, superiorly, and inferiorly can be detected. The routine use of Eklund views can be expected to improve the radiographic demonstration of such abnormalities.

Overall, mammography can be highly informative for the augmented patient. It is an excellent first study for implant evaluation. Radiography does have its limitations, however, and often additional imaging will be needed to evaluate suspected abnormalities. Ultrasound and MRI are the most useful adjunctive imaging methods and are discussed fully in Chapters 7 and 9.

REFERENCES

1. Domanskis EJ, Owsley JQ. Histological investigation of the etiology of capsule contracture following augmentation mammoplasty. *Plast Reconstr Surg.* 1976;58(6):689–693.
2. Coleman DJ, Foo ITH, Sharpe DT. Textured or smooth implants for breast augmentation? A prospective controlled trial. *Br J Plast Surg.* 1991;44:444–448.
3. Capozzi A, Pennisi VR. Clinical experience with polyurethane-covered gel-filled mammary prostheses. *Plast Reconstr Surg.* 1981;68(4):512–518.
4. Melmed EP. Polyurethane implants: a 6-year review of 416 patients. *Plast Reconstr Surg.* 1988;82(2):285–290.
5. Cocke WM, Leathers HK, Lynch JB. Foreign body reactions to polyurethane covers of some breast prostheses. *Plast Reconstr Surg.* 1975;56(5):527–530.
6. Capozzi A. Long-term complications of polyurethane-covered breast implants. *Plast Reconstr Surg.* 1991;88(3):458–461.
7. Berrino P, Galli A, Rainero ML, et al. Long-lasting complications with the use of polyurethane-covered breast implants. *Br J Plast Surg.* 1986;39:549–553.
8. Important information on breast implants. FDA Backgrounder September 1991;BG91-62.
9. FDA cautions women not to remove polyurethane-coated breast implants. *ACR Bull.* 1991;47(9):16.
10. Bostwick J III. *Plastic and Reconstructive Breast Surgery,* vol. 1. St. Louis: Quality Medical Publishing; 1990:181.
11. Steinbach BG, Hardt NS, Abbitt PL. Mammography: breast implants—types, complications, and adjacent breast pathology. *Curr Probl Diagn Radiol.* 1993; 41–86.
12. Ganott MA, Harris KM, Ilkhanipour ZS, et al. Augmentation mammoplasty: normal and abnormal findings with mammography and ultrasound. *Radiographics.* 1992;12:281–295.
13. Destouet JM, Monsees BS, Oser RF, et al. Screening mammography in 350 women with breast implants: prevalence and findings of implant complications. *AJR.* 1992;159:973–978.
14. Berger K, Bostwick J III. *A Woman's Decision. Breast Care Treatment, and Reconstruction,* 2nd ed. St. Louis: Quality Medical Publishing; 1994:166–167.
15. Ahn CY, DeBruhl ND, Gorczyca DP, et al. Silicone implant rupture diagnosis using computed tomography: a case report and experience with 22 surgically removed implants. *Ann Plast Surg.* 1994;33(6):624–628.
16. Gorczyca DP, DeBruhl ND, Ahn CY, et al. Silicone breast implant ruptures in an animal model: comparison of mammography, MR imaging, US, and CT. *Radiology.* 1994;190:227–232.
17. Ahn CY, DeBruhl ND, Gorczyca DP, et al. Comparative silicone breast implant evaluation using mammography, sonography, and magnetic resonance imaging: experience with 59 implants. *Plast Reconstr Surg.* 1994;94(5):620–627.
18. Monticciolo DL, Nelson RC, Dixon WT, et al. MR detection of leakage from silicone breast implants: value of a silicone-selective pulse sequence. *AJR.* 1994;163:51–56.

7

Ultrasonographic Evaluation of the Failing Implant

KATHLEEN M. HARRIS

Widely publicized concerns about breast implants include imaging limitations of possible obscuration of breast cancers due to the radiopacity of the implants and compaction of the parenchyma[1–7] as well as concerns over the safety of the silicone polymer itself.[8–14] Many of the concerns related to health issues are distinct from "implant failure," which is defined as loss of integrity of the elastomer shell. Nevertheless, the media attention to breast implant litigation has led physicians to refer their patients for breast imaging evaluation for possible implant rupture or because of breast symptoms such as mass, pain, or autoimmune disease.

Reliable noninvasive and inexpensive imaging techniques are required to evaluate patients who have had implants placed for augmentation or reconstruction or who have undergone direct silicone injections into their breasts. With mammography, an average of 25% of the parenchyma can be obscured by the implant[15] even with the use of implant displacement views.[16] Breast ultrasound, along with physical examination and mammography, has been shown to be valuable in assessing symptomatic breast disease in patients without implants.[17–20] For patients with implants, ultrasound can also help in evaluating the implant as a possible source of the symptoms.[21–23] Ultrasound is a valuable adjunct and can be performed by the radiologist at the same time as the mammogram with same-day differentiation of significant breast lesions from implant complications. Ultrasound can also better assess subtle implant ruptures compared with mammography or clinical examination.[24–26] Although magnetic resonance (MR) imaging is more sensitive than ultrasound in detecting intracapsular leaks,[27–29] MR imaging requires a separate appointment, is more costly, and may not be available in every community.

The true rate of implant failure is unknown. Published prevalence rates vary, depending on the method of detection employed. Destouet et al[30] reported a 5% failure rate among asymptomatic women using mammography, whereas Harris et al[25] reported a 6.5% prevalence of implant rupture noted during diagnostic imaging by mammography and ultrasound. Berg et al[28] reported a 35% implant failure rate using mammography and MR imaging. Much higher levels of implant rupture have been detected at the time of surgical explantation, with deCamera et al[31] finding 50% and Robinson et al[32] reporting 71.3% of the elastomer shells of implants disrupted. Petro et al[33] found ruptures in 7% of surgically removed implants, and Peters et al[34] found ruptures in 33% of symptomatic patients. With the increasing use of ultrasound and MR imaging, and occasionally computed tomography (CT), more subtle intracapsular leaks are being detected. An intracapsular leak is one in which the elastomer shell has failed but the surrounding fibrous capsule formed by the patient's tissues remains intact.

Although published reports show that ultrasound evaluation is useful, the number of patients reported in the radiology literature with ultrasound-detected ruptures is relatively small compared with the 1 to 2 million women with implants in the United States.[25,28,35–41] Additional reports in the plastic surgery literature of ultrasound detection of implant ruptures corroborate the findings reported in the radiology literature.[24,29,33,42] What is needed is a larger series to better determine the significance of the sonographic signs of implant failure.

The published data suggest the value of ultrasound in detection of implant failure. Additionally, ultrasound is readily available, cost effective, and can image not only the breast and implant but also the adjacent tissues where free silicone can migrate. Knowledge of the various sonographic appearances of intact implants and complications that may occur with implants will facilitate differentiation of intrinsic breast disease from implant failure.

TECHNIQUE OF PERFORMING ULTRASOUND IN IMPLANT PATIENTS

The performance of breast ultrasound in implant patients requires no special equipment. The same 7.5- to 10-MHz linear array handheld transducers that are used for imaging the breast parenchyma can also effectively image the implant and the axilla. In women with implants, the breasts tend to be more rounded, firm, and protuberant in the supine position than are the breasts of women without implants. A standoff pad (3M Company, Kitecko, St. Paul, MN) placed between the transducer and the skin enables imaging of the entire breast from the skin to the implant as well as the implant itself. This is especially important in women with minimal breast tissue overlying their implants and in women who have undergone reconstruction following mastectomy.

The anterior and lateral aspects of breast implants are easily visualized with the 7.5- to 10-MHz transducers. The posterior wall of the implant may be difficult to visualize in larger-breasted women with larger-sized implants because of the superficial focal plane of the 7.5- to 10-MHz transducers and because of artifactual posterior displacement of the silicone implant due to the slower speed of sound in silicone.[25,38] If posterior implant rupture is suspected in a larger-breasted woman, a 5-MHz transducer can be used for deeper imaging. Although 5-MHz transducers would be valuable for penetration of larger implants placed in larger breasts, there is poor anterior resolution with the 5-MHz transducers.[43] Most patients with augmentation mammoplasty are small breasted and can be imaged adequately with the 7.5-MHz transducer.[44]

Ideally, the radiologist who interprets the mammogram will also be the one who performs the ultrasound examination for correlation with mammographic and clinical findings. Because the implant itself can account for a palpable "mass,"[21,23,25] real-time ultrasound enables one to place a finger over the palpable area while visualizing whether this corresponds to an intrinsic breast lesion or to a palpable portion of the implant such as a wrinkle, bulge, or hernia, or whether it represents extruded silicone. This holds true for palpable masses in the breast as well as for sites adjacent to the breast that can be easily imaged with the real-time handheld transducer such as axillary or infraclavicular areas or superficial subcutaneous areas of the thoracic or abdominal walls.

With ultrasound examination, the entire breast overlying the implant, the implant itself, and areas adjacent to the breast can be imaged. Because silicone can enter the lymphatic system and be deposited in the axillary or infraclavicular nodes or more remotely,[25,45] we routinely scan the entire breast parenchyma, the implant, and the axillary and infraclavicular areas. The entire circumference of the implant is systematically covered, ensuring imaging of all areas, especially along the periphery of the implant where small leaks are commonly detected.

In women with capsular contracture, the breast may be quite firm and noncompliant because of the thick constricting fibrous capsule with its consequent rounding of the implant and a subsequent increase in the anterior-posterior (AP) diameter of the implant. Capsular contracture, therefore, can pose a special technical problem because it may be difficult to maintain good contact of the transducer with the rounded, firm breast. The standoff device can be used as a softer interface between the transducer and the breast, allowing better contact. By rotating the transducer to conform to the contour of the breast, and by rotating the patient medially and laterally, the entire breast can be imaged. This may be especially difficult along the periphery of the implant, particularly in the region of the inframammary fold because of the noncompliant breast.

Whenever an implant leak is suspected sonographically but cannot be imaged mammographically, a metal marker can be placed on the skin over the sonographic area of suspected extruded free silicone, and additional special mammographic views can be obtained in an effort to identify the silicone leak mammographically.

THE INTACT IMPLANT

Every implant, whether silicone or saline, is surrounded by a fibrous capsule that is formed as a response to the prosthesis and that in effect walls off the implant from the surrounding tissues.[46–49]

The envelope or elastomer shell that composes the outer layer of all implants (whether silicone or saline) consists of a semipermeable membrane of variable thickness constructed of more highly cross-linked polymer chains of polydimethylsiloxane with cross-linkages of methyl groups to create an elastic solid.[50-51] In saline-implant patients, saline is inserted within the envelope through a valve or tubing. In silicone implants, silicone gel, consisting of variably viscous molecules of less highly cross-linked polymer chains of polydimethylsiloxane, is inserted and sealed within the envelope. Double-lumen implants consist of an outer saline implant and inner silicone implant, and reverse double-lumen implants consist of an outer silicone and an inner saline implant. The inner and outer aspects of the double-lumen implants may be detected mammographically but are only rarely detected sonographically.[28] Occasionally, two implants will be placed on top of each other ("stacked" implants) to obtain larger breast size. Sonographically these two implants have an echogenic line running horizontally where the anterior implant rests on the posterior implant.

The outer surface of the implant envelope can be smooth (shiny) or rough (dull), almost most implants, whether silicone or saline, have a smooth, shiny surface. Rough-surfaced envelopes have been manufactured either by applying an outer coating of polyurethane foam or by creating a permanent textured pattern within the outer surface of the envelope. Polyurethane-coated implants and textured envelopes increase the overall surface area of the implant[52] and thus decrease the degree of formation of tight fibrous capsules that are associated with capsular contracture by changing the alignment of the fibroblasts and myofibroblasts. The polyurethane applied to the surface of the implant interdigitates with the adjacent tissues of the breast and usually cannot be imaged by either mammography or sonography. Polyurethane-coated implants are no longer manufactured because the polyurethane to some extent changes chemically into toluene diamine (TDA), which is a potentially carcinogenic substance.[53]

Sonographic Appearance of the Intact Implant

The sonographic appearance of implants was first described in 1983 by Cole-Beuglet et al.[54] Sonographically, a bright echogenic line or interface surrounds all implants, whether they are of the silicone or saline variety, or whether they are placed in the prepectoral or retropectoral positions (Fig. 7–1). This echogenic interface results from the acoustic differences between silicone and the adjacent tissues as well as from the large reflective surface of the implant, resulting in a strong echogenic signal along the entire implant periphery (Fig. 7–1A). It is unknown whether the fibrous capsule contributes to the echogenic interface between the implant and the adjacent tissues. The mammographically visible fibrous capsule is normally quite thin, measuring approximately 1 mm in thickness.[23]

Sonographically, the echogenic interface is imaged along the entire implant surface, especially anteriorly and as the implant curves posteriorly. The posterior echogenic interface (anterior to the pectoral muscle in prepectoral implants or anterior to the ribs and intercostal muscles in retropectoral implants) may be visible with smaller-volume implants placed in smaller breasts (Fig. 7–1B), but the posterior implant border may be difficult or impossible to visualize in larger-volume implants placed in larger breasts.[25,54,55] The more superficial focus of the 7.5- to 10-MHz transducers and the slower speed of sound through silicone, which displaces the far wall of the implant posteriorly, account for this difficulty. Because sound travels more slowly in silicone[25,38,56] compared with the speed at which sound travels in breast tissue, and because all ultrasound equipment assumes that the tissues have the same speed of sound, the posterior aspects of all silicone implants are artificially displaced deeper than their actual position and appear to have an increased AP diameter of 1.5 times their real size[25] (Fig. 7–1A,C,D). This phenomenon was first described by Cole-Beuglet et al[54] in 1983 and subsequently reported by Rosculet et al[38] in 1992 and by Harris et al[25] in 1993. Thus, ultrasound is limited in its ability to detect free silicone that may be situated deep to the posterior wall of larger volume implants within larger breasts. Film screen mammography also does not visualize the posterior wall of the implant. However, the posterior implant wall can be seen[57-59] with xeroradiograph images, or with special high-kVp mammograms that included the ribs[2] or with MR[2,59] or CT imaging.

Textured implants have a permanent, repetitive pattern of small grooves that can be imaged on overpenetrated mammographic views (Fig. 7–1E). Sonographically, textured implants create a multilayered echogenic interface anteriorly, usually consisting of three closely adjacent horizontal parallel lines (Fig. 7–1F). These are distinguishable from the single echogenic line that is associated with smooth-surfaced implants (Fig. 7–1B). Sonography may incidentally detect small fluid collections adjacent to implants, especially those with polyurethane coating.[60] These areas of fluid are not an indication of implant failure.

Sonographically, the internal aspects of both silicone and saline implants are anechoic compared with breast tissue (Fig. 7–1B). There are usually reverberation echoes projected within the anterior aspect of all implants (Fig. 7–1C,D). These normal reverberations are always parallel to the anterior echogenic interface and run horizontally, overlying variable amounts of the anterior aspect of the implant. Saline implants contain valves used for inflation that occasionally can be imaged sonographically as echogenic areas. Also, sometimes the tubing used to fill the saline implant can be seen as two echogenic parallel lines within a saline implant.[23]

Sonographic Appearance of Wrinkles, Folds, Bulges, and Hernias

Contour deformities of silicone and saline implants are most often not associated with implant failure, and are commonly seen as undulations of the implant surface by mammography or sonography (Fig. 7–2). *Wrinkles* or *folds* (sometimes referred to as membranes)[39] are common, as the soft pliable implant conforms to the confines of the surrounding fibrous capsule. These have been reported in over half the implants (silicone or saline) studied by Ganott et al[23] and Shestak et al[21] (Fig. 7–2B,C). Sonographically detected echogenic bands associated with wrinkles or folds extend from the periphery of the implant inward and can be seen as somewhat linear echogenic areas that change shape on orthogonal views, ie, narrower in the transverse and wider in the sagittal planes, or vice versa (Fig. 7–2D–F). Wrinkles and folds are not a sign of implant failure, but their sonographic appearance may be difficult to distinguish from the internal echoes

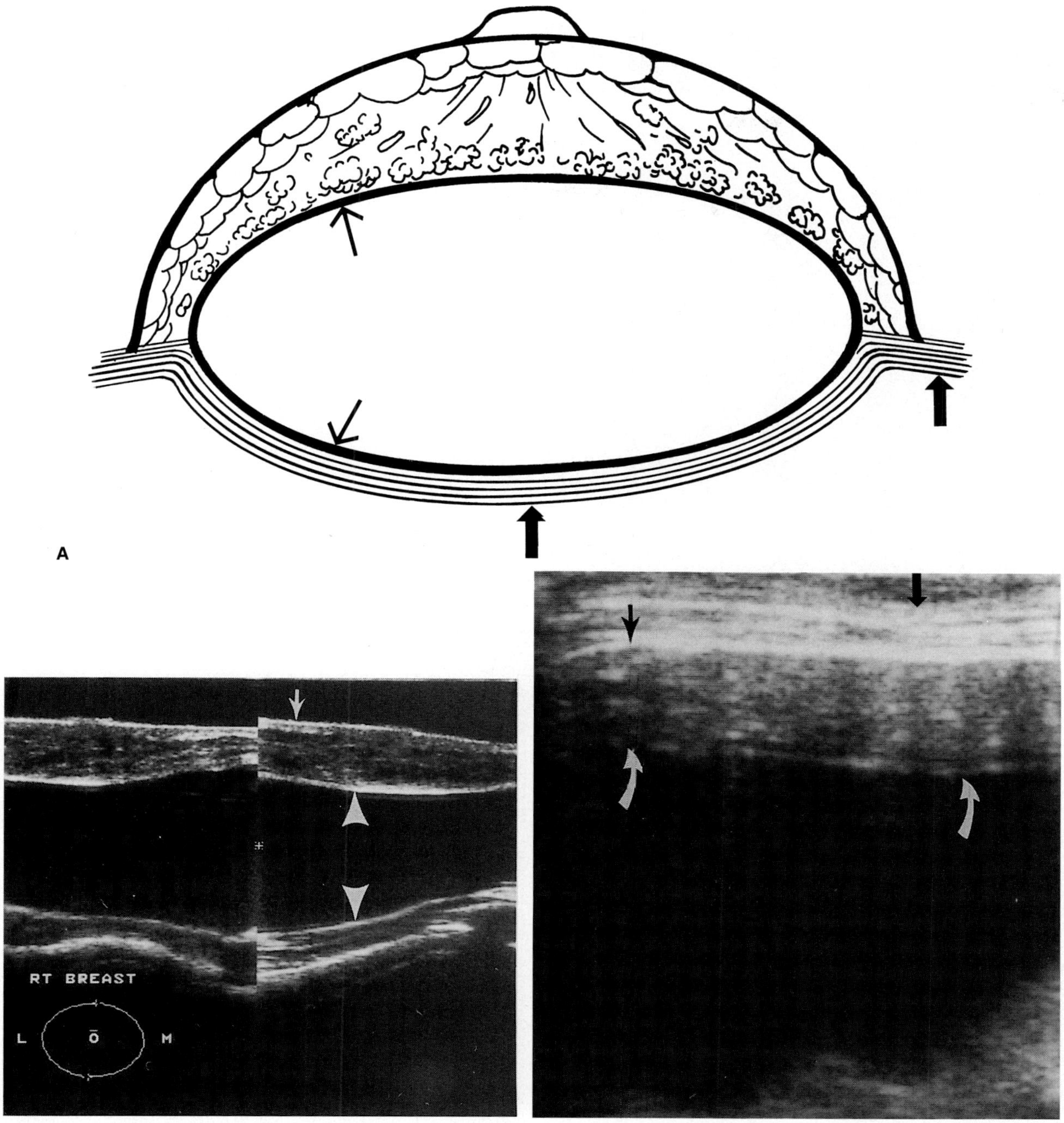

A B C

Figure 7–1. (**A**) The sonographic appearance of an intact implant, whether silicone or saline filled, consists of a thin echogenic line at the implant-tissue interface (thin arrows) that surrounds the entire implant. In silicone gel–filled implants, artifactual posterior displacement, due to the slower speed of sound in silicone, results in the implant appearing to be deeper than its actual location (thick arrows). (**B**) The interior of the intact implant (whether silicone or saline) is sonographically anechoic. In the side-by-side transverse images, note the skin line (arrow), and the underlying breast tissue. The breast-implant interface appears as an echogenic line (arrowheads) in this smooth surfaced implant. (**C**) In this silicone implant, reverberation echoes (white arrows) are seen in the anterior aspect of the implant just beneath the anterior echogenic interface (thin black arrow). Note the pectoral muscle (thick black arrow) anteriorly in this retropectoral implant. The posterior implant wall is poorly seen. *(continued)*

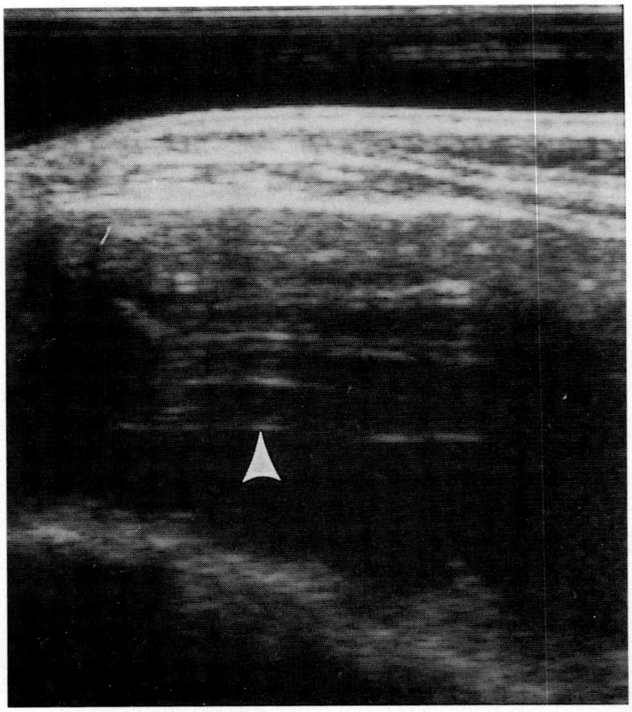

D

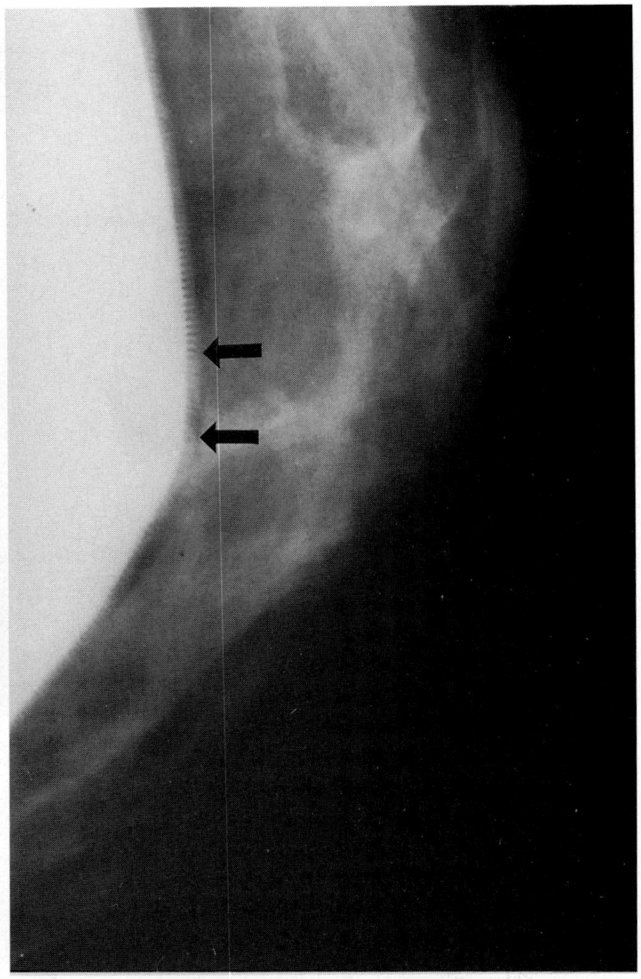

E

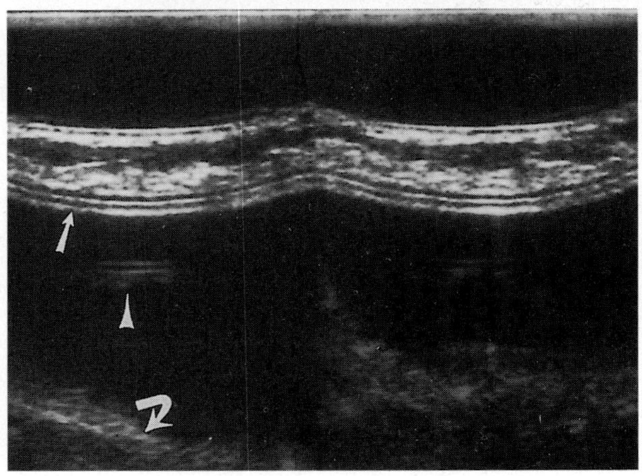

F

7–1. ***(Continued)*** (**D**) In the same patient at the same time with use of a standoff pad (Kitecko 3M Co.), the reverberation echoes appear to extend deeper into the implant (arrowhead). These added reverberation echoes are produced by the standoff pad and moved "up and down" with greater or lesser pressure applied to the handheld transducer overlying the standoff pad. This maneuver in real time helps to differentiate reverberation echoes caused by the standoff pad from the horizontal lines of a collapsed implant envelope, which would maintain a fixed position within the implant. (**E**) Textured implants (dull or rough surfaced elastomer shells) have a permanent repetitive pattern incorporated into the envelope. The striated pattern (arrows) can be seen with overpenetrated mammographic views on this closeup image of the implant. Compare with the smooth surfaced implant in Figure 7–2B. (**F**) Sonographically (side-by-side transverse images), the anterior echogenic interface of this textured implant appears as a triple line (straight arrow) sonographically compared to the single echogenic line of smooth surfaced implants (**B**). There are faint reverberation echoes associated with the anterior interface that repeat the triple lines (arrowhead). The posterior echogenic line is poorly resolved because of decreased resolution with the 7.5-MHz probe at this greater depth (curved arrow).

associated with implant rupture, accounting for some false-positive reports.[28,36,39]

A *bulge* occurs when there is an outpouching of both the intact implant and the overlying intact fibrous capsule. A *hernia* occurs when there is disruption of the fibrous capsule, allowing herniation of the intact implant through a tear in the fibrous capsule. A new fibrous capsule may form to wall off the hernia. Sonographically a bulge or a hernia can have similar appearances. In both, the sonolucent internal silicone gel within silicone implants or the saline within saline implants is continuous with the bulge or hernia, and there is no line of demarcation or area of increased echo-

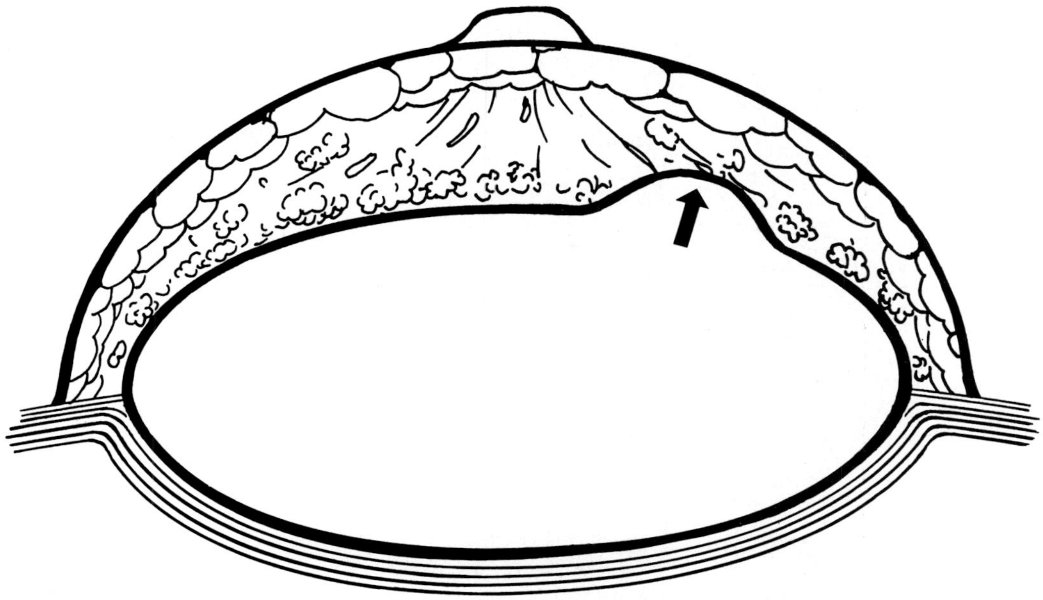

A

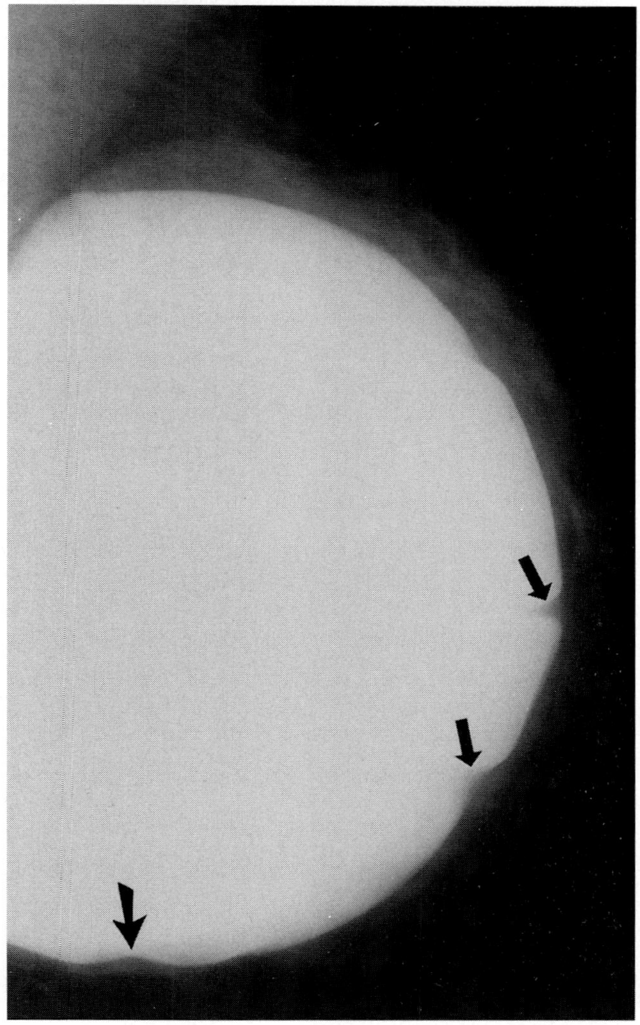

B

Figure 7–2. (**A**) Wrinkles, bulges or hernias are commonly seen, and are not a sign of implant rupture. The outpouching (arrow) of a bulge, hernia, or wrinkle maintains the thin echogenic interface between the implant and overlying tissues. The anechoic silicone or saline interior is contiguous with the contour deformity. (**B**) Wrinkles are more commonly seen in saline implants but occasionally can be seen in silicone implants, especially with more penetrated views. Wrinkles (arrows) are seen anteriorly and inferiorly within this prepectoral silicone implant on the mediolateral oblique view. This is a smooth surfaced implant. *(continued)*

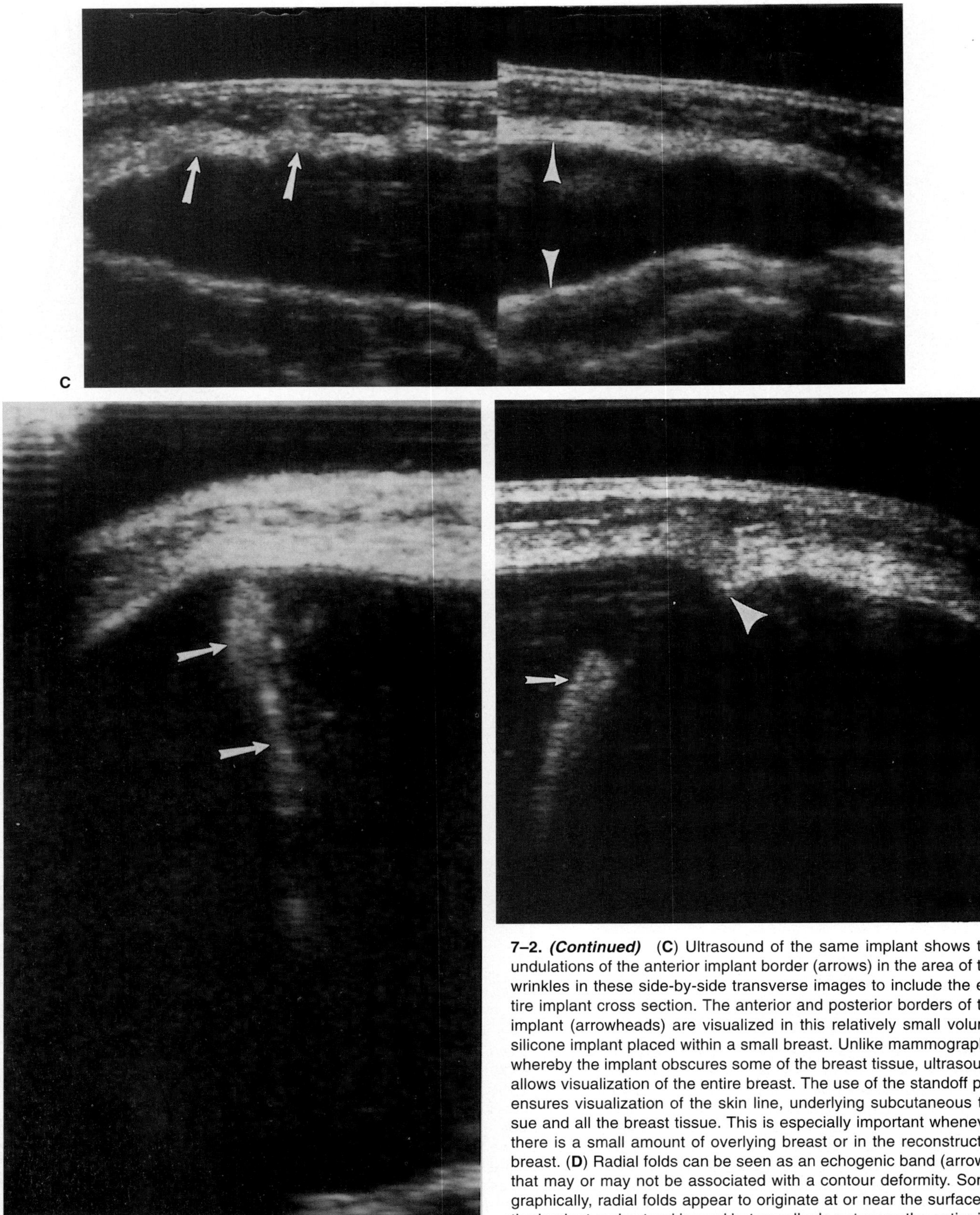

7–2. *(Continued)* (**C**) Ultrasound of the same implant shows the undulations of the anterior implant border (arrows) in the area of the wrinkles in these side-by-side transverse images to include the entire implant cross section. The anterior and posterior borders of the implant (arrowheads) are visualized in this relatively small volume silicone implant placed within a small breast. Unlike mammography, whereby the implant obscures some of the breast tissue, ultrasound allows visualization of the entire breast. The use of the standoff pad ensures visualization of the skin line, underlying subcutaneous tissue and all the breast tissue. This is especially important whenever there is a small amount of overlying breast or in the reconstructed breast. (**D**) Radial folds can be seen as an echogenic band (arrows) that may or may not be associated with a contour deformity. Sonographically, radial folds appear to originate at or near the surface of the implant and extend inward but usually do not cross the entire implant. (**E**) In the transverse projection, an indentation (arrowhead) of the anterior surface of the implant is associated with the echogenic band of a radial fold (arrow). *(continued)*

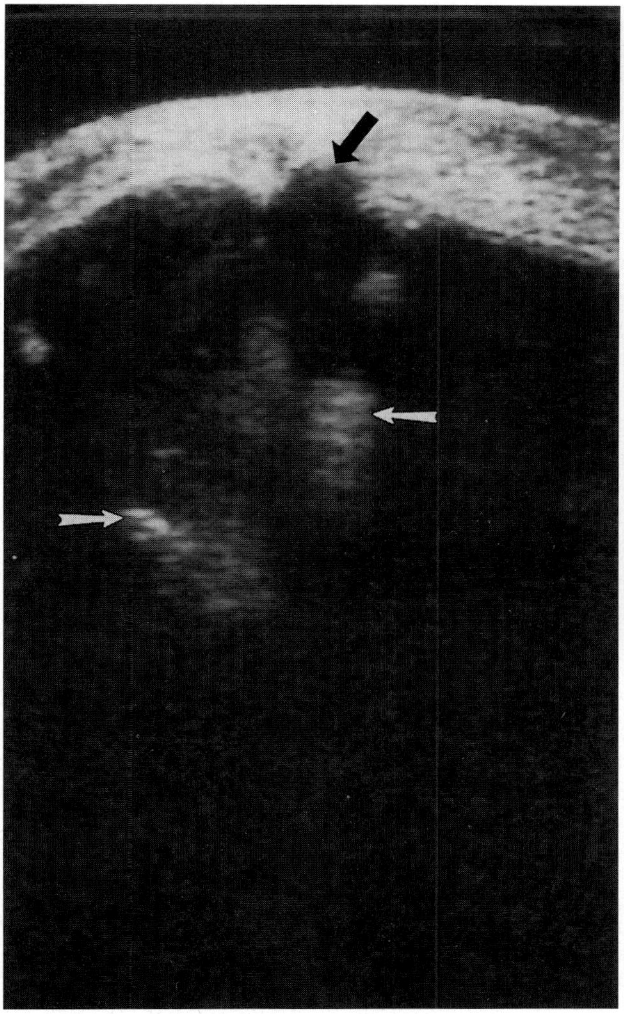

F

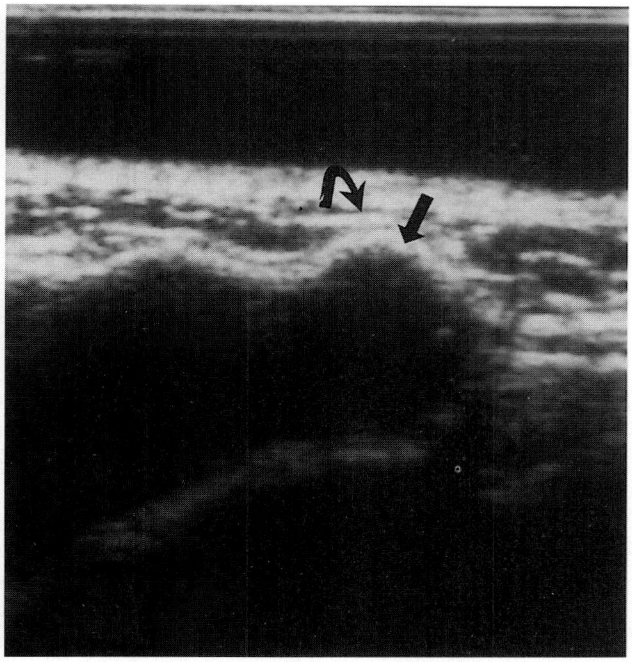

G

7–2. ***(Continued)*** (**F**) In the sagittal view of the same area, the contour deformity appears as a bulge (black arrow) and the echogenic radial fold appears wider (white arrows). Radial folds will often change in configuration between transverse and sagittal planes. In this patient with a clinical capsular contracture, ultrasound was unable to visualize the posterior implant wall because of rounding of the implant and an increased AP diameter, placing the posterior wall deeper than the penetration of the 7.5-MHz ultrasound beam. The artifactual displacement of silicone posteriorly due to the slower speed of sound in silicone also contributes to the inability to image the posterior implant wall. (**G**) The implant bulge (straight arrow), just below the skin surface (curved arrow), presented as a palpable "mass." Real-time ultrasound confirmed the implant bulge as the source of the physical finding. The bulge was soft and easily compressed with the examining finger.

genicity at the site of origin of the bulge or hernia (Fig. 7–2G). It is important to recognize that bulges or hernias are not ruptures. The contour deformities of bulges or hernias may be mammographically indistinguishable from a confined leak. Thus, false-positive diagnoses based on mammography have been reported in these cases.[61] Therefore, it is important to evaluate contour deformities sonographically to avoid overcalling these findings. A hernia may continue to enlarge and may eventually result in a rupture over time. The rupture most often occurs at the apex of the hernia and can be detected sonographically as the characteristic echogenic pattern overlying the hernia.[25] Ultrasound enables differentiation of a bulge or hernia from a rupture. A confident diagnosis of a bulge or hernia can allay patient anxiety and avoid unnecessary referral to the plastic surgeon.

■ COMPLICATIONS OF THE FIBROUS CAPSULE

Capsular Calcifications and Capsular Contracture

Two complications that involve the fibrous capsule and are unrelated to the implant itself are capsular calcification and capsular contracture. These complications are not usually diagnosed with ultrasound. Capsular calcifications, commonly associated with aging implants, are visible on overpenetrated mammographic views but are not usually detectable sonographically. Theoretically, a very thick calcific plaque within the capsule could result in shadowing, similar to any large calcific deposit. The calcific plaques, however, are usually thin and flat and are not associated with acoustic shadowing.

A diagnosis of capsular contracture is based on clinical findings of a hard, painful, protuberant, incompressible breast. Occasionally, mammography will show a thickened fibrous capsule associated with rounding of the implant in patients who have a clinical diagnosis of capsular contracture.[23] Implants (silicone or saline) are normally oval, with the flatter surface parallel to the chest wall. A tight fibrous capsule will cause rounding of the implant as the fibrous capsule squeezes the implant into a smaller space. Subsequent increase in the AP diameter of the implant can be detected clinically as a firm, protuberant breast, mammographically as a rounded implant, and sonographically as an increased AP diameter. Sonographically, the thickened fibrous capsule cannot be imaged but the rounded, firm noncompliant implant with an increased AP diameter can be technically challenging (see discussion of technique, above).

Implant Failure

Implant failure has been defined in many ways ranging from frank disruption or disintegration of the implant envelope with significant amounts of silicone gel extruded into the breast or with the gel remaining within the confines of the fibrous capsule. Other definitions include excessive amounts of "gel bleed" without an associated small tear of the envelope. Collections of silicone gel without a rupture have been variously referred to in the literature as "excessive gel bleed," "thick gel bleed," "gel leakage," and "profound gel bleed."[24,25,28,32,34,62–64] When tears occur in the elastomer shell, there can be a range of findings from no collapse of the envelope with small tears to envelope collapse with large tears. With associated tears in the fibrous capsule, findings can range from a confined leak to gross extrusion of silicone into the tissues. Subtle failure may be detected only at surgical explantation, when a sticky surface of the implant is found without a discernible tear or with a very small tear of the envelope. On the other hand, one can also find at surgery, gross tears or complete disintegration of the envelope resulting in free silicone gel contained within the fibrous capsule.

Gel Bleed

The less viscous and less highly cross-linked polymer chains of the silicone gel filling can readily pass through spaces between the more highly cross-linked polymer chains of the silicone elastomer envelope, resulting in the phenomenon of microscopic "gel bleed."[65] To a greater or lesser extent, gel bleed occurs through the intact elastomer shell (envelope) of all silicone gel–containing implants. The formation of the fibrous capsule that surrounds all implants may be in part a response to the gel bleed.[66] In the majority of cases the surrounding fibrous capsule confines the less viscous silicone gel polymers that have traversed the microscopic spaces of the elastomer shell. In some cases, however, microscopic droplets of silicone gel can gain access to the lymphatic system and be deposited in remote sites.[25] In such cases, free silicone can be identified outside the confines of the fibrous capsule, not secondary to an implant rupture, but due solely to excessive gel bleed. Small amounts of free silicone in axillary nodes resulting from gel bleed can be identified by ultrasound as a characteristic echogenic "snowstorm" pattern. This pattern is specific for small microglobules of silicone gel mixed within the tissues, whether these result from gel bleed or from implant failure. Although gel bleed is most often detected serendipitously by sonography in nodes of asymptomatic women, clinically evident silicone lymphadenopathy that resulted from excessive gel bleed alone (unassociated with implant rupture) has been reported.[25] Implant replacement may be indicated whenever excessive gel bleed becomes clinically symptomatic, as in the case of palpable axillary adenopathy. Thus, excessive gel bleed that results in a leak of silicone outside the confines of the fibrous capsule can be a form of implant failure.[32] With ultrasound, there are no criteria for identifying excessive gel bleed when it is unassociated with a rupture[28] and remains confined by the fibrous capsule. MR imaging, however, can depict "excessive" or "thick" gel bleed as the "noose" sign or "inverted teardrop" sign when it is the only finding.[28,67] There are conflicting opinions in the literature about whether asymptomatic excessive gel bleed as the only finding constitutes implant failure if it remains confined to the fibrous capsule. Gel bleed found serendipitously by MR imaging or as a thick sticky material overlying the implant at the time of surgical explantation is categorized as implant failure by Berg et al[28] and by Robinson et al[32] but not by Reynolds et al.[68] Microscopic amounts of gel bleed, which occurs in all silicone implants, is not a sign of implant failure and cannot be imaged by MR or by ultrasound.

■ SONOGRAPHIC SIGNS OF IMPLANT FAILURE

Various types of complications from implants have been described in this text and commentators have advocated both different terminologies as well as approaches to such complications.[69–81]

Although, as noted above, the number of published cases of sonographically detected implant ruptures is small,[25,28,35–41] the literature reports two major categories of sonographic features of implant rupture. The first category relates to echoes within the implant itself, such as horizontal or oblique lines, diffuse homogeneous echoes, or bizarre echo patterns. The second category of sonographic features relates to echoes outside the implant in the form of a characteristic echogenic "snowstorm." The same patient may have signs of both internal echoes associated with intracapsular rupture and the echogenic "snowstorm" pattern associated with extracapsular rupture.

Complicated Internal Echoes and Horizontal Lines

Diffuse or complicated echogenic patterns within the implant have been described as sonographic signs of implant failure (Fig. 7–3). Diffuse homogeneous *internal echoes* throughout the implant,[28,35,40] linear or curvilinear *horizontal lines* within the implant,[36,39,41] and *complicated bizarre echogenic patterns* extending across the entire implant[40,41] have been reported as signs of implant rupture that have been mainly associated with the intracapsular variety. In 1989 vanWingerden and vanStaden[41] first suggested that dense linear echoes representing invaginations of the prosthesis could be a sign of implant rupture. Also, a discrepancy in the AP diameters between the ruptured and intact implants

A

B

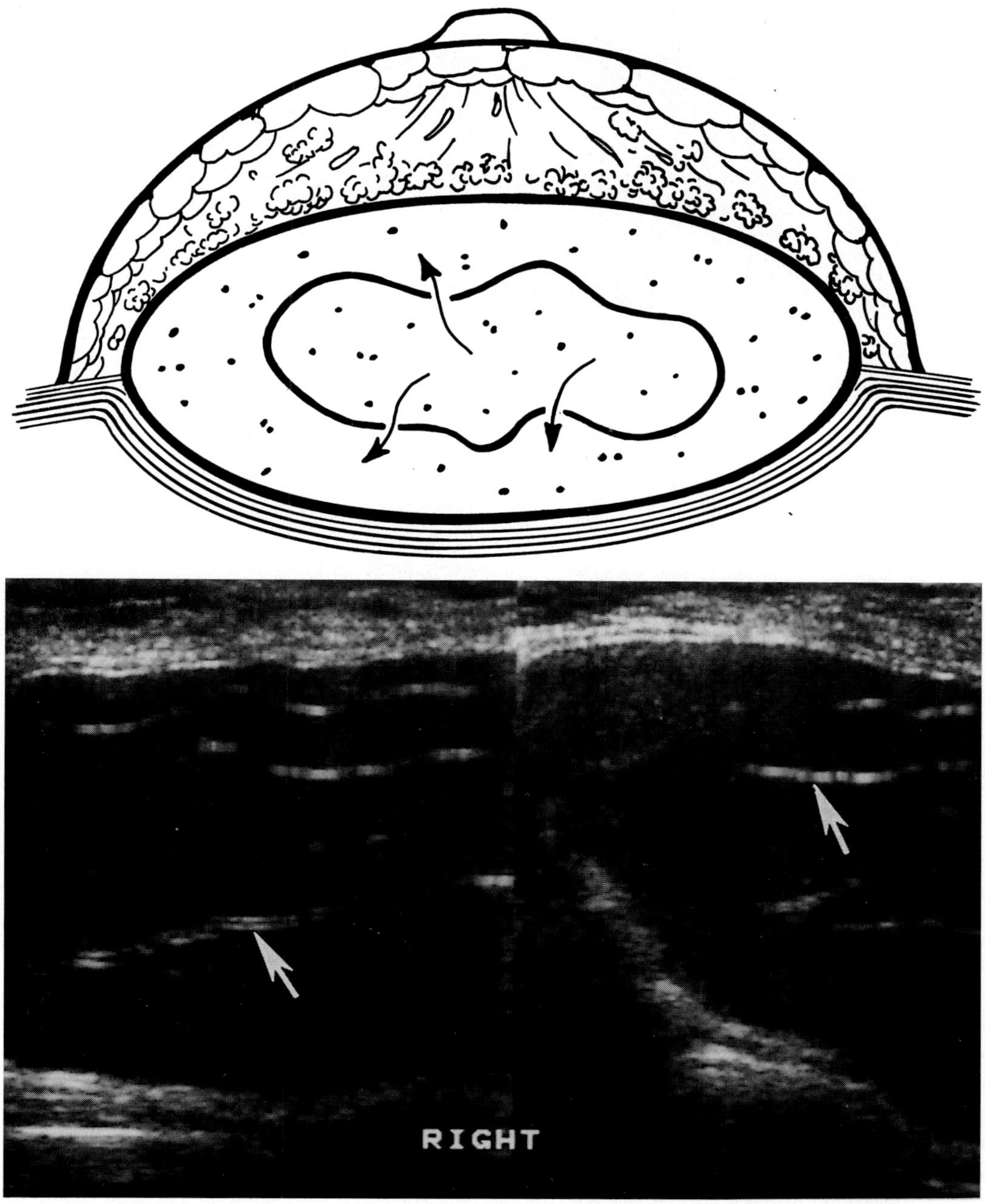

Figure 7–3. (**A**) An intracapsular leak occurs when silicone gel escapes through tears in the elastomer shell but is confined by the surrounding fibrous capsule. The elastomer shell (or envelope) can collapse inwardly as the gel escapes. Concomitantly, echoes appear within the silicone gel. (**B**) Sonographically, the collapsed shell can be seen as parallel horizontal or curvilinear lines (arrows) called "doublets" or the "stepladder" sign, which can occur throughout the implant. These must be distinguished from anterior reverberation echoes or radial folds. *(continued)*

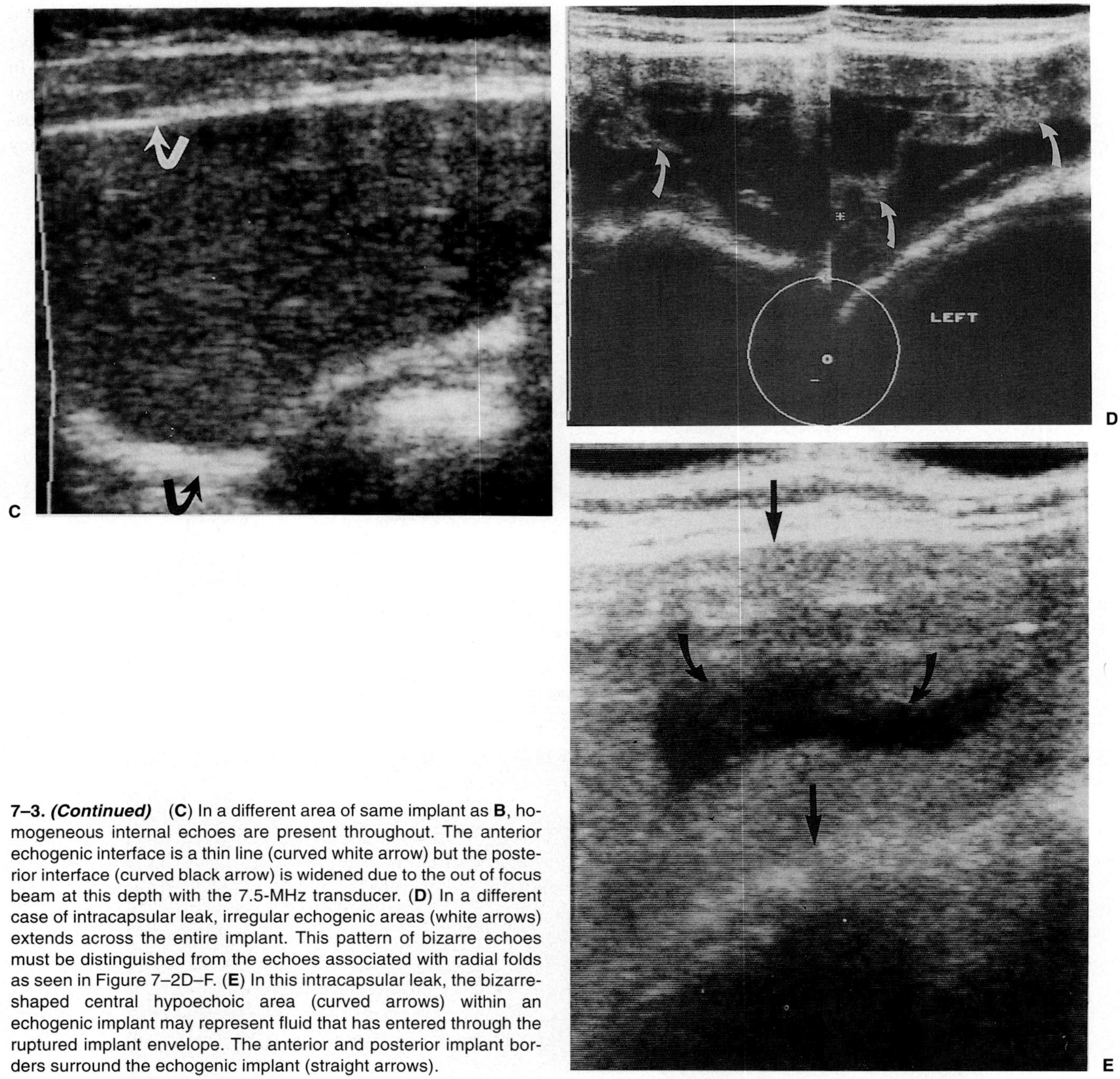

7–3. ***(Continued)*** (**C**) In a different area of same implant as **B**, homogeneous internal echoes are present throughout. The anterior echogenic interface is a thin line (curved white arrow) but the posterior interface (curved black arrow) is widened due to the out of focus beam at this depth with the 7.5-MHz transducer. (**D**) In a different case of intracapsular leak, irregular echogenic areas (white arrows) extends across the entire implant. This pattern of bizarre echoes must be distinguished from the echoes associated with radial folds as seen in Figure 7–2D–F. (**E**) In this intracapsular leak, the bizarre-shaped central hypoechoic area (curved arrows) within an echogenic implant may represent fluid that has entered through the ruptured implant envelope. The anterior and posterior implant borders surround the echogenic implant (straight arrows).

was noted with the ruptured implant having a relatively smaller AP diameter.[41] In 1991 Levine and Collins[40] described different patterns of implant ruptures; some ruptures produced echoes extending across the entire implant while others resulted in complicated echoes described as "echogenic confusion." In 1993 Berg et al[39] described internal echoes and parallel horizontal lines called "doublets" as well as complicated internal echoes. DeBruhl et al[36] described similar horizontal internal lines as the "stepladder" sign and postulated that these lines correspond to the collapsed silicone envelope surrounded by silicone gel that remains contained within the fibrous capsule. These straight or curvilinear horizontal lines (Fig. 7–3A,B) are analogous to the "linguine sign" detected during MR imaging by Gorczyca et al[27,82] in cases of implant rupture. Although the stepladder sign is highly specific for the collapse of the implant envelope, it was only found in less than half (43%) of surgically proven ruptures. Likewise, implants can rupture without collapse of the envelope so that absence of the stepladder sign does not exclude a rupture. In 1994 Caskey et al[35] found low-level homogeneous echoes (Fig. 7–3C) to be the most reliable sign of implant rupture but also noted horizontal parallel internal lines in some cases, with a combination of both internal echoes and horizontal lines being a reliable indicator of rupture. Berg et al[28] found the combination of the stepladder sign and/or moderate-to-marked low-level echoes within the gel to be present in only 26 of 40 ruptured implants with a sensitivity of 65% and specificity of 57%.

The majority of failed implant cases reported in the literature with the patterns of diffuse or complicated internal echoes and short segments of horizontal parallel lines have represented intracapsular ruptures at the time of surgical removal (explantation). Everson et al[37] reported 22 patients with ruptured implants with 21 of these being intracapsular and only 1 extracapsular. DeBruhl et al[36] reported 20 ruptured implants with 16 being intracapsular and 4 extracapsular. Caskey et al[35] reported 21 proven ruptures with 20 being intracapsular and 1 being extracapsular. Ahn et al[29] reported 21 ruptures with 18 intracapsular and 3 extracapsular. Berg et al[28] in 1995 reported on another 40 proven ruptures with 31 being intracapsular and 9 being extracapsular.

There are reports of false-positives and false-negatives associated with the above-described signs of intracapsular rupture. DeBruhl et al[36] found a sensitivity of 70% and a specificity of 92% based on 20 ruptured implants, with 16 being intracapsular. Of DeBruhl's 16 intracapsular ruptures, 3 were false positives and 6 were false-negatives. Everson et al[37] evaluated mammography, ultrasound, CT and MRI, based on 22 ruptured implants, 21 of which were intracapsular, and found mammography to be the least accurate, with sensitivity of 23% and a specificity of 98%; ultrasound had a sensitivity of 59% and a specificity of 79%; CT and MRI were both found to be more reliable with a sensitivity of 82% and specificity of 88% for CT, and for MRI a sensitivity of 95% and a specificity of 93%. Reynolds et al[68] reported sensitivities and specificities of the three imaging modalities in 13 patients respectively as follows: mammography 69% and 82%; ultrasound 54% and 64%; MR imaging 69% and 55%. Berg et al[28] reported greater accuracy for gross ruptures when MR imaging was used (sensitivity 98%) but less accuracy with leakage associated with excessive gel bleed where there was no evidence of rupture or with minimal rupture where the envelope did not collapse (sensitivity 50%). The overall specificity for an intact implant was 91%, suggesting that MR imaging is useful in excluding implant failure. With ultrasound, the sensitivity was 65%, which included ruptures as well as "excessive gel bleed" or "leakage" of small amounts of silicone without a rupture.[28] The specificity with ultrasound was 57% for predicting an intact implant.[28] In Berg et al's study, the "stepladder" sign as an isolated sonographic finding was present in only 4 of 28 cases of rupture and was present in 1 of 54 intact implants, for a sensitivity of 42% and specificity of 98%. Moderate-to-marked low-level echoes within the gel as the only finding were present in 21 of 40 ruptures and in 4 of 28 cases of minimal leakage, but were also seen in 10 of 54 intact implants, with a sensitivity of 52% and specificity of 81%.[28] Malone et al[83] have found low-level internal echoes to be common in intact polyurethane-coated implants. Therefore, as an isolated finding, low-level echoes may be an unreliable sign of implant failure.[28]

False-positive diagnoses of implant rupture occur when reverberation artifacts, folds, wrinkles, or proteinaceous fluid within the implant are mistaken for intracapsular leaks.[28,35,36,39] Reverberation artifacts are normally present in the anterior aspect of implants parallel to the anterior echogenic interface and are seen overlying approximately one fourth to one half of the volume of the implant, depending somewhat on the implant size (Fig. 7–1C,D) and whether or not a standoff pad is used.

Sonographically, wrinkles or folds create echoes in a "linear" pattern that originate from the surface of the implant, and radiate into the interior of the implant, but usually do not extend across the entire implant (Fig. 7–2D–F). It may be difficult in some cases, however, to distinguish the echoes associated with wrinkles or folds from the linear echoes of intracapsular leakage that usually extend across the entire implant (Fig. 7–3D).

False-positives are reported with MR imaging as well. Berg et al[28] reported three false-positives when folds were mistaken for minimal leakage. This was described as the "noose" sign or "teardrop" sign.

Proteinaceous materials or small fluid collections may traverse an intact implant envelope, probably through the same small openings that allow small silicone molecules to exit. These materials create a complex pattern of internal echoes that may be present in intact implants as well as those with disruption (Fig. 7–3E). In double-lumen implants, silicone from a ruptured inner silicone implant can mix with the saline of the outer implant and vice versa, causing a bizarre, complex pattern of internal echoes. A history of the type of implant will prevent the radiologist from mistaking implant failure for a type of single-lumen implant whereby saline has been injected into the silicone for size adjustment. In addition, a history could aid in differentiating silicone implants that have been injected with steroids or antibiotics at surgery to decrease inflammation in order to diminish capsular contracture formation.[28,64]

False-negative diagnoses of implant rupture occur with the loss of the integrity of the envelope, allowing small amounts of silicone gel to spread out evenly over the outer surface of the envelope without causing the envelope to collapse inwardly. Sonographically, false-negative intracapsular leaks appear similar to the normal anechoic intact implant.

Because of false-positives related to the difficulty of distinguishing the echogenic pattern of normal variations from intracapsular leaks, in our clinical practice we recommend MR imaging for confirmation whenever an intracapsular leak is suspected by ultrasound. Weizer et al,[42] however, found no added diagnostic benefit in using the combined results from MR imaging and ultrasound. No test or combination of tests is 100% accurate, however, and there have been false-positives and false-negatives reported with MRI as well.[27] Ahn et al[29] has reported that mammography is the least reliable test for intracapsular rupture, with MR imaging being the most reliable, followed by ultrasound. Weizer et al,[42] however, found no diagnostic advantage of MR imaging over ultrasound for correctly diagnosing implant rupture.

Echogenic "Snowstorm" Pattern and Associated Hypoechoic "Masses"

The characteristic echogenic "snowstorm" pattern of free silicone is a reliable sign of extracapsular leakage, whether it is confined to the area adjacent to the implant and sealed off by a new fibrous response as in a confined leak (Fig. 7–4) or whether it is located anywhere in the body (Fig. 7–5) as a result of implant rupture or from silicone injections into the breast. This sign is present only when silicone has mixed with the tissues and will not be present in isolated intracapsular leakage. By sonography, the characteristic echogenic pattern occurs when microglobules of silicone mix with the tissues of the body. This pattern was first described in 1980 by Barlow et al,[45] who reported an echogenic appearance of silicone granulomas in the inguinal area in a patient whose silicone had migrated following direct silicone injections into her breasts. Rosenbaum et al[84] in 1981, Cole-Beuglet et al[54] in 1983, and Herzog[73] in 1989 described a similar echogenic appearance with nonpenetration and scattering of sound associated with silicone granulomas in women who had undergone direct silicone injections for augmentation. In 1991 the echogenic sonographic appearance of silicone granulomas resulting from implant rupture was described by Levine and Collins[40] as "echogenic confusion." Rosculet et al[38] in 1992 characterized the sonographic appearance of ruptured implants as "echogenic noise" but also noted occasional hypoechoic "masses" either alone or associated with the echogenic areas. In 1993, Harris et al[25] described the highly echogenic pattern of free silicone within the tissues as a "snowstorm" pattern with loss of all detail posteriorly. This characteristic highly echogenic pattern of free silicone within the tissues is a reliable sign specific for silicone that has escaped from the confines of the fibrous capsule. This sign was present in 24 of the 25 cases reported by Harris et al[25] and in 17 of the 19 cases reported by Rosculet et al.[38]

The sonographic appearance of free silicone in the tissues consists of a characteristic highly echogenic pattern of scattered and reverberating echoes with loss of all detail of the underlying structures as the echogenicity is propagated posteriorly (Figs. 7–4A,C and 7–5A–C,E).[25,85] The area of echogenicity has a well-defined anterior margin but a poorly defined posterior margin, appearing as a "snowstorm." With a confined leak (Fig. 7–4) the echogenic pattern originates adjacent to the periphery of the implant with echoes propagated posteriorly, and appearing as if the echoes were within the implant as the "noise" continues posteriorly until it dissipates. When the free silicone within the breast overlies the

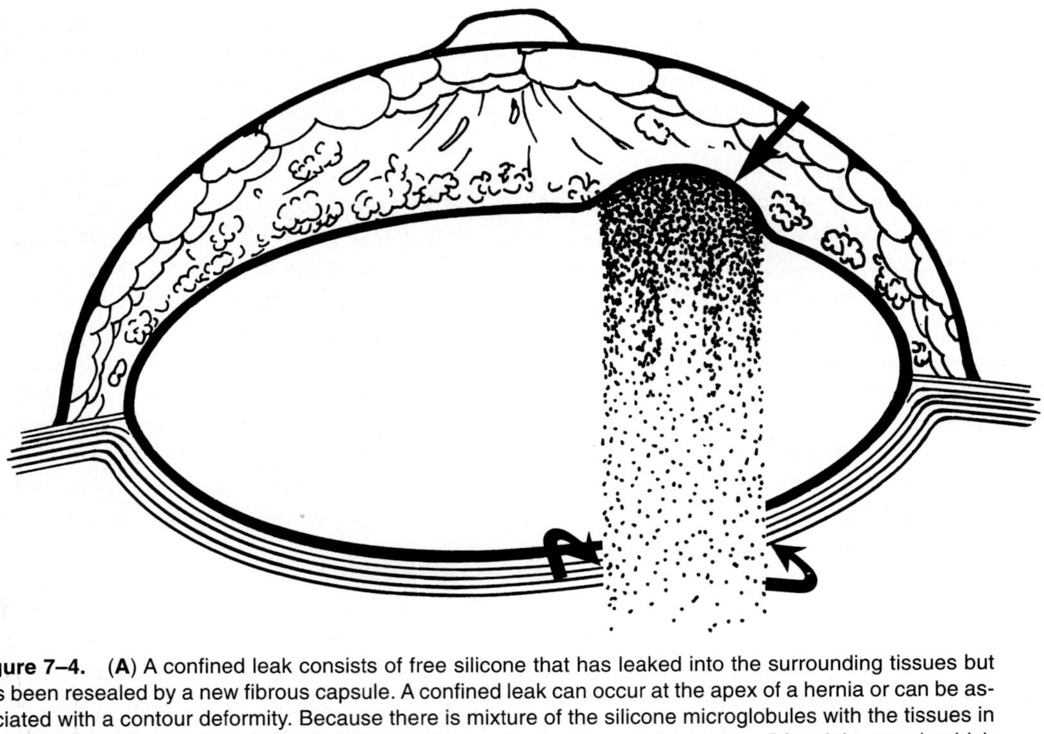

A

Figure 7–4. (**A**) A confined leak consists of free silicone that has leaked into the surrounding tissues but has been resealed by a new fibrous capsule. A confined leak can occur at the apex of a hernia or can be associated with a contour deformity. Because there is mixture of the silicone microglobules with the tissues in a foreign body granulomatous reaction, there is the resultant echogenic "snowstorm" (straight arrow), which overlies the implant and obliterates the tissues posteriorly (curved arrows). *(continued)*

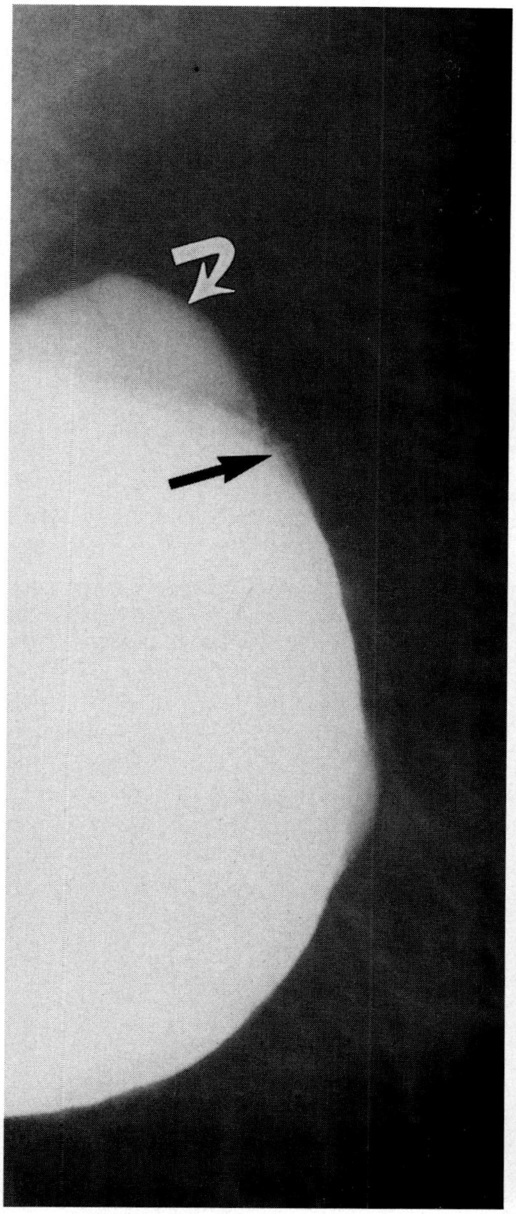

B

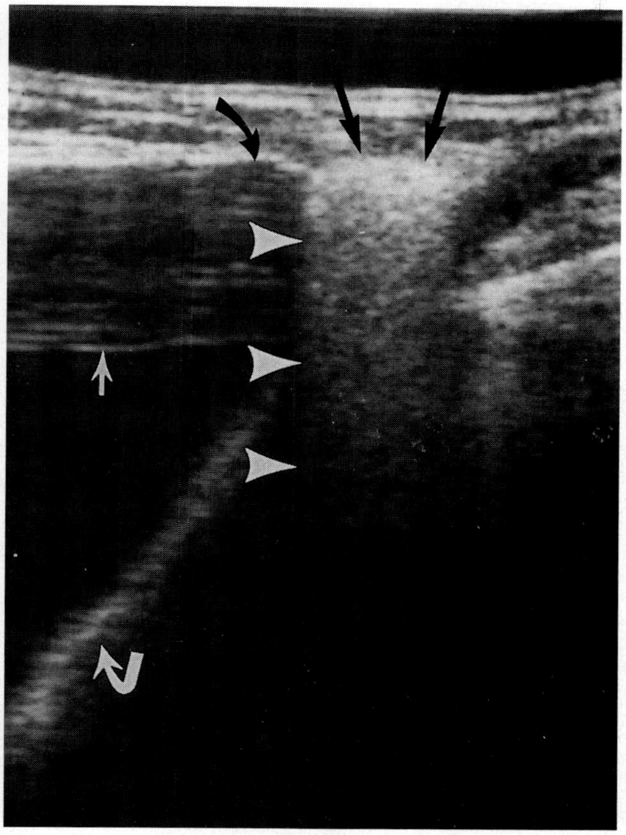

C

7–4. *(Continued)* (**B**) A confined leak may be indistinguishable from a bulge or hernia mammographically. In this patient the confined leak (curved arrow) is smoothly marginated but has a slightly lower density compared with the adjacent implant. The calcified fibrous capsule is disrupted (black arrow). A new fibrous capsule that is not calcified confines the small rupture, giving it a smooth contour. (**C**) Ultrasound evaluation of contour deformities can differentiate a bulge or hernia (Fig. 7–2G) from a confined leak. The confined leak is seen along the superolateral aspect of the silicone implant. The echogenic snowstorm (straight black arrows) originates at the same level as the anterior echogenic line (curved black arrow) of the implant. Note the propagation of echogenic "noise" with loss of all detail posteriorly until the noise dissipates (arrowheads). Also note the horizontal anterior reverberation echoes (straight white arrow). The lateral edge of the implant is seen as it extends posteriorly (curved white arrow).

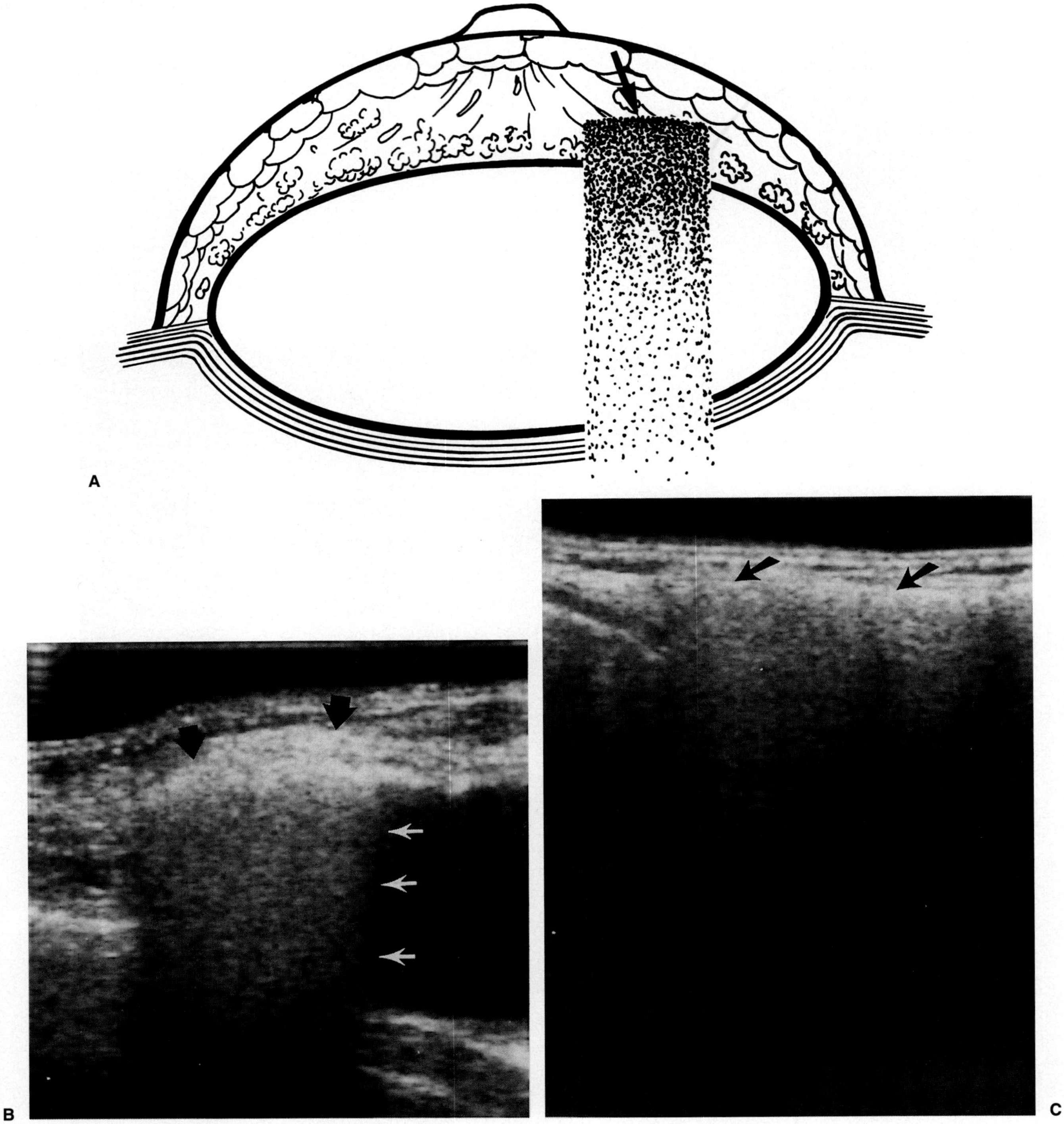

Figure 7–5. (**A**) Free silicone within the breast, axilla, or elsewhere in the body has a characteristic sonographic echogenic pattern with a well-defined anterior border (arrow) and obliteration of all the underlying structures as the echogenic "noise" is propagated posteriorly. Note the obliteration of the anterior and posterior echogenic implant interfaces as well as the underlying tissues posterior to the implant. The echoes overlie the implant but appear as if they were within the implant. Also note the sharp lateral margins of the echogenic "snowstorm" as the echogenic noise is propagated posteriorly. (**B**) With a standoff pad used to visualize the skin and subcutaneous tissues, the echogenic snowstorm originates just under the skin (black arrows). The echogenic pattern obliterates the underlying tissues and the lateral margin of the implant with the noise propagated posteriorly until it dissipates. Note the "squaring off" of the lateral aspect of the implant by the straight lateral margin of the snowstorm (white arrows). (**C**) In areas remote to the implant, the echogenic pattern appears as the characteristic snowstorm extending from the subcutaneous area anteriorly (arrows) with the noise propagated posteriorly causing loss of detail of all the underlying structures. *(continued)*

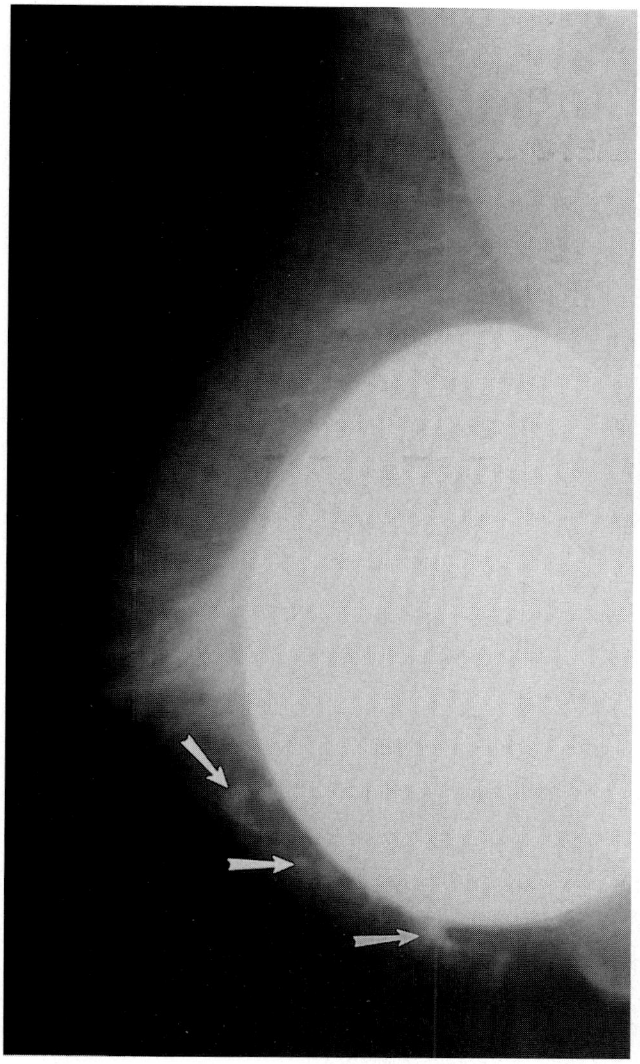

D

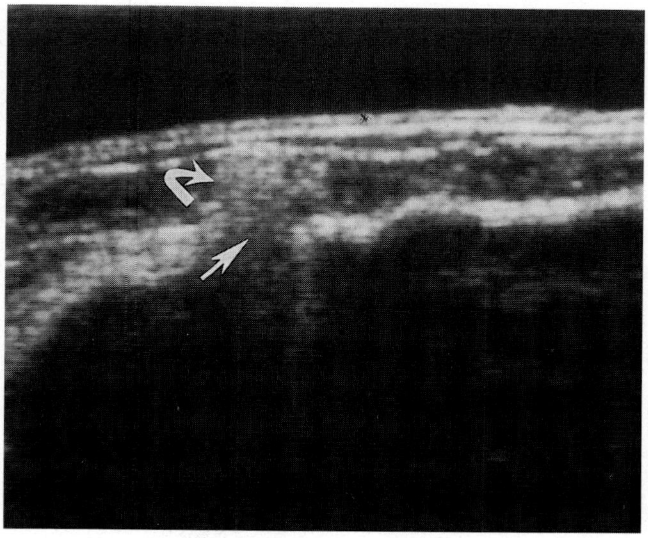

E

7–5. ***(Continued)*** (**D**) Multiple small nodules (arrows) are present in the inferior aspect of the right breast adjacent to the prepectoral silicone implant on the mediolateral oblique view. The nodules are mammographically indeterminate as to whether they represent true intrinsic breast lesions or silicone granulomas. (**E**) Ultrasound reveals a small echogenic snowstorm (curved arrow) with obliteration of the underlying anterior echogenic implant interface (straight arrow), compatible with a silicone granuloma associated with an extracapsular leak. Multiple small silicone granulomas accounted for the nodules seen mammographically. *(continued)*

implant, there is an associated obliteration of all underlying detail including the breast-implant interface and the underlying implant (Fig. 7–5A–C,E) in the region of the "snowstorm." The identical highly echogenic pattern with loss of detail posteriorly is also detected when free silicone is present in axillary nodes, corresponding to silicone lymphadenopathy.

Rubin et al[36] have attributed the characteristic echogenic pattern of free silicone to the small size of the silicone droplets (on the order of a wavelength) as well as to phase aberration caused by the sound waves encountering small droplets of silicone, which have a slower speed of sound (997 m/sec) compared with the adjacent tissue, which has a faster speed of sound (1540 m/sec).[56] An acoustic mismatch occurs when the beam encounters microscopic globules of silicone mixed within the tissue. This results in loss of coherence of the beam, with destruction of the beam focus, which ultimately destroys the image, resulting in loss of all detail.[73,87] Rubin et al[86] attribute the "noise" to coherent and incoherent summing of out-of-phase backscatter with no true signal remaining. This pattern is unique to free silicone in tissues and differs from the typical "dirty shadow" ascribed to gas in the abdomen.[88]

Harris et al[25] and Lopez[85] point to a number of factors that contribute to the echogenic pattern, including the small size of the silicone droplets, the acoustic impedance mismatch between silicone microglobules and the surrounding tissues, and the large number of silicone microglobules acting as reflecting surfaces.[85,89] Further research is needed to establish the actual physical factors that contribute to the echogenic "snowstorm" that is a signature for free silicone microglobules mixed within tissue.

Hypoechoic areas or "masses" representing larger cohesive collections of silicone are sometimes noted in the vicinity of the characteristic echogenic pattern (Fig. 7–6A,B,D).

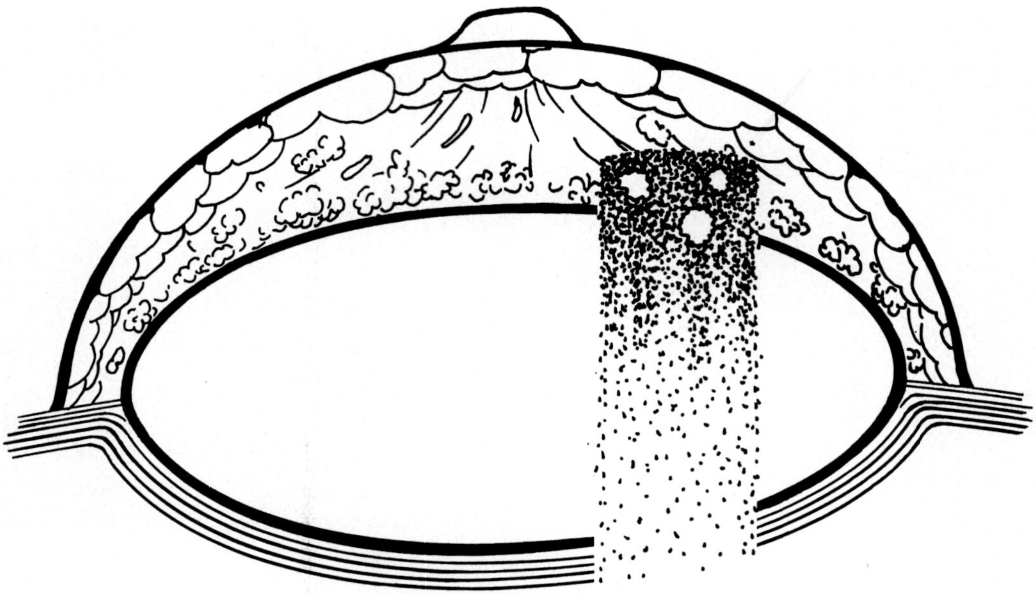

A

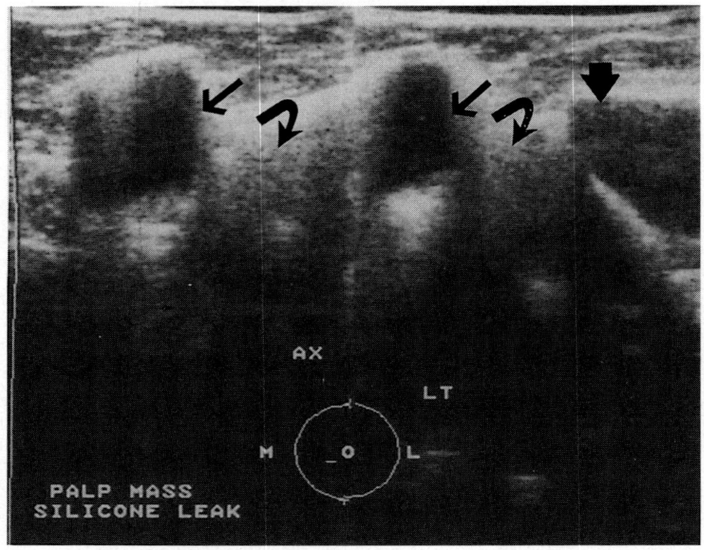

B

Figure 7–6. (**A**) Larger confluent globules of silicone can appear as hypoechoic "masses," which are usually associated with the area of echogenicity. These hypoechoic areas of larger globules of cohesive silicone transmit the sound similar to a "miniature" implant. Conversely, the surrounding microscopic globules of free silicone reflect and reverberate the sound. The resultant mismatch of acoustic velocities of multiple small microscopic silicone droplets mixed within tissue accounts for the characteristic "snowstorm" pattern. (**B**) Orthogonal views on a split screen demonstrate a large hypoechoic mass (straight arrows) representing a large globule of cohesive silicone, which transmits the sound as a miniature implant. This mass is within the vicinity of the characteristic echogenic snowstorm (curved arrows). This patient presented with palpable masses corresponding to the implant rupture. Note the edge of the lower inner aspect of the left implant (thick short arrow). *(continued)*

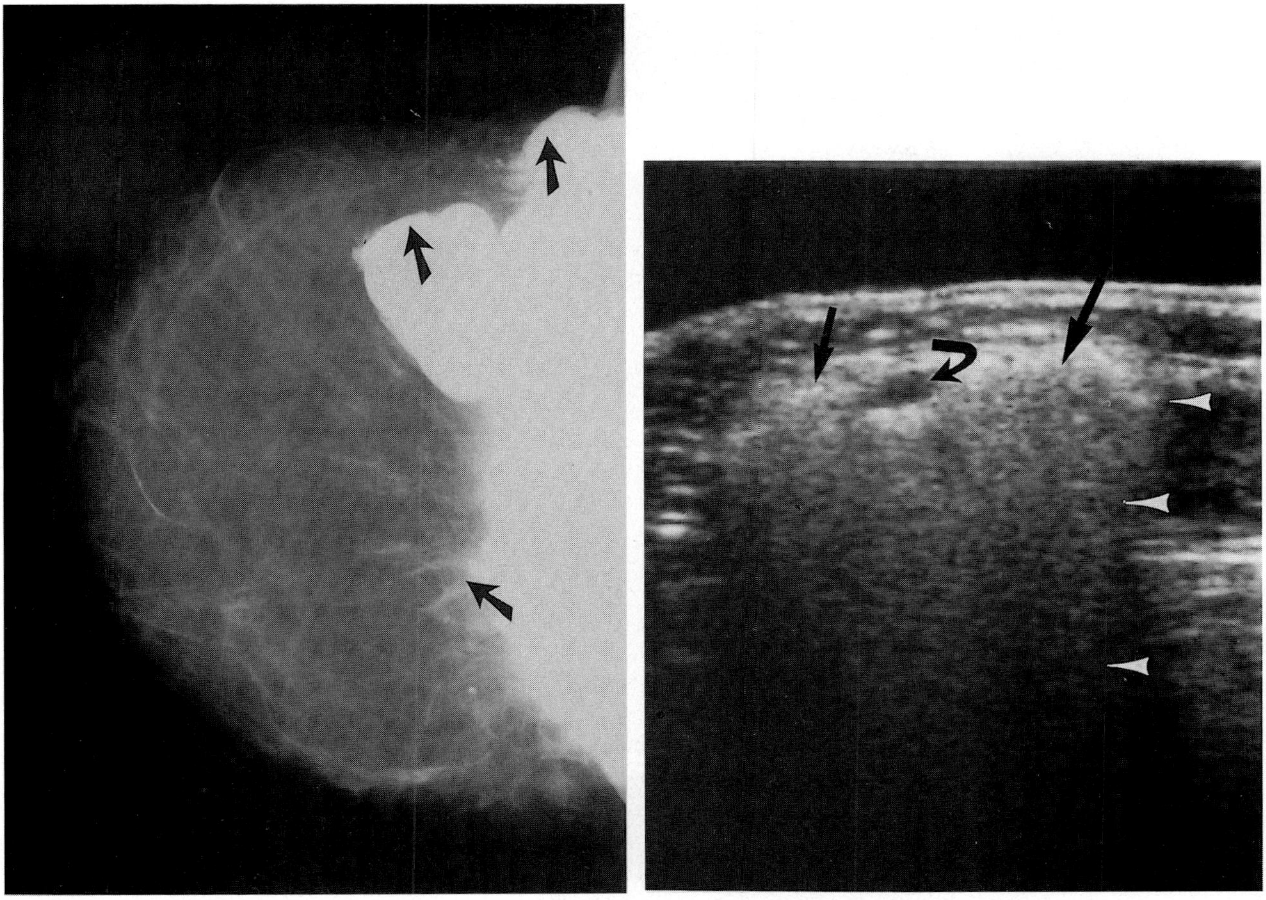

C D

7–6. *(Continued)* (**C**) Craniocaudal mammographic view of the same patient reveals the extruded silicone (arrows) that presented as palpable masses. Despite the obvious leak mammographically, ultrasound was valuable in determining the extent of the leak, with silicone extending into the subcutaneous tissues of the upper abdomen. (**D**) Hypoechoic masses (curved arrow) may be relatively small compared to the surrounding echogenic area (straight arrows). Note the surrounding echogenic snowstorm pattern with a well-defined anterior margin (straight arrows) and loss of all detail of the underlying structures. The posteriorly propagated noise gradually dissipates (arrowheads). *(continued)*

Less frequently, hypoechoic "masses" can be an isolated finding (Fig. 7–6E). Rosculet et al[38] reported hypoechoic "masses" associated with the echogenic pattern in 10 of 17 cases and as the only sign of free silicone in two cases of rupture. Leibman and Sybers[90] reported sonolucent masses in areas of echoes associated with loss of definition of posterior breast parenchyma in two cases after silicone breast injections. Larger conglomerates or globules of cohesive silicone gel can appear as hypoechoic "masses" and act sonographically as a "miniature implant" with uniform transmission of sound. These larger collections of cohesive silicone are not associated with loss of detail of structures behind the "mass" because the beam remains coherent. It is helpful to place a metal marker on the skin over an isolated sonographic "mass" that may not be associated with the echogenic "snowstorm" pattern and to obtain special mammographic views to correlate the sonographic finding with a possible silicone granuloma mammographically (Fig. 7–6F). MR imaging can confirm whether an isolated hypoechoic "mass" represents a collection of silicone (Fig. 7–6G). Ultrasound-guided aspiration of material from the "mass" does not usually yield a diagnosis because the silicone is dissolved to some extent by the chemicals used for processing the slides. The cytopathologists are unable to diagnose free silicone but can infer its presence if foreign body giant cells containing vacuoles within their cytoplasm are identified within the cytologic specimen. Special energy dispersive x-ray analysis is necessary to detect elemental silicon, which is present in silicone gel.[48,76,80]

The sonographic snowstorm pattern is attributed to imaging the small droplets of silicone (on the order of the size of a wavelength) within the granulomatous reaction of the for-

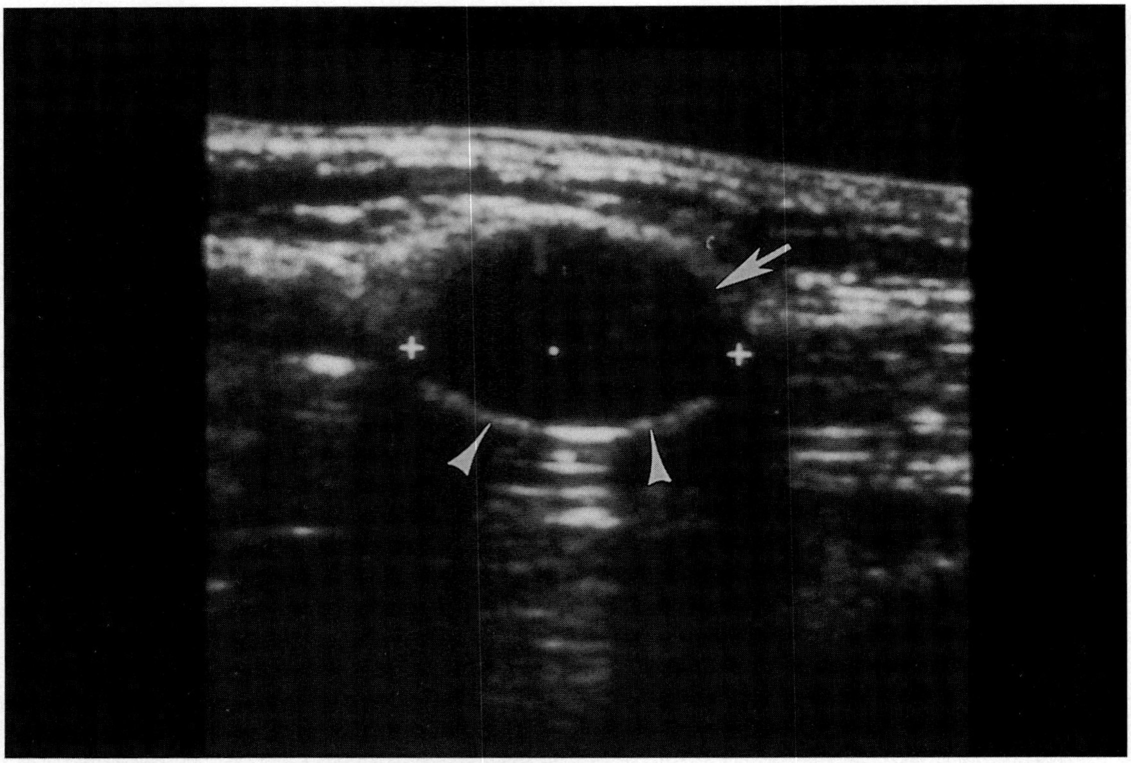

E

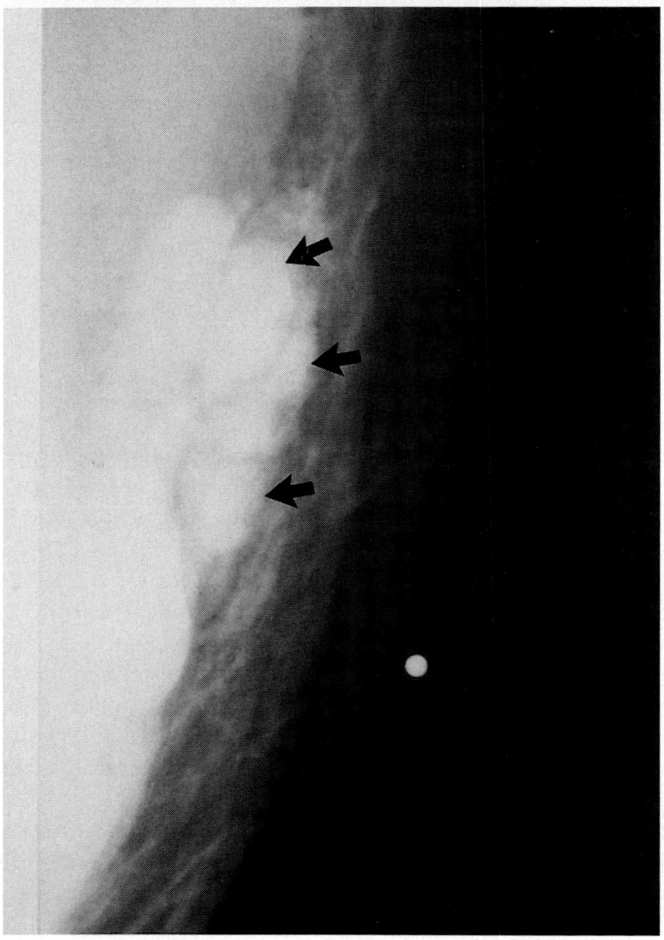

F

7–6. ***(Continued)*** (**E**) This patient had a history of a previously ruptured silicone implant that had been surgically replaced with a new silicone implant. Residual cohesive silicone globules in the anterior chest wall with the sonographic appearance of hypoechoic masses (arrow) were seen at the 12 o'clock position. Note the echogenic posterior boundary of the cohesive silicone globule (arrowheads), which acts like a miniature implant. (**F**) A metal marker was placed over the hypoechoic "masses" seen at ultrasound and a tangential mammographic view reveals multiple radiopaque masses having the appearance of silicone (arrows). *(continued)*

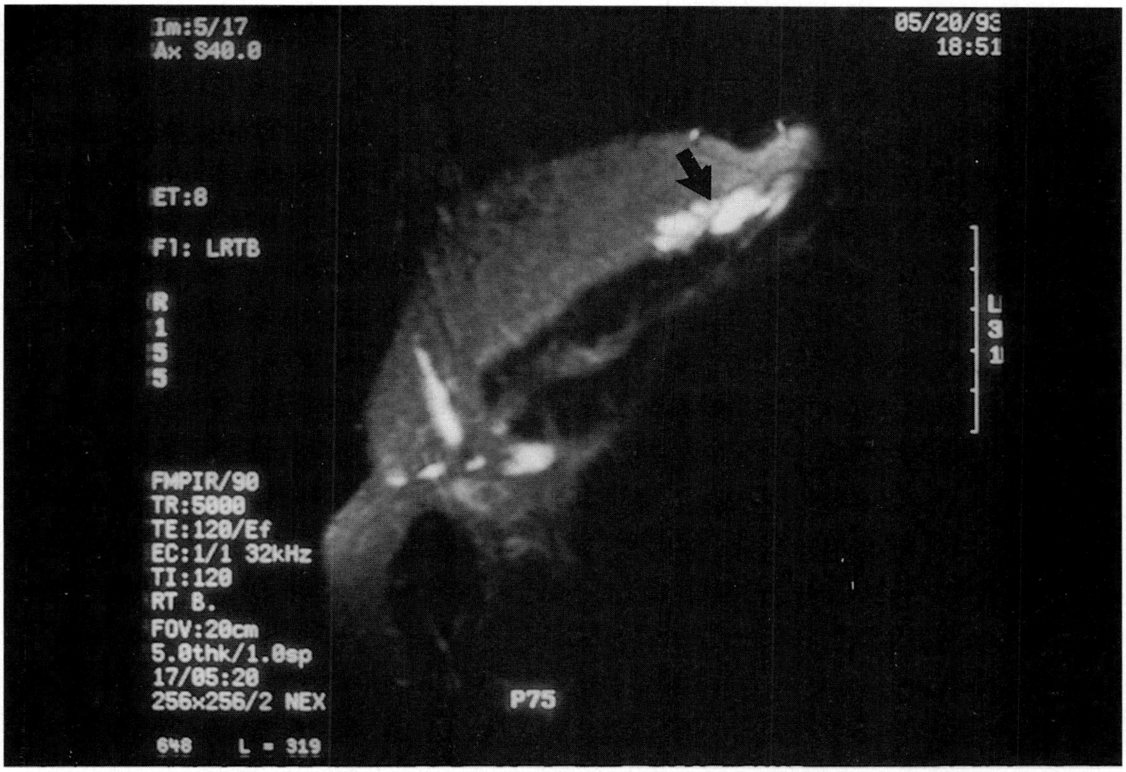

G

7–6. ***(Continued)*** (G) MR imaging with special pulse sequences for silicone confirms that the masses represent collections of silicone within the anterior chest wall (arrow).

eign body giant cell inflammatory response to silicone gel within the tissues of the body.[91] Silicone gel is phagocytized by scavenger macrophages in an attempt to surround and "engulf" the silicone microglobules while fibroblasts attempt to wall off the foreign material[25,46] (Fig. 7–7). The result is analogous to a mixture of "oil" droplets (silicone microglobules) in "water" (body tissues containing giant cells and fibroblasts), which accounts for the characteristic echogenic appearance of free silicone wherever it is found, whether in the breast, axilla, chest wall, or beyond. By physical examination or by mammography, a silicone granulomatous mass may be nonspecific. Because of the characteristic echogenic pattern detected with ultrasound, however, silicone granulomas (related to the implant) can be differentiated from pathologic lesions arising in the breast or axilla (unrelated to the implant). Because of the associated fibrous reaction it may be impossible to surgically remove all the silicone once it is within scar tissue.[92]

Ultrasound is very sensitive in detecting small amounts of free silicone. MR imaging has greater difficulty in detecting small quantities of silicone, perhaps because of partial volume averaging of the silicone microglobules mixed within the granulomatous tissues. In our experience, small quantities of silicone within axillary nodes detected by ultrasound have not been detectable by MR imaging.[93] Ahn et al,[29] however, illustrate one case with silicone gel extravasation into the axilla detected with MR imaging.

Harris et al[25] found physical examination to be the least reliable method of detecting silicone leaks, missing half of a set of cases that were later surgically confirmed. Mammographic detection was more reliable than was clinical examination but failed to detect 6 of 20 leaks. Ultrasound was the most sensitive, detecting all but one surgically confirmed leak. Ahn et al[29] described a positive "squeeze test" performed by clinical examination that could suggest a ruptured implant.

■ IMPLANT-ASSOCIATED LYMPHADENOPATHY

Silicone lymphadenopathy can result from silicone gel bleed or from a silicone implant rupture[77,80,94] (Fig. 7–8). Microglobules of silicone can enter the lymphatic system and be deposited in the axillary or infraclavicular nodes and de-

(text continues on page 97)

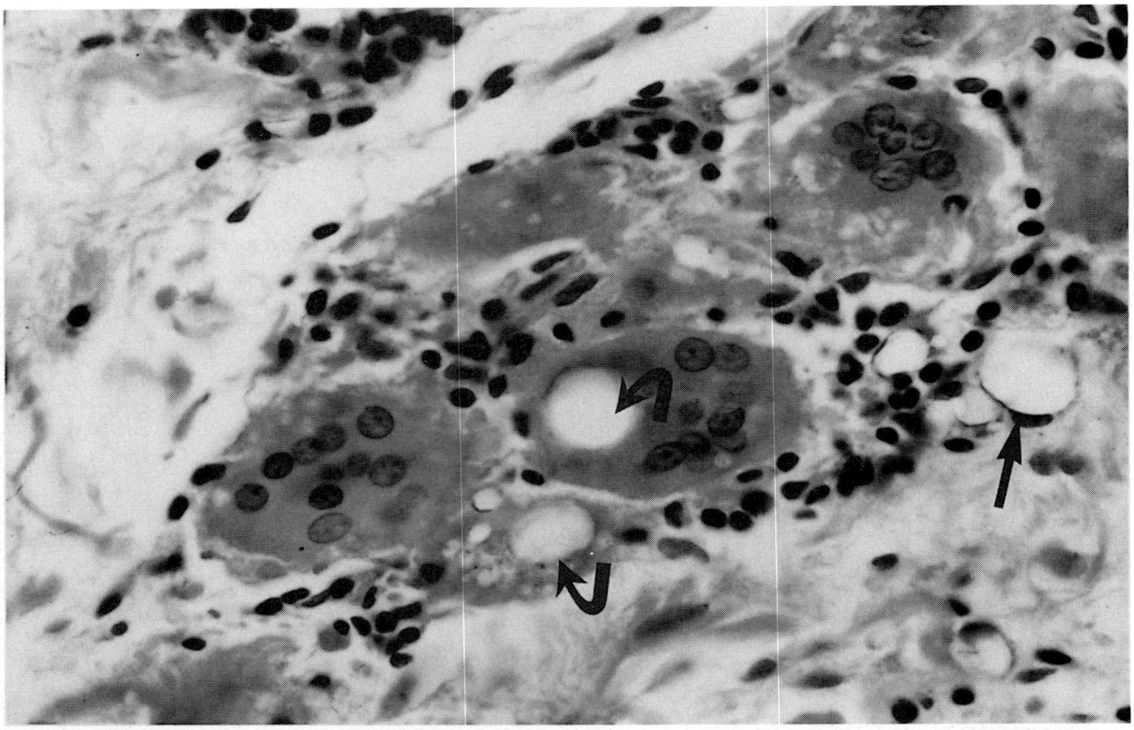

A

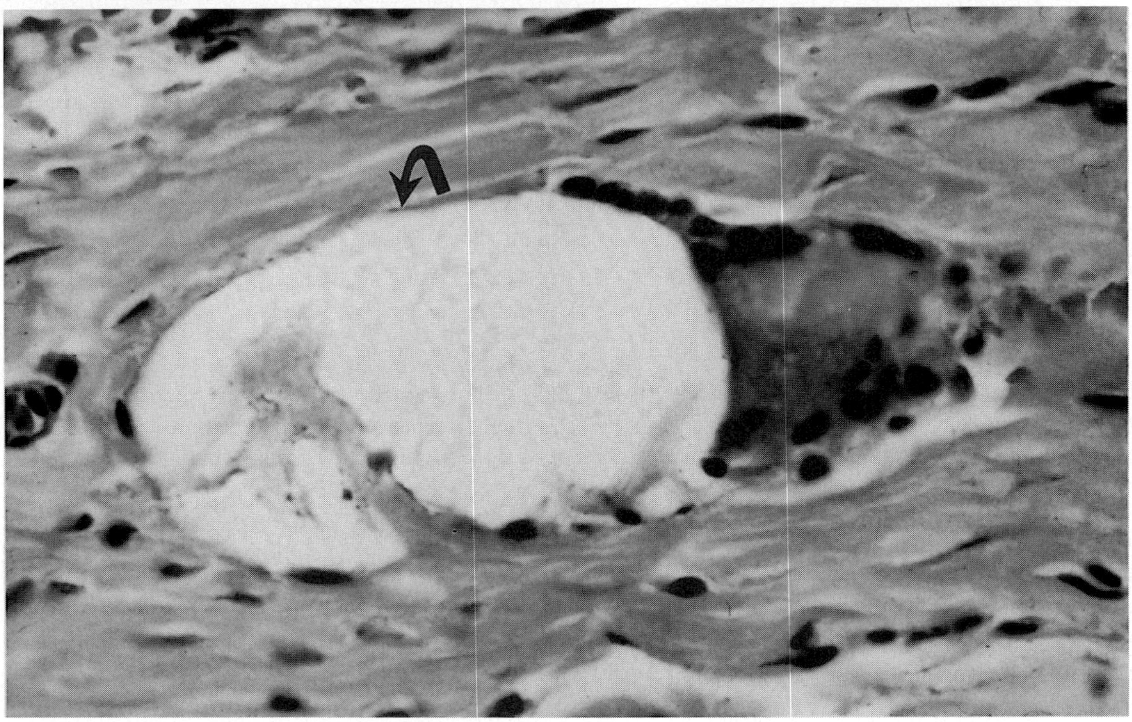

B

Figure 7–7. (**A**) Histologic sections illustrate the small size of the silicone microglobules within tissue that account for the characteristic "snowstorm" pattern seen sonographically. Histologic section of breast tissue (hematoxylin-eosin stain; original magnification ×200) in a case of extracapsular silicone rupture. The silicone microglobules are seen as empty vacuoles within the cytoplasm of the giant cells (curved arrows) and within the fibrous tissue (straight arrow) and inflammatory cells of the foreign body giant cell reaction. (**B**) High power of a single macrophage that has engulfed a silicone microglobule (curved arrow) (magnification ×400).

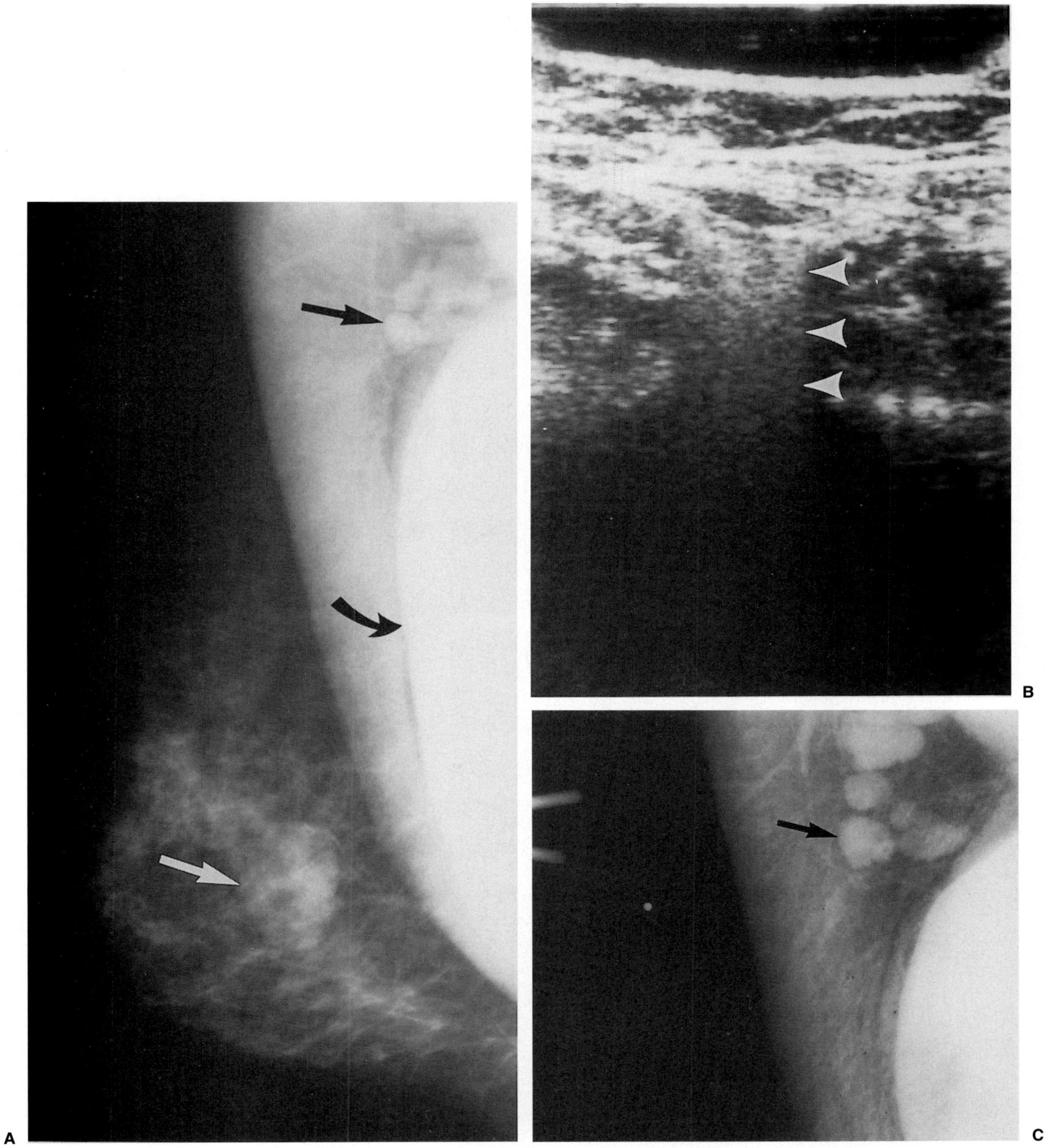

Figure 7–8. (**A**) Mediolateral oblique view reveals the retropectoral silicone implant (curved black arrow), a circumscribed oval breast mass (white arrow), and normal appearing axillary nodes (straight black arrow). Ultrasound was subsequently performed to evaluate the right breast mass, which was a simple cyst. (**B**) Ultrasound of the axilla reveals the subtle echogenic "snowstorm" associated with silicone lymphadenopathy (arrowheads). This was found serendipitously at the time of the breast ultrasound. (**C**) A metal marker has been placed on the skin overlying the sonographic area of the echogenic snowstorm within the axilla. In the special axillary view, the nodes (arrow) do not appear to contain radiopaque silicone. Ultrasound can better detect small quantities of free silicone within nodes than mammography. *(continued)*

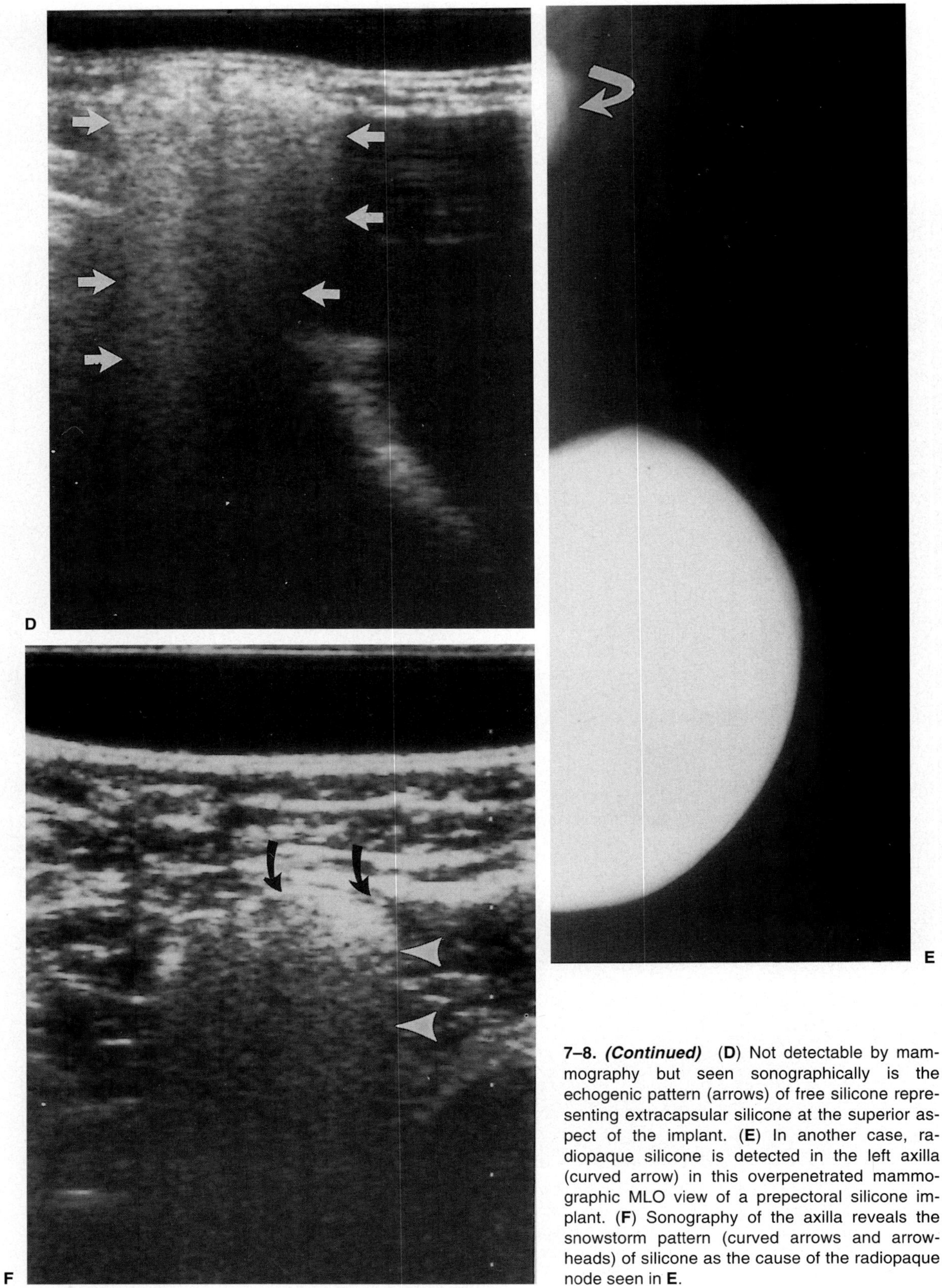

7–8. ***(Continued)*** (**D**) Not detectable by mammography but seen sonographically is the echogenic pattern (arrows) of free silicone representing extracapsular silicone at the superior aspect of the implant. (**E**) In another case, radiopaque silicone is detected in the left axilla (curved arrow) in this overpenetrated mammographic MLO view of a prepectoral silicone implant. (**F**) Sonography of the axilla reveals the snowstorm pattern (curved arrows and arrowheads) of silicone as the cause of the radiopaque node seen in **E**.

tected sonographically (Fig. 7–8B). Small quantities of silicone (Fig. 7–8C) may be insufficient to increase the radiodensity of axillary nodes mammographically, although larger volumes of silicone will increase nodal radiopacity (Fig. 7–8E). However, ultrasound is sensitive in detecting even small amounts of silicone in lymph nodes (Fig. 7–8B,F). Silicone lymphadenopathy is most often detected serendipitously in asymptomatic women during ultrasound examination of the axilla but may rarely present as a clinically palpable node[25] or as arm paresthesias. Nodes containing microscopic globules of silicone have the same sonographic characteristic echogenic "snowstorm" pattern as does free silicone in the breast. The prevalence of free silicone in the axillary nodes of women with breast implants is unknown. Asymptomatic silicone lymphadenopathy found serendipitously at the time of ultrasound examination is rarely biopsied for confirmation, since axillary dissection is a major surgical procedure with possible sequelae of arm swelling or nerve damage. There is, therefore, little proof in the literature of surgical confirmation of silicone within axillary nodes.[77,80,94]

Polyurethane from polyurethane-coated implants can also enter the lymphatic system and result in axillary lymphadenopathy, which is most often asymptomatic but can occasionally be clinically apparent. Polyurethane adenopathy appears mammographically similar to enlarged reactive axillary nodes that are usually present bilaterally. Mammographically, polyurethane is not radiopaque and therefore the nodes appear enlarged but are not radiodense. While the sonographic echogenic "snowstorm" pattern has been detected within the axillary nodes in patients with polyurethane-coated silicone gel implants, it has not been established whether or not polyurethane particles could be contributing to the characteristic echogenic pattern in a similar manner to the silicone microglobules.

■ INDICATIONS FOR ULTRASOUND OF IMPLANT PATIENTS

The same indications for performing breast ultrasound apply to implant patients, except that complications related to the implant enter into the differential diagnosis. The indications include:

- Breast mass: mammographically or clinically detectable
- Axillary mass: mammographically or clinically detectable
- Deformed or changing implant
- Mammographically detected rupture of silicone implants
- Symptomatic patient
- History of breast trauma
- Aging implants
- Preoperative, intraoperative, and postoperative evaluation
- Evaluation of silicone in remote sites
- Postexplantation evaluation for residual silicone or postoperative hematoma/seroma
- Evaluation of the explanted implant for the plastic surgeon: a potential use in selected cases.

Breast Mass

Clinically occult breast masses detected mammographically as well as clinically evident masses could represent true breast lesions[95,96] or could be related to the implant (Figs. 7–9 and 7–10). Implant-related findings such as bulges, hernias, valves, prominent folds, or silicone granulomas may be evident mammographically or may be palpable, especially in women with little overlying breast tissue. Mammographically and by clinical examination it may be difficult to differentiate an intrinsic breast mass such as a carcinoma from a silicone granuloma. Ultrasound can differentiate a true breast mass[96,97] associated with benign or malignant breast disease (Fig. 7–9A,B,E,F) from free silicone in the tissues as the cause of the mass[25] (Fig. 7–9C,D). Despite the addition of implant displacement views mammographically, breast masses can be obscured, especially those near the tissue-prosthesis interface.[16,21] Ultrasound, however, can better evaluate breast lesions in implant patients since all the breast tissue lies anterior to the implant.[21] In the case of prepectoral implants the breast tissue is anterior to the implant, and with retropectoral implants the pectoral muscle lies anterior to the implant. Sonography is useful to confirm, characterize, or localize mammographically suspected lesions that are seen in only one view or are poorly seen because of compaction of the tissues associated with suboptimal compression. Real-time ultrasound allows direct palpation with visual correlation.

Axillary Mass

Axillary adenopathy detected by mammography or by clinical examination could represent metastatic carcinoma, lymphoma, benign reactive lymph nodes, or silicone lymphadenopathy.[25,80] Ultrasound can distinguish lymphadenopathy unrelated to the implants from silicone lymphadenopathy because of the characteristic "snowstorm" appearance of the free silicone microglobules in the nodes.[25] Clinically significant silicone lymphadenopathy from gel bleed can occur in the absence of implant rupture.

Deformed or Changing Implant

Ultrasound imaging can evaluate the mammographically deformed implant[23] or the implant that is exhibiting a changing

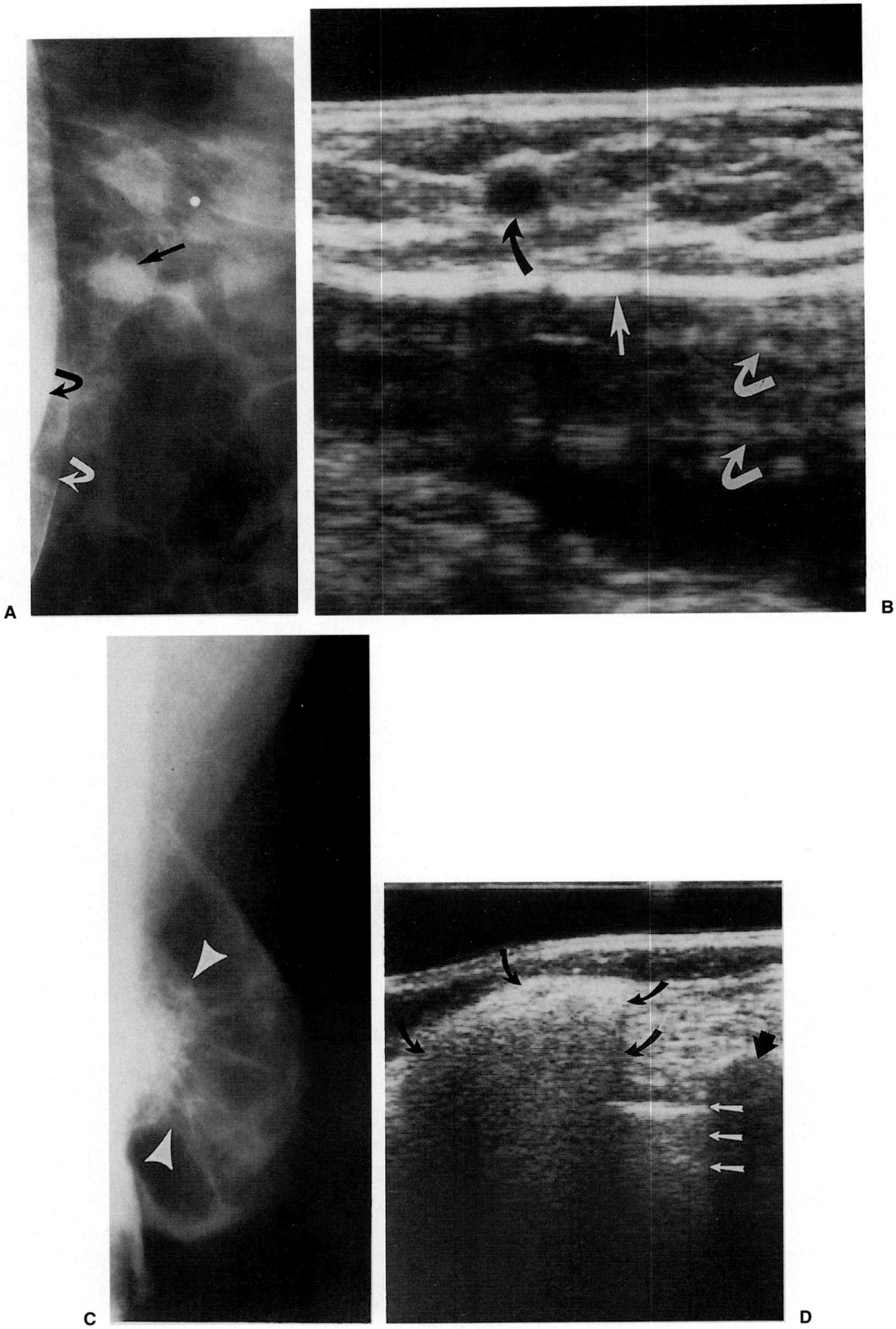

Figure 7–9. (**A**) This patient was seen for a second opinion because of a breast mass detected mammographically in another facility, for which surgical excision was advised. There is a smooth marginated circumscribed mass (straight arrow) in a closeup of the implant displacement view. The metal marker had been placed on the skin over a hypoechoic mass detected by ultrasound to confirm that the sonographic and mammographic findings were the same lesion. Note the double-lumen prepectoral implant with the outer saline (curved white arrow) and inner silicone (curved black arrow) implants. *(continued)*

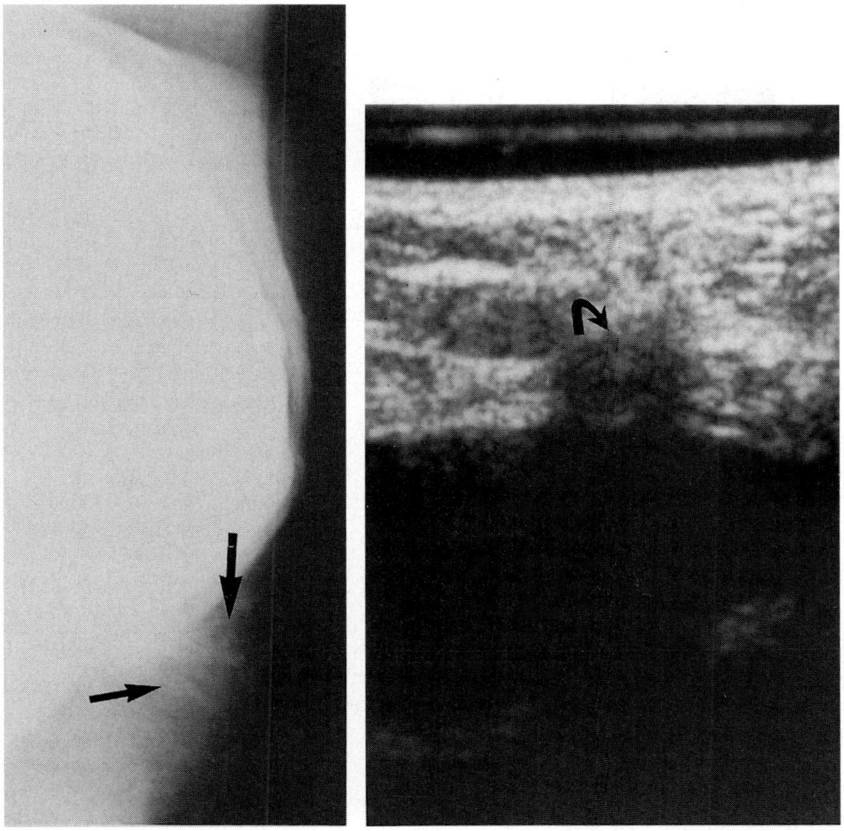

E F

7–9. *(Continued)* (**B**) Ultrasound reveals the small hypoechoic mass that was thought to be a cyst, but, because of its small size (5 mm), did not fulfill all the criteria of a simple cyst (black arrow). Subsequent ultrasound-guided fine-needle aspiration successfully decompressed this cyst, thus averting unnecessary surgery. The anterior echogenic interface of the implant (straight white arrow) and reverberation echoes within the implant (curved white arrows) are noted. The outer saline implant cannot be distinguished from the inner silicone implant sonographically. (**C**) This patient presented with a spiculated left breast mass (arrowheads) on the MLO view. There was marked breast deformity following previous surgical explantation for a clinically ruptured silicone implant. The differential for the spiculated mass was carcinoma versus silicone granuloma. (**D**) Ultrasound reveals the characteristic echogenic appearance of free silicone, which corresponded to the "spiculated mass" (curved black arrows). Note the rib (thick black arrow) and rib interspace (white arrows). The echogenic space between the ribs is distinguishable from the characteristic echogenic pattern of free silicone. At surgery, silicone granulomatous tissue was the cause of the spiculated mass. There was no evidence of carcinoma. (**E**) This 53-year-old postmastectomy patient had a 13-year-old retropectoral silicone implant that had been placed for reconstruction. A new palpable thickening inferior to the implant was noted by the patient and corresponded to an area of architectural distortion adjacent to the implant inferiorly in the MLO view (arrows). (**F**) At ultrasound, an irregularly marginated hypoechoic mass (curved arrow) with acoustic shadowing was detected adjacent to the implant, which was suggestive of malignancy. At surgery there was a chest wall recurrence of an infiltrating ductal carcinoma with "invasion" of the implant.

configuration or position over time (Fig. 7–11). Additionally, the patient may be aware of a change in the contour, consistency, or position of one or both implants despite mammographic stability. Ultrasound can evaluate contour deformities by differentiating a wrinkle, bulge, or hernia from an implant rupture[25] or can detect a fluid collection adjacent to an implant that could present as a changing contour mammographically. Fluid collections associated with implants, especially common with polyurethane-coated implants, are an incidental finding unassociated with implant rupture.[60]

Mammographically Detected Rupture of Silicone Implants

In the case of mammographically detected rupture, ultrasound can evaluate the extent of the spread of free silicone.[25] The entire breast and adjacent areas (axilla, infraclavicular area, anterior chest wall) can be imaged by ultrasound. Mammography is limited by the radiopacity of the implant,[71] which can obscure the adjacent breast tissue in the periprosthetic area, the most common location for small confined leaks.

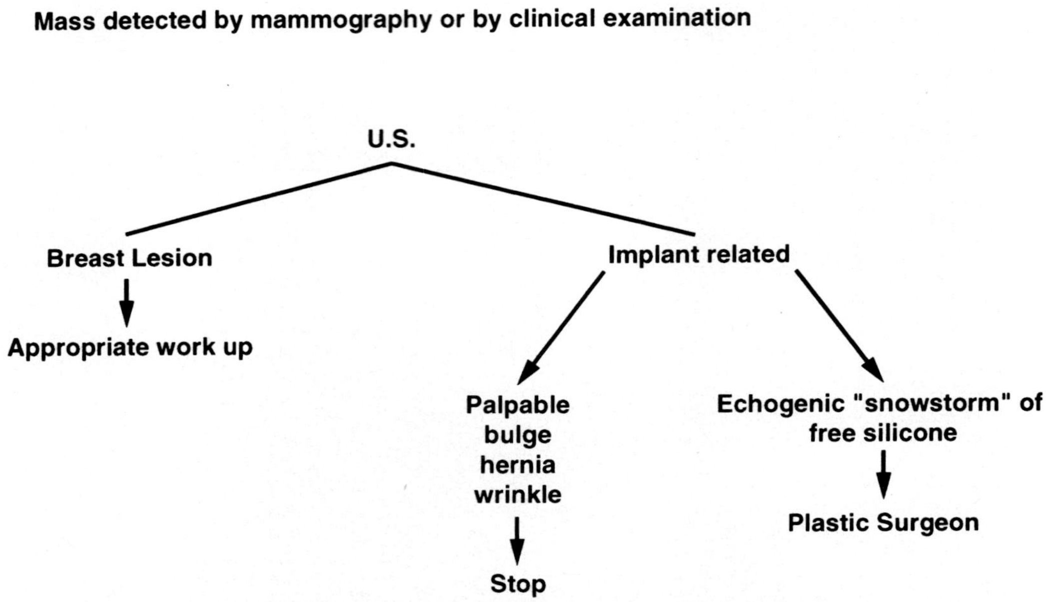

Figure 7–10. Algorithm: masses detected by clinical examination or by mammography can be evaluated by ultrasound. True intrinsic breast lesions can be distinguished from implant related "masses," which could be bulges, hernias, wrinkles, or silicone granulomas associated with implant rupture. Superficially situated silicone granulomas may be palpable in the breast, axilla, or elsewhere in the body.

Ultrasound can better localize a leak seen in only one mammographic view. Placement of a metal marker on the skin over the "snowstorm" pattern detected sonographically can facilitate obtaining special extra mammographic views in an attempt to visualize the leak in orthogonal views.

Whenever sonography identifies a rupture in one implant, ultrasound evaluation of the contralateral implant is recommended for detection of a possible unsuspected asymptomatic rupture.[25] This information enables preoperative planning for either unilateral or bilateral explantation. Because the potential for leakage in the contralateral implant increases as the implants age,[25,32] plastic surgeons often elect to replace the implants bilaterally. The cosmetic results and the patient's wishes also enter into the decision for unilateral or bilateral explantation with or without replacement.

Symptomatic Patient

Ultrasound evaluation is indicated in the clinically symptomatic patient (Fig. 7–12). Symptoms may include new onset

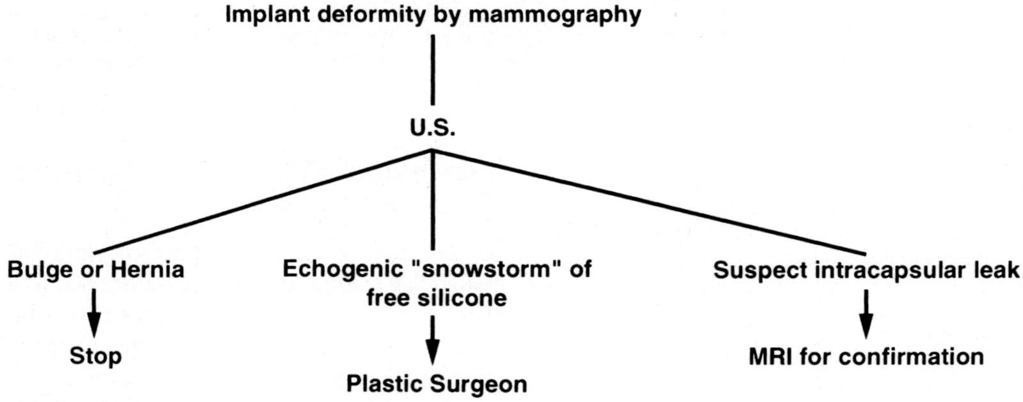

Figure 7–11. Algorithm: implant deformities can be evaluated with ultrasound to distinguish a bulge or hernia from extracapsular implant rupture including confined leaks.

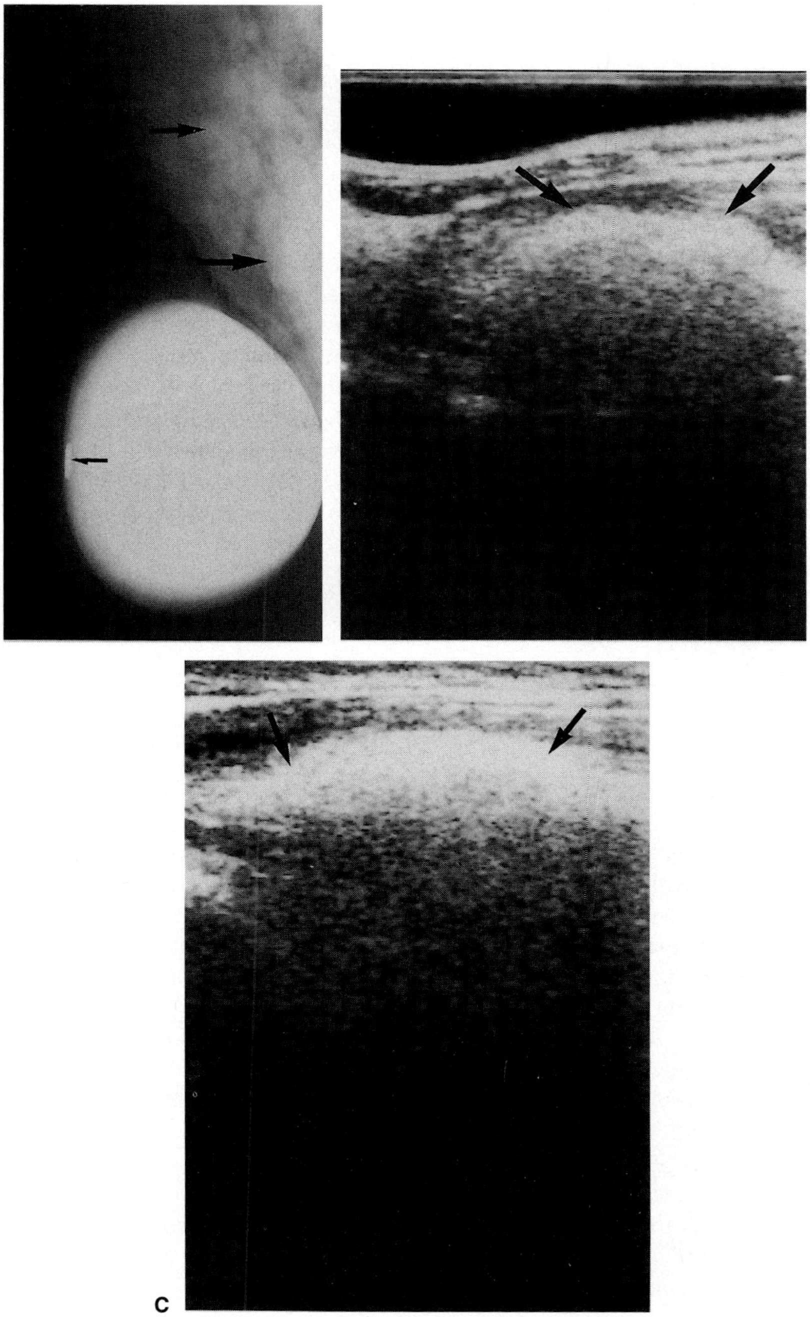

A B C

Figure 7–12. (**A**) This patient presented with pain and paresthesias of the right arm subsequent to an implant rupture that occurred years earlier. A new silicone prepectoral implant is in place. Extensive free silicone is present within the pectoral muscle (long black arrows) on the mediolateral oblique view. The radiodense area along the anterior margin of the implant presumably is a Dacron patch (short black arrow). (**B**) The echogenic "snowstorm" is present in the right axilla (arrows) of the same patient. (**C**) Corresponding to a subtle palpable "fullness" in the right infraclavicular area is the echogenic pattern of free silicone (arrows) confirming migration of silicone to the infraclavicular nodes. Presumably, encasement of the brachial plexus due to the fibrous reaction to the free silicone has resulted in the patient's right arm symptoms. Silicone in the infraclavicular area and within the pectoral muscle was subsequently confirmed with MR imaging. The axillary silicone, however, was not detectable by MRI.

of breast pain; hardening or increasing firmness of the implant; painful lump in the breast, axilla, abdominal wall,[98] or upper extremity[81]; arm paresthesias[99]; or symptoms of autoimmune disease.[100] Breast pain could be associated with fibrocystic changes but implant complications can also produce pain. Arm paresthesias may be secondary to entrapment of the brachial plexus by the fibrosis associated with silicone granulomas.[99] Capsular contracture is associated with painful, firm, protuberant breasts.[101–103] Occasionally a new onset of symptoms of pain or a change of consistency of the implant can be associated with an intracapsular leak or a confined leak, which results in thickening and constriction of the fibrous capsule. Silicone granulomas associated with free silicone in the tissues of the breast, axilla, or chest wall can present as hard, painful masses and can be diagnosed by their characteristic echogenic pattern sonographically. Ultrasound can identify fluid collections (hematomas or seromas) adjacent to an implant that may present as a painful mass. A fluid collection may take the shape of the implant if it is situated between the fibrous capsule and the implant and may not be distinguishable by mammography. Patients with symptoms of possible implant rupture or of autoimmune disease may be referred by their physician or perhaps by their lawyer for ultrasound evaluation for possible implant failure.

History of Breast Trauma

When there is a history of breast trauma, ultrasound examination of the breast and the implant can identify implant rupture as well as associated findings such as hematoma or seroma. Any blunt or sharp direct force to the breast,[71,72] for example, ski accidents, seat-belt injuries in auto accidents, falls, stab wounds, as well as inadvertent intraoperative damage, can result in a ruptured implant.

Closed capsulotomy, a procedure performed by the plastic surgeons to correct the symptoms of capsular contracture, can result inadvertently in implant rupture.[104] In this procedure, the plastic surgeon externally squeezes the breast forcefully between two hands in order to create tears in the fibrous capsule, thus providing more room for the implant and relieving the symptoms of round, hard, painful breasts.[105] In some cases, however, the silicone envelope can also tear, resulting in the extrusion of free silicone through ruptures in both the implant envelope and the fibrous capsule.[104] Closed capsulotomy was commonly performed in the past, but reports of ruptures following this procedure[104,106–108] have resulted in its discontinuation. Many women give a past history of having had closed capsulotomy procedures one or multiple times. Peters et al[34] reported that half the patients with implant ruptures had a history of previous closed capsulotomy procedures. It is uncertain whether subtle leaks found serendipitously with ultrasound or MR imaging could have resulted from the force exerted during previous closed capsulotomy procedures.

Although rare, mammography was reported to cause implant rupture in one case.[109] Therefore, extreme care must be taken to avoid vigorous compression of the breast over the implant.[16,110] Compression should be just enough to hold the breast in place to prevent motion whenever the implant is included in the standard mediolateral oblique and craniocaudal views. Compression is applied only to the breast tissue anterior to the implant during the implant displacement views (craniocaudal and mediolateral oblique views where the implant is displaced posteriorly).[16] Because the risk of inadvertent rupture at the time of the implant displacement views is minimal, obtaining written informed patient consent prior to performing mammography has not been advocated.[110] The radiologist must be aware, however, of the potential for rupturing an implant, especially older implants, or for converting an unsuspected asymptomatic intracapsular rupture into an extracapsular rupture.[110]

Aging Implants

Ruptures can occur in aging implants without a history of trauma.[25,32] Tears in the envelope can occur at areas of stress such as wrinkles, bulges, or hernias.[101] It may be that the elastomer shell can develop spontaneous tears, which may result from disintegration over time.[10,32] The average age for implant leakage has been reported to be 10.7 years for unilateral leakage and 15.7 years for simultaneous bilateral leakage.[25] Berg et al[39] found the mean age for rupture to be 13.4 years for all implants, but the implants placed for reconstruction ruptured at 8.8 years on the average compared with an average of 16 years for implants placed for augmentation. Caskey et al[35] reported ruptures on an average of 15.8 years for augmentation and 9.7 years for reconstruction. Rosculet et al[38] found the average age for implant rupture to be 13 years with a range of 6 to 20 years. Peters and Pugash[111] found the mean time of diagnosis of rupture after implant insertion to be 8.5 years, with a range of 2.0 to 18 years.

Robinson et al[32] believe that disruption is directly related to the length of time since implantation and reported a disruption rate of 63.5% at the time of surgical explantation. They defined "disruption" as the breakdown of the integrity of the silicone envelope as manifested by either frank rupture or by severe silicone gel bleed that has extended over 12 inches, or a combination of both. They believe that most implants will lose their integrity between 8 and 14 years, resulting in either intracapsular or extracapsular leaks. The optimal interval for performing ultrasound in the search for asymptomatic intracapsular or extracapsular leakage has not been determined. Because of reports of ruptures in aging implants,[25,39] there may be a role for ultrasound surveillance of silicone implants in a search for asymptomatic ruptures after 10 years or more in augmented breasts or after 8 years in reconstructed breasts. As yet, however, screening for asymptomatic ruptures in older implants has not been widely advocated. The reason for the accelerated time of implant failure associated with reconstruction may be related to subtle trauma, because there is minimal overlying tissue between the skin and the implant when compared with the larger amount of overlying tissue in the augmented breast.

Preoperative, Intraoperative, and Postoperative Evaluation

Whenever a decision has been made for surgical explantation based on symptoms of pain, autoimmune disease, or because of the patient's wishes based on "silicone-induced anxiety," the implants can be evaluated preoperatively by ultrasound as well as by MR imaging. The preoperative information can alert the plastic surgeon to intracapsular rupture or to the location of any extracapsular free silicone.[24]

Intraoperatively, ultrasound can direct the surgeon to areas of free silicone that may not be visible because of encasement within fibrous granulomatous tissue.[112] Same-day ultrasound-directed preoperative marking of the skin with a Magic Marker over areas of subcutaneous silicone can facilitate their precise localization and removal.

Postoperative residual silicone can be differentiated from intrinsic lesions arising in the breast by the characteristic "snowstorm" pattern of silicone. In the case of a previous rupture where a new silicone implant has been inserted, however, it is impossible to distinguish old residual silicone from a possible rupture of the new implant. Stability of the amount of extruded silicone over time is an indication of prior old silicone granulomas, whereas increasing areas occupied by the free silicone would suggest a new rupture. MR imaging can better evaluate the new implant for integrity in this clinical setting. In cases of prior explantation for rupture where a new implant has not been inserted, Caskey et al[113] found ultrasound to be more effective than MR or mammography in detecting residual silicone in the breast (Fig. 7–9C,D).

Avoiding unnecessary surgical biopsies is important in implant patients because of the added risk of puncturing the implant at the time of surgery. Ultrasound-guided aspiration biopsies can help to avoid surgical procedures for cytologically confirmed benign lesions.

Evaluation of Silicone in Remote Sites

Distant migration of silicone causing siliconomas has been reported.[45,81,98,114,115] Ultrasound is valuable in identifying free silicone that may have migrated to sites remote from the breast (Fig. 7–12).[25,80] Ultrasound of the axilla and infraclavicular areas can be performed at the same time as the breast ultrasound examination. The recumbent patient can elevate the ipsilateral arm to facilitate scanning of the axilla and can lower the ipsilateral arm for easier access to the infraclavicular area and anterior superior chest wall. Real-time ultrasound can image superficially palpable silicone granulomas that have migrated into the arm, anterior aspects of the thorax, or anterior abdomen, or even to the inguinal areas.[45]

Postexplantation Evaluation for Residual Silicone or Postoperative Hematoma/Seroma

After explantation, mammography[116] and ultrasound can aid in the diagnosis of postoperative hematomas, seromas, or residual silicone (Fig. 7–9C,D). At the time of implant removal, there are two surgical options: capsulotomy or capsulectomy.[117]

Surgical capsulectomy can consist of either total removal of the fibrous capsule along with the underlying implant or partial capsulectomy with a portion of the capsule remaining. Capsulectomy requires a lengthy surgical procedure performed under general anesthesia during which the surgeon meticulously dissects between the adjacent tissues and the underlying fibrous capsule in order to preserve as much breast tissue as possible while avoiding entering the fibrous capsule or implant.

In surgical capsulotomy, the fibrous capsule is incised and the implant is removed. A new implant can be inserted into the space within the original fibrous capsule. If the implant is not replaced, the collapsed fibrous capsule is left in place within the tissues. In the latter scenario, the surgeon might scar the inner surface of the capsule with electrocauterization to encourage the capsule walls to become adherent. Hemorrhage or serous fluid, however, can accumulate within the residual fibrous capsule, resulting in either clinically or mammographically detectable "masses," which are often smoothly marginated, taking the shape of the confines of the remaining fibrous capsule. Hematomas or seromas usually occur in the immediate postoperative period and could be mistaken mammographically for residual silicone if there is a large volume of fluid because of its radiopacity (Fig. 7–13). Hematomas or seromas could also be mistaken for a breast mass on physical examination. Capsulotomy is a simpler and quicker procedure than capsulectomy and can be performed under local anesthesia. Mammographically, the residual collapsed fibrous capsule can appear as bilateral soft tissue masses with or without associated calcifications in the retroglandular or retropectoral positions.[118] There has been one reported case of "mesh-like" calcifications seen mammographically, which are presumed to represent a foreign-body response to residual polyurethane[118] that remained within the breast following explantation. Sonographically, the collapsed fibrous capsule could appear as an echogenic area if it contains residual silicone or it could mimic a breast mass. Hematomas or seromas can also occur following an open surgical biopsy in implant patients[119] and can also be an incidental complication related to augmentation or reconstruction. Reactive fluid is commonly seen around intact polyurethane-coated or textured-surfaced single-lumen silicone implants.[60]

Evaluation of the Explanted Implant for the Plastic Surgeon: A Potential Use in Selected Cases

At surgery, on gross inspection, the surgeon may fail to identify a focally confined leak when the overlying fibrous capsule is removed along with the implant, especially if the fibrous capsule is adherent to the underlying implant. Because a new fibrous capsule can form to confine a leak, the plastic surgeon cannot see the free silicone by observing the outer surface of the "intact" fibrous capsule prior to capsulotomy. Ultrasound examination of the surgically removed implant that is still within its "intact" overlying fibrous capsule may allow identification of the specific focal area of the underlying confined implant rupture that was detected by ultrasound preoperatively. A subsequent meticulous dissection, with removal of the fibrous capsule in the area of the confined leak, can improve identification of the underlying tear in the implant envelope and the free silicone outside the envelope but within the fibrous capsule. This is not advocated in all cases of explantation but could be valuable in selected difficult cases where correlation of the preoperative sonographic findings with the findings of the explanted implant within the "intact" overlying fibrous capsule is warranted. In difficult cases, this can prevent a false-positive diagnosis by the surgeon who might call such a scenario negative without the radiologist to localize the specific area of the confined leak by ultrasound, which would allow the surgeon to confirm a true positive leak.

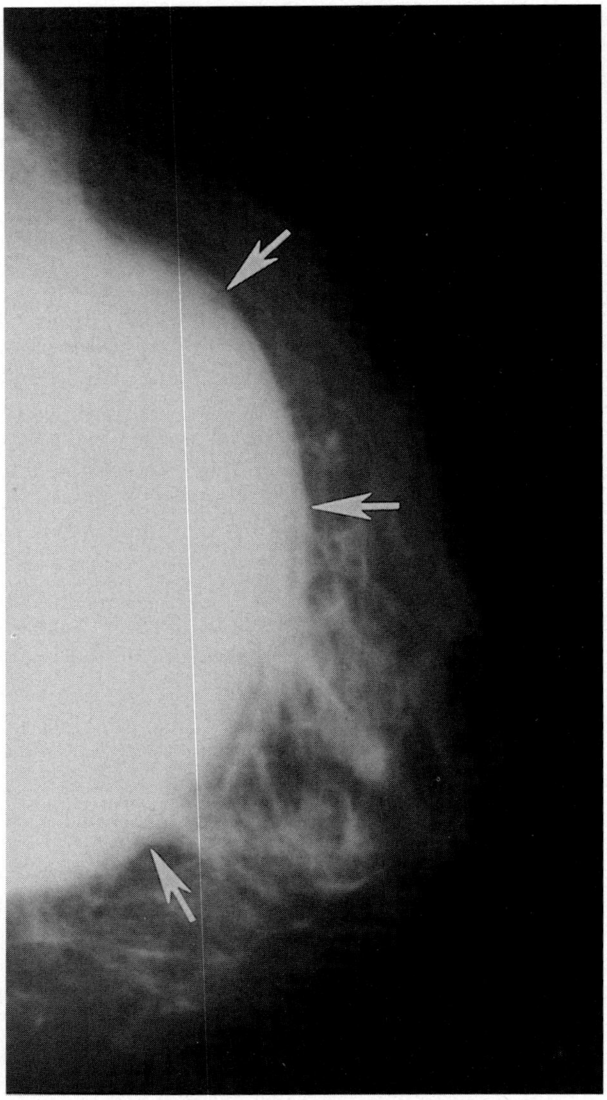

A

Figure 7–13. (**A**) Several days following bilateral capsulotomy and explantation of silicone implants, the patient noted a large painful left breast mass. Mammography revealed a large, smoothly marginated, well-circumscribed, high-density oval "mass" taking the configuration of an implant (arrows). Compression was suboptimal because of the severe breast pain. *(continued)*

■ LIMITATIONS OF ULTRASOUND IN IMPLANT PATIENTS

There are limitations of breast ultrasound in implant evaluation, including difficulty in differentiating normal internal echoes from the echoes associated with intracapsular rupture, loss of anatomic detail of the tissues underlying the echogenic "snowstorm," and difficulties in visualizing the chest wall deep to the implant.

Specifically, there are difficulties in

- differentiating intracapsular leaks from nonspecific internal echoes produced by folds, wrinkles, proteinaceous materials, and reverberation echoes;
- identifying the posterior implant interface with the posterior chest wall and free silicone posterior to the implant;
- evaluating patients who have had direct silicone injections into the breast tissue for augmentation;
- determining the integrity of a new implant when residual silicone granulomas from a previous rupture overlie the new implant;
- determining the exact anatomic structures containing the free silicone;
- identifying small quantities of silicone between the intact fibrous capsule and the envelope when the envelope has not collapsed;
- imaging the inner and outer envelopes of a double-lumen implant.

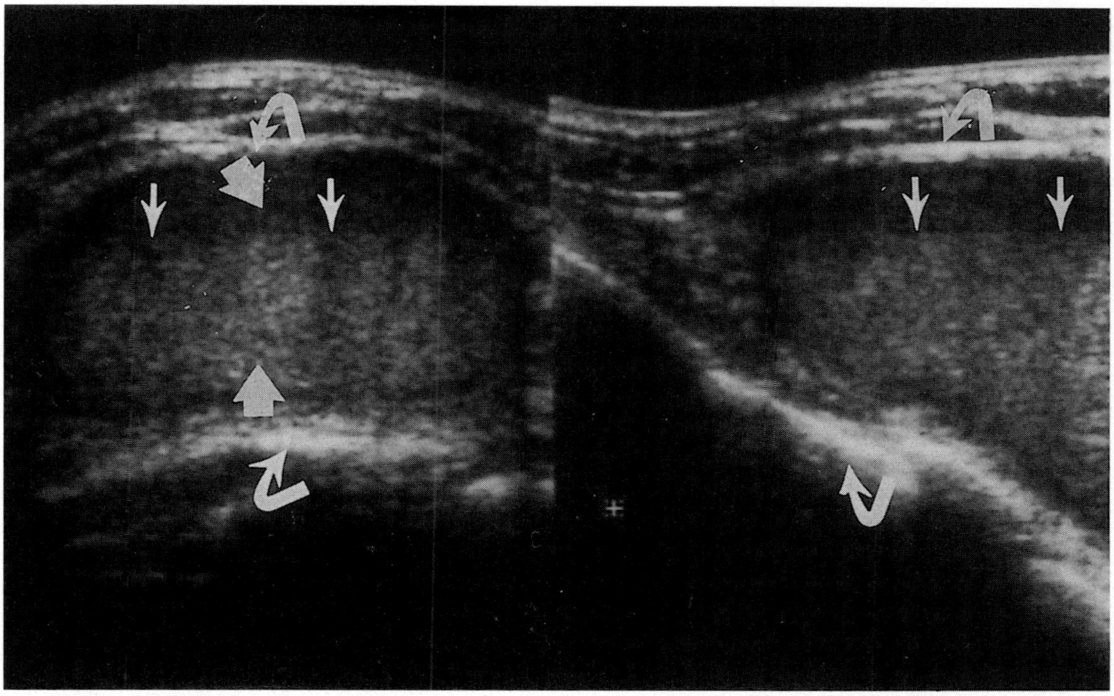

B

7–13. *(Continued)* (**B**) At ultrasound, a large fluid collection was noted (thick arrows) mimicking an implant in the side-by-side transverse and sagittal projections. The fluid collection is confined by the residual fibrous capsule that remained following the capsulotomy and explanation (curved arrows). A fluid level (straight arrows) is associated with layering of serosanguineous fluid consisting of different densities. Because of the acutely painful mass, three separate ultrasound-guided fine-needle aspirations were performed to relieve the symptoms as fluid continued to accumulate over a period of 2 weeks. The hematoma subsequently resolved and the patient has had no further symptoms.

As noted above, identification of intracapsular rupture by ultrasound can be difficult because of similar sonographic appearances of reverberation echoes, folds, and proteinaceous material as compared with the horizontal and curvilinear lines of the collapsed envelope and homogeneous internal echoes associated with intracapsular leakage.

Ultrasound evaluation of the posterior wall of the implant and the area behind the implant is limited in larger breasts with larger size implants.

When a woman has undergone direct silicone injections, the resultant characteristic echogenic pattern of free silicone obliterates all detail posteriorly, making it impossible to evaluate the breast sonographically. All detail of a coexistent breast mass in such a case would be lost because of the overlying echogenic snowstorm.

It is difficult to evaluate a new implant whenever there is residual silicone within the breast from an old rupture. Silicone granulomas from a prior rupture can overlie the new implant, with the resultant echogenic pattern obliterating portions of the new implant, making it difficult to evaluate for possible subsequent leakage.

Because the echogenic pattern of free silicone obliterates all detail posteriorly, the underlying structures are obliterated by the overlying echogenic snowstorm. Thus, there is a loss of anatomic detail of all the structures posterior to the free silicone, whether in the breast, axilla, or elsewhere.

Loss of integrity of the silicone envelope, allowing silicone gel to leak through but still remain confined to the fibrous capsule, may or may not produce enfolding of the envelope upon itself. Ultrasound cannot detect small amounts of free silicone confined between the fibrous capsule and the uncollapsed envelope. MR imaging, however, can detect small amounts of gel on the outer surface of the envelope. Both false-positive and false-negative cases, however, have been reported with sonography as well as with MR imaging in cases of intracapsular leakage.[27–29,35,36]

Both mammography and MR can image the outer saline and inner silicone compartments of double-lumen implants. Ultrasound, however, cannot usually distinguish the two separate envelope surfaces and therefore cannot evaluate for collapse of the outer saline implant.[28,120]

RELATIVE ADVANTAGES AND DISADVANTAGES OF ULTRASOUND AND MR IMAGING: OBSERVATIONS OF THE AUTHOR

Although no definitive statement can be made about the appropriate use(s) of ultrasound and/or MR imaging until more data are acquired, some observations can be made based on present knowledge and experience.

Because of its availability and relative low cost, ultrasound is our first choice after mammography whenever implant integrity is questioned. Ultrasound is reliable in detecting free silicone microglobules outside the confines of the fibrous capsule or within a thickened fibrous capsule in the case of a walled-off, confined leak. The echogenic snowstorm is a highly specific sign of free silicone microglobules within the tissues. In our experience the detection of the snowstorm is evidence enough of implant failure and the patient is referred to their plastic surgeon. Ultrasound (US) is less reliable, however, in differentiating the various patterns of internal echoes commonly seen with intact implants from the echoes representing intracapsular leaks. For this reason, whenever we suspect an intracapsular leak based on sonographic signs, we suggest obtaining an MR examination for confirmation. Thus we use US first and reserve MR imaging for selected cases.

The choice of modality (US vs. MRI) will depend on the experience of the individual radiologist and on the availability of US or MR equipment. Preferences of the plastic surgeon may influence choice as well.

Breast ultrasound is user dependent and less reproducible than MR imaging. The radiologist who performs the ultrasound examination records static images but should base the final interpretation on the "real-time" findings. It is not recommended that the radiologist make a diagnosis based on static images taken by someone else if the radiologist has not also personally performed the real-time ultrasound because the static images may not include the diagnostic areas.

Ultrasound seems to have an advantage over MR imaging in its ability to detect very small amounts of free silicone that are mixed within the tissues because of the characteristic echogenic snowstorm pattern. The "dilution" affect of partial volume averaging may limit detection of very small quantities of silicone mixed within the tissues by MR imaging.[93] Areas of lymphatic drainage in the infraclavicular and axillary regions can be evaluated with the real-time handheld transducer at the time breast ultrasound is performed. MR imaging performed for implant evaluation is limited to the area encompassed by the breast coil. The axillary and infraclavicular nodal areas are not routinely included within the field of the breast coil, and if a body coil is used, artifacts can degrade the image. Prior knowledge of the location of silicone in remote areas based on ultrasound findings is needed to customize the MR examination.

Ultrasound has a disadvantage in that the echogenic snowstorm obliterates all detail posteriorly. Therefore, MR imaging better displays the exact anatomic location of silicone and its relationship within muscle groups, around nerves, or within the chest wall.

Ultrasound cannot differentiate whether an isolated hypoechoic mass is a globule of silicone or a cyst. Ultrasound-guided aspiration biopsy yielding silicone gel may not be recognized by the cytopathologist because the gel is dissolved by the chemicals during the slide preparation. MR imaging can confirm silicone within an isolated hypoechoic "mass" detected by ultrasound utilizing silicone-selective pulse sequences.

Small fluid collections adjacent to an implant are not a sign of implant rupture.[27,60] Magnetic resonance can better image small fluid collections adjacent to an implant but these are also detectable with ultrasound.

CONCLUSION

Sonographic evaluation of implants is an important adjunct to mammography whenever implant rupture is suspected by history, physical examination, or equivocal mammographic findings.

Breast ultrasound is valuable in differentiating a bulge or hernia from a confined leak that may have similar mammographic features. Because of the signature echogenic pattern of free silicone microglobules mixed within tissues, ultrasound can reliably identify extracapsular leaks, even in remote locations or even with small quantities of free silicone. Ultrasound imaging can aid in the differentiation of a true breast lesion (cyst or solid) from a silicone granuloma. This is especially valuable whenever there is a question of carcinoma versus a silicone granuloma as a cause of a mass detected by mammography or by clinical breast examination. Likewise, ultrasound can differentiate pathologic adenopathy associated with disease from silicone lymphadenopathy. Ultrasound better defines the extent of a leak into the surrounding tissues than does mammography or clinical examination. Clinically occult ruptures, especially the intracapsular variety, or small leaks confined to the area of the implant are better detected by ultrasound than by mammography. Mammography, however, can better evaluate the integrity of the saline outer lumen of a double-lumen implant.[28]

There is a learning curve in recognizing the sonographic signs of implant failure.[25,70] To avoid false-positive findings, strict criteria must be followed. In the areas of the characteristic intense echogenic snowstorm with extracapsular silicone there is always accompanying loss of detail posteriorly, due to the echogenic "noise." Free silicone overlying the implant obliterates the echogenic breast-implant interface, with propagation of the echoes posteriorly. The echogenic area between the ribs must be distinguished from the echogenic pattern of free silicone in the tissues (Fig. 7–9D). The characteristic echogenic snowstorm is a signature that correlates closely with free silicone within the tissues and does not require confirmation with MR imaging. To avoid false-negatives, a meticulous search of the breast and axilla as well as a careful analysis of the implant is recommended. In the radiology literature a number of authors have reported false-positives and false-negatives (discovered at surgical explantation) based on preoperative predictions of implant rupture using ultrasound criteria.[25,28,35,36,39,83,121] Provided the correct techniques and criteria are adhered to, however, ultrasound is the method of choice for initial evaluation of implant integrity.[122]

Because of the overlap in the sonographic appearances of the echogenic areas within intact implants compared with the echogenicity associated with intracapsular leakage, confirmation with MR imaging may be valuable before recommending surgical explantation based on sonographic features alone. If intracapsular leakage is suspected by both ultrasound and MR imaging, a more confident diagnosis can be made.

Signs of Implant Rupture by Ultrasound

Reliable signs of intracapsular rupture:

- Double parallel lines, called "doublets" or "stepladder" sign
- Diffuse low-level echoes throughout the implant
- Bizarre patterns or complicated echoes occupying a large area of the implant
- Echogenic bands that cross the entire implant.

Reliable sign of extracapsular free silicone:

- Characteristic echogenic "snowstorm" with or without associated hypoechoic "masses."

Unreliable signs of implant rupture:

- Contour deformity (wrinkles, bulges, or hernias)
- Reverberation echoes within the anterior aspect of the implant
- Radial folds emanating from the implant surface, extending inward but not traversing the entire implant
- Periprosthetic fluid collections.

Hernias, bulges, wrinkles, radial folds, or associated seromas are not a sign of implant rupture.

The appropriate intervals for surveillance for implant failure and the choice of the most effective imaging modality or combination of modalities is as yet unknown. For women at the age appropriate for breast cancer screening, whenever implant failure is suspected, mammography supplemented with sonography constitutes the most cost-effective initial study, followed by MR imaging for findings that remain equivocal.[62] Ultrasound and MR imaging have an advantage over mammography or CT scanning for younger women because of the absence of ionizing radiation. In searching for occult implant failure, initial evaluation with ultrasound by an experienced radiologist may be more cost effective and convenient compared with MR imaging or CT scanning. Combining the imaging techniques of mammography, ultrasound, and MR imaging can improve accuracy in assessing ambiguous findings. Each imaging modality has advantages and limitations.

Ultrasound, after the initial learning curve, can reliably assess for possible implant rupture and can be used to reassure an anxious patient that her implants are intact, with a confidence level of 87%.[24]

Further studies with larger numbers of women are needed to better establish the sensitivity and specificity of mammography, ultrasound, and MR imaging to determine the most accurate and cost-effective methods for detecting free silicone in the tissues and occult tears in the silicone envelope.

REFERENCES

1. Deapen DM, Pike MC, Casagrande JT, et al. The relationship between breast cancer and augmentation mammoplasty: an epidemiologic study. *Plast Reconstr Surg.* 1986;77:361–367.
2. Heywang SH, Eiermann W, Bassermann R, et al. Carcinoma of the breast behind a prosthesis: comparison of ultrasound, mammography and MRI (case report). *Comput Radiol.* 1985;9:283–286.
3. Silverstein MJ, Gierson ED, Gamagami P, et al. Breast cancer diagnosis and prognosis in women augmented with silicone gel-filled implants. *Cancer.* 1990;66:97–101.
4. Gumucio CA, Pin P, Young VL, et al. The effect of breast implants on the radiographic detection of microcalcification and soft-tissue masses. *Plast Reconstr Surg.* 1989;84:772–778.
5. Mitnick JS, Harris MN, Roses DF. Mammographic detection of carcinoma of the breast in patients with augmentation prostheses. *Surg Gynecol Obstet.* 1989;168:30–32.
6. Young VL, Lund H, Destouet J, et al. Effect of breast implants on mammography. *South Med J.* 1991;84:707–714.
7. Berkel H, Birdsell DC, Jenkins H. Breast augmentation: a risk factor for breast cancer? *N Engl J Med.* 1992;326:1649–1653.
8. Kessler DA. Proceedings of the General and Plastic Surgery Devices Panel Meeting, U.S. Department of Health and Human Services Food and Drug Administration Hearings, February 18, 1992.
9. McGrath MH, Burkhardt BR. The safety and efficacy of breast implants for augmentation mammoplasty. *Plast Reconstr Surg.* 1984;74:550–566.
10. Blair P. A staff report. In: The FDA's Regulation of Silicone Breast Implants. Dec. 30, 1992. Washington, DC: U.S. Government Printing Office, 1993:24.
11. Kessler DA. The basis of the FDA's decision on breast implants. *N Engl J Med.* 1992;326:1713–1715.
12. vanNunen SA, Gatenby PA, Bosten A. Post-mammoplasty connective tissue disease. *Arthritis Rheum.* 1982;25:694–697.
13. Vargo J, Schumacher HR, Jimenez SA. Systemic sclerosis after augmentation mammoplasty with silicone implants. *Ann Intern Med.* 1989;111:377–382.

14. Sahn EE, Garen PD, Silver RM, Maize JC. Scleroderma following augmentation mammoplasty: report of a case and review of the literature. *Arch Dermatol.* 1990;126:1198–1202.
15. Handel N, Silverstein MJ, Gomagomi P, et al. Factors affecting mammographic visualization of the breast after augmentation mammaplasty. *JAMA.* 1992;268:1913–1917.
16. Eklund GA, Busby RC, Miller SH, et al. Improved imaging of the augmented breast. *AJR.* 1988;151:469–473.
17. Jackson VP, Rothchild PA, Kreipke DL, et al. The spectrum of sonographic findings of fibroadenoma of the breast. *Invest Radiol.* 1986;154:1196–1197.
18. Heywang SH, Lipsit ER, Glassman LM, et al. Specificity of ultrasonography in the diagnosis of benign breast masses. *J Ultrasound Med.* 1984;3:453–461.
19. Fornage B, Toubas O, Deshayes JL. Role of real-time sonography in the assessment of breast disease: a review of 200 cases. *Radiology.* 1985;148:813–817.
20. Dempsey PJ. The importance of resolution in clinical breast sonography. *Ultrasound Med Biol.* 1988;14:43.
21. Shestak KC, Ganott MA, Harris KM, et al. Breast masses in the augmentation mammoplasty patient: the role of ultrasound. *Plast Reconstr Surg.* 1993;92(2):209–216.
22. Leibman AJ, Kruse B. Breast cancer: mammographic and sonographic findings after augmentation mammoplasty. *Radiology.* 1990;174:195–198.
23. Ganott MA, Harris KM, Ilkhanipour ZS, et al. Augmentation mammoplasty: normal and abnormal findings by mammography and ultrasound. *Radiographics.* 1992;12:281–295.
24. Liston JC, Molata CM, Varma S, et al. The role of ultrasound imaging in the diagnosis of breast implant rupture: a prospective study. *Br J Plast Surg.* 1994;47:477–482.
25. Harris KM, Ganott MA, Shestak K, et al. Silicone implant rupture: detection with US. *Radiology.* 1993;187(3):761–768.
26. Skolnick AA. Ultrasound may help detect breast implant leaks. *JAMA.* 1992;267(6):786.
27. Gorcyzca DP, Sinha S, Ahn CY, et al. Silicone breast implants in vivo: MR imaging. *Radiology.* 1992;185:407–410.
28. Berg WA, Caskey CI, Hamper UM, et al. Single and double-lumen silicone breast implant integrity: prospective evaluation of MR and US criteria. *Radiology.* 1995;197:45–52.
29. Ahn CY, DeBruhl ND, Gorczyca DP, et al. Comparative silicone breast implant evaluation using mammography, sonography, and magnetic resonance imaging: experience with 59 implants. *Plast Reconstr Surg.* 1994;94(5):620–627.
30. Destouet JM, Monsees BS, Osar RF, et al. Screening mammography in 350 women with breast implants: prevalence and findings of implant complications. *AJR.* 1992;159: 973–978.
31. deCamera DL, Sheridan JM, Kammer BA. Rupture and aging of silicone gel breast implants (abstr). Plastic Surgery Forum: 60th Annual Scientific Meeting, Seattle, 1991. Arlington Heights, IL: American Society of Plastic and Reconstructive Surgeons; 1991:244.
32. Robinson OG Jr, Bradley EL, Wilson DS. Analysis of explanted silicone implants: a report of 300 patients. *Ann Plast Surg.* 1995;34(1):1–6.
33. Petro J, Klein S, Naizi Z, et al. Evaluation of ultrasound as a tool in the follow-up of patients with breast implants: a preliminary prospective study. *Ann Plast Surg.* 1994;32: 580–587.
34. Peters W, Keystone E, Smith D. The factors affecting the rupture of silicone-gel implants. *Ann Plast Surg.* 1994;32:449–451.
35. Caskey CI, Berg WA, Anderson ND, et al. Breast implant rupture: diagnosis with ultrasonography. *Radiology.* 1994;190: 819–823.
36. DeBruhl ND, Gorczyca DP, Ahn CY, et al. Silicone breast implants: US evaluation. *Radiology.* 1993;189:95–98.
37. Everson LI, Parontainen H, Detlie T, Stillman AE, et al. Diagnosis of breast implant rupture: imaging findings and relative efficacies of imaging techniques. *AJR.* 1994;163:57–60.
38. Rosculet KA, Ideka DM, Forrest ME, et al. Ruptured gel-filled silicone breast implants: sonographic findings in 19 cases. *AJR.* 1992;159:711–716.
39. Berg WA, Caskey CI, Hamper UM, et al. Diagnosing breast implant rupture with magnetic resonance imaging, ultrasound, and mammography. *Radiographics.* 1993;13:1323–1336.
40. Levine RA, Collins TL. Definitive diagnosis of breast implant rupture by ultrasonography. *Plast Reconstr Surg.* 1991;87:1126–1128.
41. vanWingerden JJ, vanStaden MM. Ultrasound mammography in prostheses-related breast augmentation complications. *Ann Plast Surg.* 1989;22:32–35.
42. Weizer G, Malone RS, Netscher DT, et al. Utility of magnetic resonance imaging and ultrasonography in diagnosing breast implant rupture. *Ann Plast Surg.* 1995;34:352–361.
43. vanWingerden JJ. Definitive diagnosis of breast implant rupture by ultrasonography: instrumentation and user requirements. *Plast Reconstr Surg.* 1989;6:1182.
44. Levine RA, Collins TL. Reply to vanWingerden correspondence. *Plast Reconstr Surg.* 1989;6:1183.
45. Barlow RE, Torres WE, Sones PJ Jr, et al. Sonographic demonstration of migrating silicone. *AJR.* 1980;135:170–171.
46. Kossovsky N, Papasian N. Mammary implants: clinical reviews. *J Appl Biomaterials.* 1992;3:239–242.
47. Brody GS. Fact and fiction about breast implant "bleed." *Plast Reconstr Surg.* 1977;60:615–616.
48. Rudolph R, Abraham J, Vecchione T, et al. Myofibroblasts and free silicone around breast implants. *Plast Reconstr Surg.* 1978;62:185–196.
49. Kossovsky N, Heggers JP, Robson MC. The bioreactivity of silicone. *CRC Crit Rev Biocompat.* 1987;3:53–85.
50. Callahan T. Rupture, tensile strength and liquid silicone bleed. Presented to the General and Plastic Surgery Devices Panel Meeting, U.S. Department of Health and Human Services Food and Drug Administration Hearing, February 18, 1992.
51. Braley S. The chemistry and properties of the medical-grade silicones. *J Macromol Sci Chem.* 1970;4:529–544.
52. Hester TR, Nahai F, Bostwick J, et al. A five-year experience with polyurethane-covered mammary prostheses for treatment of capsular contracture, primary augmentation mammoplasty, and breast reconstruction. *Clin Plast Surg.* 1988;15: 569–584.
53. Rheinstein PH, Hoffman FA. Update on breast implants. FDA perspective. *Am Fam Physician.* 1991;44:2227–2229.
54. Cole-Beuglet C, Schwartz G, Kurtz A, et al. Ultrasound mammography for the augmented breast. *Radiology.* 1983;146: 737–742.
55. Jellins J, Kossoff G, Reeve T. Detection and classification of liquid-filled masses in the breast by gray scale echography. *Radiology.* 1977;125:205–212.
56. *Table of Ultrasonic Properties.* Richmond, WA: Metro Tek; 1982.
57. Jensen SR, Mackey JK. Xeromammography after augmentation mammoplasty. *AJR.* 1985;144:629–633.
58. McNamara MP Jr, Kahn LA, Blum AH, et al. Mammographic evaluation of breast implants for rupture: radiologic-pathologic correlation. (Abstr RSNA). *Radiology.* 1992; 185(suppl):113.

59. Cohen IK, Scheflan M. The value of xeromammography for ruptured breast implants (letter). *Plast Reconstr Surg.* 1982; 69:898.
60. Berg WA, Caskey C, Chang BW, et al. Fluid collections around breast implants: prevalence and clinical implications (abstr). *AJR.* 1993;160:127.
61. Smith DS. False-positive radiographic diagnosis of breast implant rupture: report of two cases. *Ann Plast Surg.* 1985;14: 166–167.
62. Samuels JB, Rohrich RJ, Weatherall MD, et al. Radiographic diagnosis of breast implant rupture: current status and comparison of techniques. *Plast Reconstr Surg.* 1995;96:865–877.
63. Dowden RV. Definition of terms for describing loss of gel from breast implants (letter). *AJR.* 1993;160:1360.
64. Berg WA, Anderson ND, Zerhouni EA. MR imaging of the breast in patients with silicone breast implants: normal postoperative variants and diagnostic pitfalls. Pictorial essay. *AJR.* 1994;163:575–578.
65. Wilkerson P. The chemistry of silicone gel. Presented to the General and Plastic Surgery Devices Panel Meeting. U.S. Department of Health and Human Services Food and Drug Administration Hearings, February 18, 1992.
66. Barker DE, Retsky MI, Schultz A. "Bleeding" of silicone from bag-gel breast implants, and its clinical relation to fibrous capsule reaction. *Plast Reconstr Surg.* 1978;61:836– 841.
67. Mund DF. Farria DM, Gorczyca DP, et al. MR imaging of the breast in patients with silicone-gel implants: spectrum of findings. Pictorial essay. *AJR.* 1993;161:773–778.
68. Reynolds HE, Buckwalter KA, Jackson VP, et al. Comparison of mammography, sonography, and magnetic resonance imaging in the detection of silicone gel breast implant rupture. *Ann Plast Surg.* 1994;33:247–255.
69. Leibman AJ, Kossoff MB, Kruse BD. Intraductal extension of silicone from a ruptured breast implant. *Plast Reconstr Surg.* 1991;89:546–547.
70. Gorczyca DP, DeBruhl ND, Ahn CY, et al. Silicone breast implant ruptures in an animal model: comparison of mammography, MR imaging, US and CT. *Radiology.* 1994;190:227–232.
71. Anderson B, Hawtof D, Alani H, et al. The diagnosis of ruptured breast implants. *Plast Reconstr Surg.* 1989;84:903–907.
72. Theophelis LG, Stevenson TR. Radiographic evidence of breast implant rupture. *Plast Reconstr Surg.* 1986;78:673–675.
73. Herzog MP. Silicone granulomas: detection by ultrasonography (letter). *Plast Reconstr Surg.* 1989;84:856–857.
74. Shestak K. Personal communication. University of Pittsburgh Medical Center, Pittsburgh, PA, 1995.
75. Heggers JP, Kossovsky N, Parsons RW, et al. Biocompatibility of silicone implants. *Ann Plast Surg.* 1983;11:38–45.
76. Travis WD, Balogh K, Abraham J. Silicone granulomas: report of three cases and review of the literature. *Hum Pathol.* 1985;16:19–27.
77. Rivero MA, Schwartz D, Miles C. Silicone lymphadenopathy involving intramammary lymph nodes: a new complication of silicone mammaplasty. *AJR.* 1994;162:1089–1090.
78. Shermis RB, Adler DD, Smith DJ Jr, et al. Intraductal silicone secondary to breast implant rupture, an unusual mammographic presentation. *Breast Dis.* 1990;3:17–20.
79. Mendelson EB. Silicone implants present mammographic challenge. *Diagn Imaging Sept.* 1992;136:70–76.
80. Truang LD, Cartwright J Jr, Goodman MD, et al. Silicone lymphadenopathy associated with augmentation mammoplasty: morphologic features of nine cases. *Am J Surg Pathol.* 1988;12:484–491.
81. Huang TT, Blackwell SJ, Lewis SR. Migration of silicone gel after the "squeeze technique" to rupture a contracted breast capsule. *Plast Reconstr Surg.* 1978;60:277–280.
82. Gorczyca DP, DeBruhl ND, Mund DF, et al. Linguine sign at MR imaging: Does it represent the collapsed silicone implant shell? *Radiology.* 1994;191:576–577.
83. Malone RS, Schwartz LA Jr, Lambi N, et al. Pitfalls in US evaluation of patients with silicone gel breast implants. (Abstr RSNA). *Radiology.* 1994;193(suppl):177.
84. Rosenbaum JL, Bernardino ME, Thomas JL, et al. Ultrasonic findings in silicone-augmented breasts. *South Med J.* 1981; 74:455–458.
85. Lopez H. Personal communication. Center for Devices and Radiological Health, Food and Drug Administration, 1995.
86. Rubin JM, Helvie MA, Adler RS, et al. US appearance of ruptured silicone breast implants (letter). *Radiology.* 1994;190: 583–584.
87. Trahey GE, Feiburger PD, Ng G, et al. The impact of acoustic velocity variations on target detectability in ultrasound imaging of the breast. *Invest Radiol.* 1991;9:782–791.
88. Rubin JM, Adler RS, Bude RO, et al. Clean and dirty shadowing at US: a reappraisal. *Radiology.* 1991;181:231–236.
89. Harris KM, Ganott MA, Skolnick ML. Response to letter of Rubin JM (letter). *Radiology.* 1994;190:584.
90. Leibman AJ, Sybers R. Mammographic and sonographic findings after silicone injection. *Ann Plast Surg.* 1994;33: 412–414.
91. Cruz G, Gillooley JF, Waxman M. Silicone granuloma of the breast. *NY State J Med.* 1985;85:599–601.
92. McGunalge D. Gel recovery and extractable chemicals. Presented to the General and Plastic Surgery Devices Panel Meeting, U.S. Department of Health and Human Services Food and Drug Administration Hearings, February 18, 1992.
93. Davis P. Personal communication. University of Pittsburgh Medical Center, Pittsburgh, PA, 1995.
94. Hausner RJ, Schoen FJ, Mendez-Fernandez MA, et al. Migration of silicone gel to axillary lymph nodes after prosthetic mammoplasty. *Arch Pathol Lab Med.* 1981;105:371– 372.
95. Stavros AT, Thickman D, Rapp CL. Solid breast nodules: use of ultrasonography to distinguish between benign and malignant lesions. *Radiology.* 1995;196:123–134.
96. Steinbach BG, Hardt NS, Abbitt PL. Breast implants, common complications, and concurrent breast disease. *Radiographics.* 1993;13:95–118.
97. Fornage BD, Sneige N, Singletary S. Masses in breasts with implants: diagnosis with US-guided fine needle aspiration biopsy. *Radiology.* 1994;191:339–342.
98. Capozzi A, DuBou R, Pennisi VR. Distant migration of silicone gel from a ruptured breast implant. *Plast Reconstr Surg.* 1980;62:302–303.
99. Brem RF, Tempany CM, Zerhouni EA. MR detection of breast implant rupture. *J Comput Assist Tomogr.* 1992;16: 157–159.
100. Peters W. Silicone breast implants and autoimmune connective tissue disease. *Ann Plast Surg.* 1995;34:103–109.
101. Burkhardt B. Breast implants: a brief history of their development, characteristics, and problems. In: Gant TD, Vasconez LO, eds. *Postmastectomy Reconstruction,* 2nd ed. Baltimore: Williams and Wilkins; 1988:68–83.
102. Bostwick J III. *Aesthetic Breast Surgery in Plastic and Reconstructive Breast Surgery,* vol 1. St. Louis: Quality; 1990: 131–292.
103. Guthrie R, Schwartz G. *Reconstructive and Aesthetic Mammoplasty.* Philadelphia: Saunders; 1989:97–215.
104. Aposos J, Pope TL. Silicone granuloma following closed capsulotomy of mammary prostheses. *Ann Plast Surg.* 1985; 14:403– 406.

105. Baker JL, Bartles RJ, Douglas WM. Closed compression technique for rupturing a contracted capsule around a breast implant. *Plast Reconstr Surg.* 1976;58:137–141.
106. Gruber RP, Jones HW. Review of closed capsulotomy complications. *Ann Plast Surg.* 1981;6:271–275.
107. Nelson GD. Complications of closed compression after augmentation mammoplasty. *Plast Reconstr Surg.* 1980;66: 71–73.
108. Eisenberg HV, Bartels R. Rupture of a silicon bag-gel breast implant by closed compression capsulotomy. *Plast Reconstr Surg.* 1977;59:849–850.
109. Howes OR. Collapse of a breast implant after mammography (letter). *AJR.* 1990;154:1345.
110. Bassett LW, Brenner RJ. Considerations when imaging women with breast implants. *AJR.* 1992;159:979–981.
111. Peters W, Pugash R. Ultrasound analysis of 150 patients with silicone gel breast implants. *Ann Plast Surg.* 1993;31:7–9.
112. Conant EF, Piccoli CW, Forsberg F, et al. Intraoperative US guidance for removal of free silicone from ruptured breast implants. (Abstr RSNA). *Radiology.* 1994;193(suppl):178.
113. Caskey CI, Berg WA, Homper UM, et al. Detection of silicone after removal of ruptured breast implants: US evaluation. (Abstr RSNA). *Radiology.* 1994;193(suppl):178.
114. Mason J, Apisarnthararax P. Migratory silicone granuloma. *Arch Dermatol.* 1981;117:366–367.
115. Persillin ST, Vogler JB, Bozis PW, et al. Detection of migratory silicone pseudotumor with use of magnetic resonance imaging. *Mayo Clin Proc.* 1992;67:891–895.
116. Hayes MK, Gold RH, Bassett LW. Mammographic findings after the removal of breast implants. Pictorial essay. *AJR.* 1993;160:487–490.
117. Soo MS, Kornguth PJ, Goergiade GS, Sullivan DC. Seromas in residual fibrous capsules after explantation: mammographic and sonographic appearances. *Radiology.* 1995;194: 863–866.
118. Stewart NR, Monsees BS, Destouet JM, et al. Mammographic appearance following implant removal. *Radiology.* 1992;185:83–85.
119. Mendelson EB. Evaluation of the post-operative breast. *Radiol Clin North Am.* 1992;185:83–85.
120. Stomper PC, Mazurchuk RV, Tsangaris TN. MRI appearance of double-lumen saline-silicone breast implants. *Breast Dis.* 1994;7:53–57.
121. Palmon LU, Foshager MC, Everson LI, et al. US of ruptured breast implants: sensitivity of snowstorm appearance. (Abstr RSNA). *Radiology.* 1994;193(suppl):177.
122. vanWingerden JJ. Letter. *N Engl J Med.* 1993;328:733.

8

Computed Tomography Evaluation of the Failing Implant

LENORE I. EVERSON

In the early 1990s the Food and Drug Administration (FDA), followed closely by the media, began questioning the safety of silicone gel implants for breast augmentation. The literature reported sporadic reports of patients developing autoimmune-like symptoms and, in some cases, full-blown autoimmune disease in patients who had breast augmentation with silicone gel implants.[1–6] Other complications that were associated with silicone breast implants included rupture and leakage, fibrous contracture, and localized pain. The intense interest in the potential complications of silicone breast implants led many plastic surgeons and radiologists to further investigate the roles of the different imaging modalities in evaluation of silicone breast implants. Mammography, ultrasonography, magnetic resonance (MR) imaging, and computed tomography (CT) were evaluated and compared in their abilities to detect silicone implant ruptures.

Computed tomography in the evaluation of the integrity of silicone breast implants was first investigated in the late 1980s. Two case reports were published in 1988 describing the detection of silicone implant rupture by CT. Scott et al[7] described the incidental detection of a silicone breast implant rupture on a patient being imaged for an unrelated condition. The authors described CT as clearly depicting a collapsed implant envelope. A second case report of CT evaluation of a collapsed silicone implant was mentioned by Anderson et al[8] in 1988, when discussing breast implant evaluation by clinical examination.[9,10] In spite of these case reports, most radiologists and plastic surgeons elected not to use CT as a method for implant evaluation because of the radiation exposure. The vast majority of breast implant patients are young women who seek augmentation for cosmetic reasons, and the radiation exposure was felt to be unwarranted.

It was in our quest to find the best modality available to evaluate the integrity of silicone breast implants that we felt the need in the early 1990s to revisit the issue of using CT to evaluate breast implant integrity. To our surprise, and to the surprise of others, CT was both sensitive and specific in the evaluation of silicone prostheses.[11] Other studies confirmed our results. In an animal study comparing the different imaging modalities, Gorczyca et al[12] found that CT could detect intracapsular implant ruptures as well as MR imaging. There was no statistically significant difference between CT or MR imaging in the detection of intracapsular silicone implant rupture. Extracapsular implant ruptures were not evaluated in this study.[12]

Prior to the studies of CT imaging of silicone implants, there were early investigations of using CT to evaluate for breast tumors in the 1970s when a prototype CT unit of the breasts was developed. However, these early units demonstrated very early, poor spatial resolution and poor soft tissue differentiation. The only successful results were reported by Chang et al[13,14] when they began using contrast-enhanced CT scans to evaluate for breast disease. Chang's original study was performed in 1978 using a General Electric CT/M dedicated breast CT scanner. Thirty-one malignant lesions were detected in 28 patients from a pool of 655 patients. All 31 lesions were histologically proven.

Patients at this time were placed prone in a canvas table containing an aperture for the dependent breast. The breast was suspended in position within a water bath. Scans were performed from the chest wall to the nipple without contrast. Subsequently the patient was placed in the sitting position and received an infusion of 300 mL of diatrizoate meglumine and then repositioned in the water bath and rescanned. The carcinomas that were detected measured from 2 mm in size to 9 cm. These breast cancers were detected because the cancers demonstrated early enhancement over the fibroglandular tissue. This enhancement was measured by taking the difference between CT measurements of the fibroglandular tissue pre- and postcontrast. The average contrast enhancement at that time for proven cancers was 34, or 6.8% increase in density. The results of this study were promising. The problem with the CT scanning, however, was that early enhancement was not specific for breast cancer. Many benign breast diseases such as fibroadenomas, hyperplasia without atypia, inflammation, and sclerosing adenosis also showed early contrast enhancement. These results parallel the results now being demonstrated in contrast-enhanced magnetic resonance of the breast. That is, the enhancement is related to angiogenesis of blood cells that can be developed because of carcinoma, but also can be developed for other inflammatory problems in the breast, and although sensitive for breast disease, it is not very specific.

Subsequently, Gisvold et al[15] at the Mayo clinic examined 724 patients using physical examination, mammography, and CT using a scanner designed for evaluation of the breast. Sixty malignant lesions were found. Ten percent were missed by mammography, 32% were missed by non–contrast-enhanced CT, and 8% by both. Among the cases where CT was supplemented by 50 mL of 75% contrast material, only 16% of the lesions were missed by CT. Among cases where 300 mL of 30% contrast materials were used, only 5% of the lesions were missed by CT. Twenty-two percent of the malignant lesions detected in both series were occult. It is also important to note that, of the 45 benign lesions suspected, 68% were suspicious by mammography and 56% with CT.

The characteristics of malignant breast tumors on CT mirrored those of conventional screening mammography. Breast tumors were associated with soft tissue masses, usually with irregular borders that could or could not be associated with calcifications. Tumors were also represented by clusters of calcifications, asymmetric density, and architectural distortion. However, benign lesions could and did mimic the physical appearance of tumors as well as the enhancement characteristics of tumor, and a definitive diagnosis could not be made by imaging alone. Although CT screening of the breast could diagnose malignant lesions with a high degree of accuracy, it was not significantly better than mammography. There were too many false-positive results with a variety of benign lesions, and it was decided that CT was not suitable for routine screening of asymptotic women, especially because of the high cost, risk of contrast material infusion, and risk of radiation exposure. Following this study, very little work was done with CT in the diagnosis of breast cancers by diagnostic radiologists, and most of the subsequent studies on CT evaluation of the breast was done by radiation oncologists.

Although CT evaluations of the breasts failed as a diagnostic examination for early breast cancers, the excellent visualization of the chest wall and axilla made it an excellent modality for evaluation of local and regional breast cancer recurrences. The first reports of this usage were made by Lindfors et al[16] in 1985. They found that CT was superior to physical examination in evaluation of regional and local breast cancer recurrence. Of the 33 patients seen with clinical evidence of chest wall recurrence, 16 (48%) had areas of disease visible by CT that were not clinically expected. Although mammography can be helpful in evaluation of recurrence in the region of lumpectomy, it is somewhat limited because of the reactive tissue from the surgery and the radiation. In addition, mammography cannot visualize the chest wall and it is limited in its visualization of the axilla. These areas both were better evaluated by CT. Several reports followed this initial study, demonstrating similar results, and CT soon became a staple of radiotherapy treatment planning for breast cancer.

In summary, the history of CT evaluation of breast disease began in the late 1970s. It was, and is still considered, not specific enough in the evaluation of early breast cancer detection to justify the cost and radiation exposure. However, it has excelled as a modality for preradiation treatment of breast cancers and for follow-up or recurrence. It is therefore mostly used as a treatment modality in breast disease by the therapeutic radiation oncologists. The remainder of this chapter describes our experiences in the evaluation of silicone breast implants using CT.

■ CT IMAGING TECHNIQUES

Patient positioning is important for acquiring optimal CT images of the breast. However, the patient must also be comfortable on the CT gantry so that motion is kept to a minimum. During our initial studies, we tried to mimic the position of the MR imaging. The patients were originally placed prone in the CT gantry, but this position was too cumbersome. Pillows had to be placed around the patients breasts, and it was too difficult to maintain this position for very long. Subsequently, the patients were placed in the gantry supine, similar to how most radiologists scan patients for a regular chest CT examination. This position assured us of minimal motion artifact and was much more comfortable for our patients. Images obtained in this position were diagnostic. Axial 5 mm contiguous images are obtained with 5 mm collimation. No intravenous contrast is used.

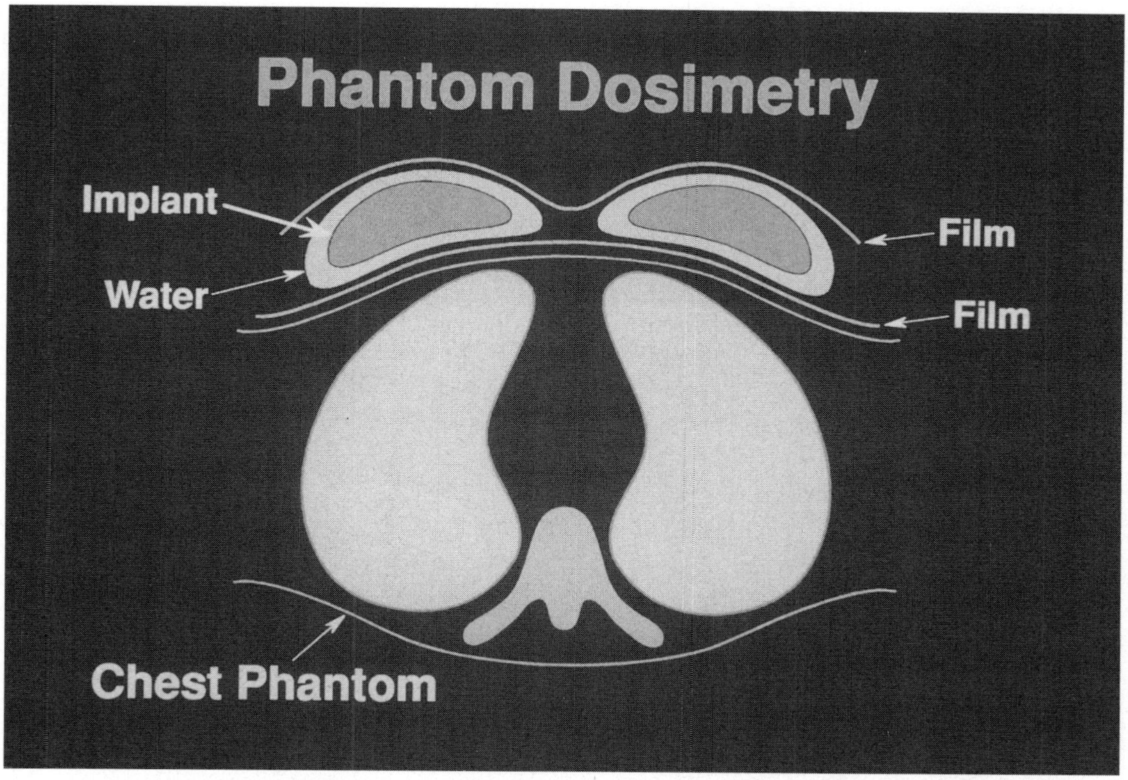

Figure 8–1. Phantom dosimetry was performed to mimic a patient with subglandular silicone breast implants. Standard CT of the chest with 280 mAs and 120 kVp yields a mean glandular dose of 1.15 cGy. Lowering the mAs alone to 85 mAs yielded a significantly lower glandular dose of 0.350 cGy, similar to the mean glandular dose in a two-view screening mammogram.

We initially used the same parameters as we used for CT scanning of the chest: mAs of 280 and a kVp of 120. To reduce both the radiation and the cost, we limited the examination to the region of the breasts and axilla, unless there was a reason to perform an examination of the entire chest. We also explored ways to reduce the mean glandular dose that was absorbed. Experimental CT studies were performed on a humanoid phantom (Rando, Alderson Research Lab CT) modified to contain silicone breast implants. The mean glandular dosage to the phantom was measured by film dosimetry (Fig. 8–1). The average glandular dosage when an mAs of 280 was used was 1.15 cGy. When the mAs was reduced to 85, the glandular dose was reduced to 0.350 cGy. This dose is equivalent to a two-view screening mammogram.

Although the dose was now felt to be acceptable, there was still a question of whether the images would be diagnostic. Therefore, 15 patients agreed to be imaged twice by CT, once with the regular parameters and then with the low-dose parameters. Although some resolution was lost, the images had enough adequate information for interpretation. We currently use the lower dosage of radiation for CT imaging of women with silicone implants (Fig. 8–2).

■ CT IMAGING FINDINGS

An intact silicone implant, either subglandular or subpectoral in location, is characterized by a homogeneous, gray density with a surrounding high-density ring. The ring was felt to represent the envelope of the implant with calcific deposits. This was later proven by evaluating a new implant by CT scanning, which showed the envelope to be not visible (Fig. 8–3). This correlates well with the literature.[6]

Signs of intracapsular implant rupture on CT consist of collapse of the white ring into the silicone gel center (Fig. 8–4). An irregular contour of the implants raises suspicion of

(text continues on page 117)

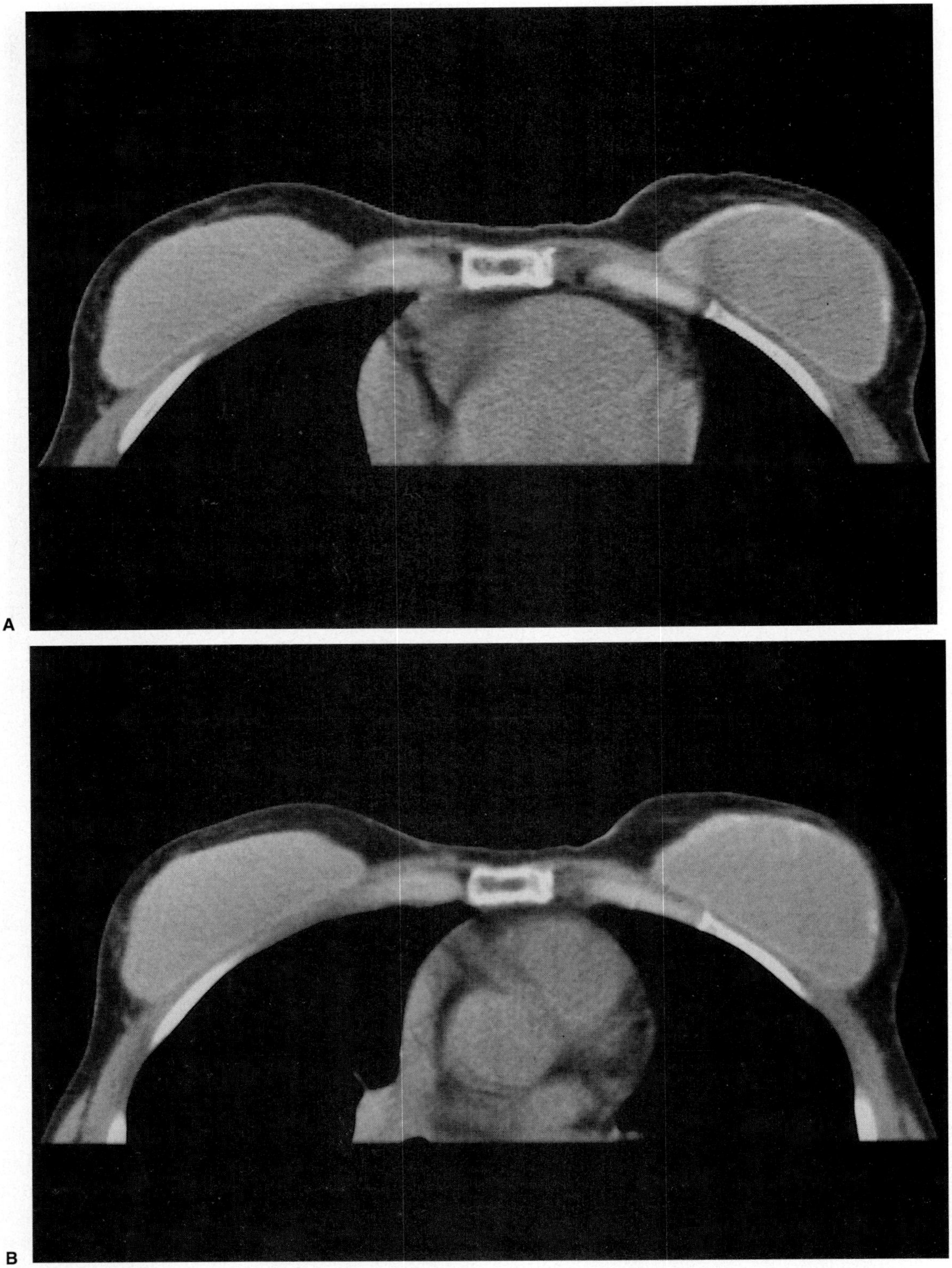

Figure 8–2. (**A**) CT scan of a patient with subglandular, single-lumen, silicone implants. Normal parameters of a 280 mAs and 120 kVp were used. Note the distinct white ring surrounding the implant, which represents the implant envelope with calcific deposits. (**B**) CT scan of the same patient as in **A**, but with an mAs of 85. The envelope ring is less distinct, but still is of diagnostic quality.

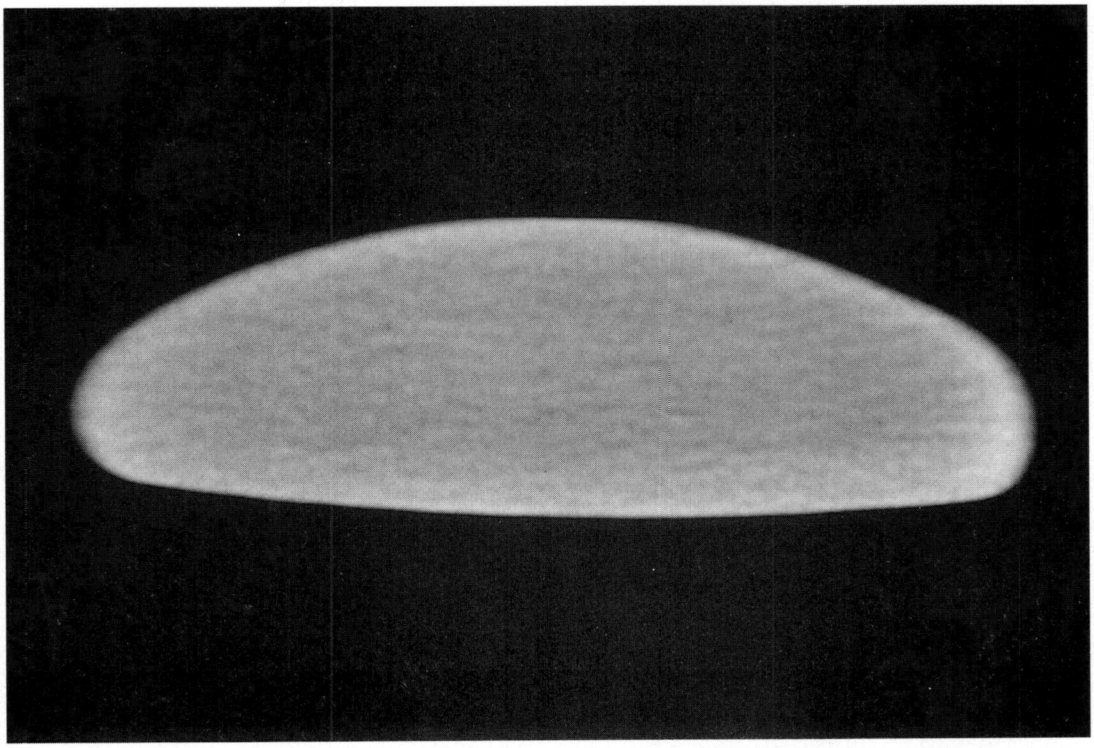

Figure 8–3. CT scan of single-lumen, silicone implant. No high-density ring is present. The implant needs to be in vivo for the calcium deposits to settle on the envelope.

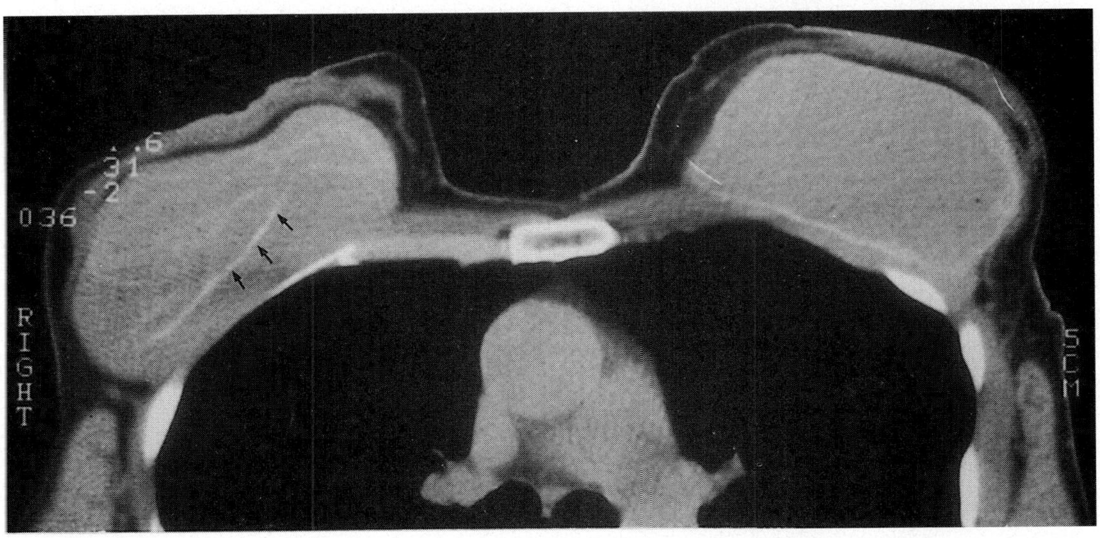

A

Figure 8–4. (**A**) CT scan of bilateral, single-lumen implants. The right breast demonstrates an intracapsular rupture, with a "linguine sign" similar to the MR appearance of intracapsular rupture. *(continued)*

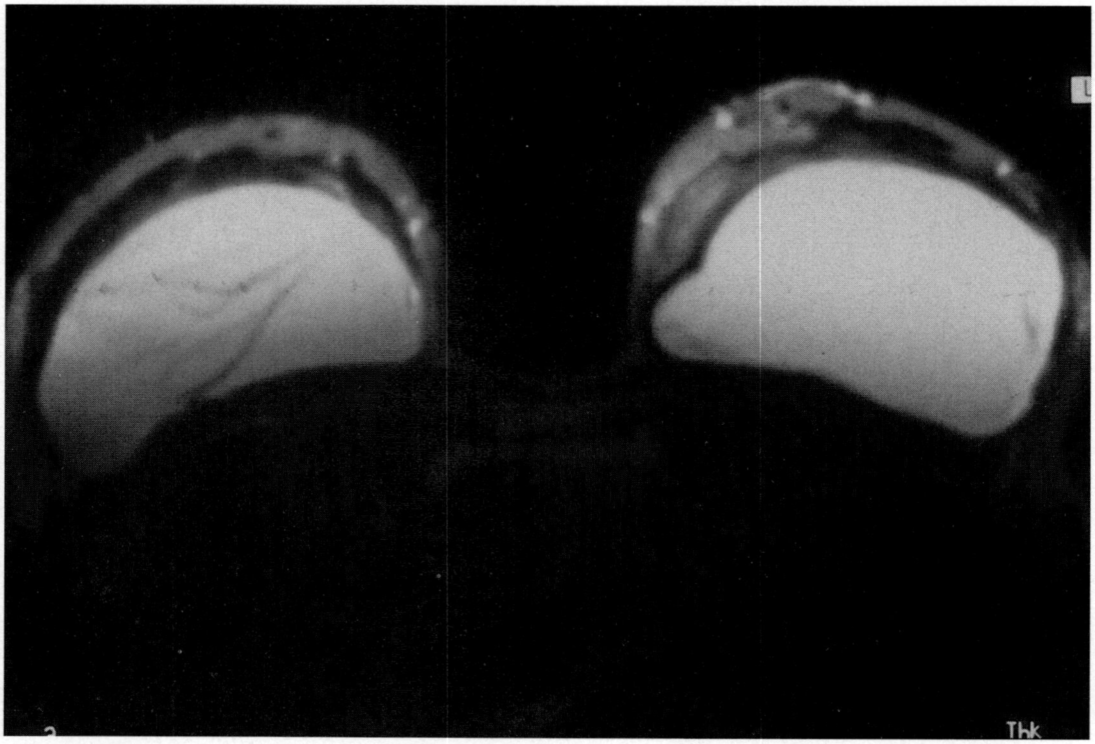

B

8–4. ***(Continued)*** (**B**) MR demonstrating the classic "linguine sign" of intracapsular rupture on the same patient as in **A**. Note also on MR the continuous dark signal fibrous capsule that restricts silicone gel migration.

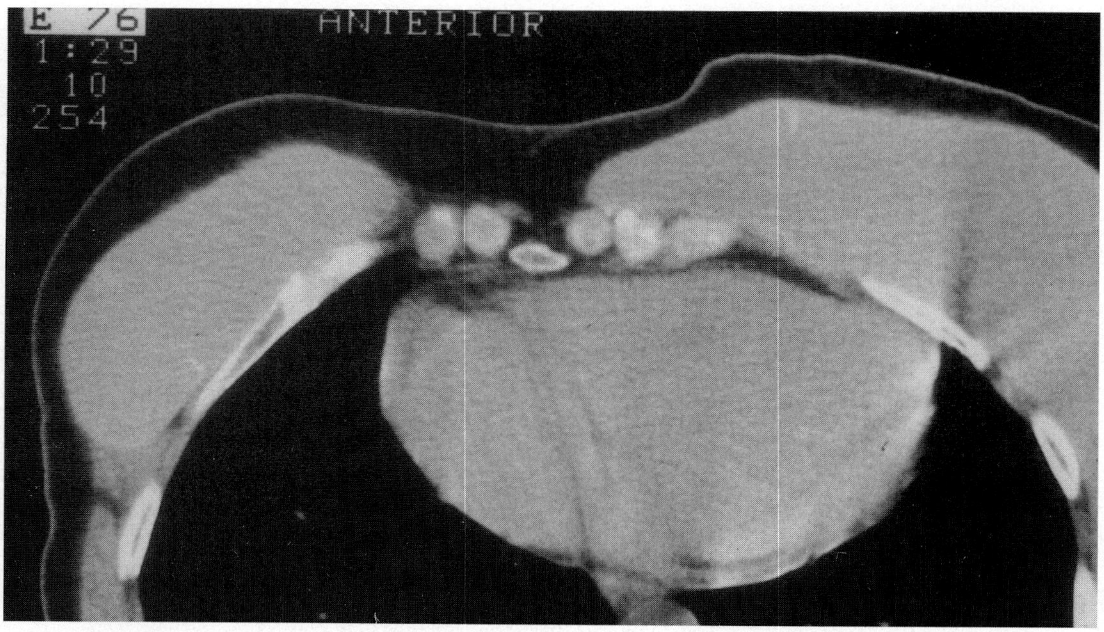

Figure 8–5. Extracapsular rupture on the left breast implant. Note the contour deformity with axillary migration of silicone gel.

A

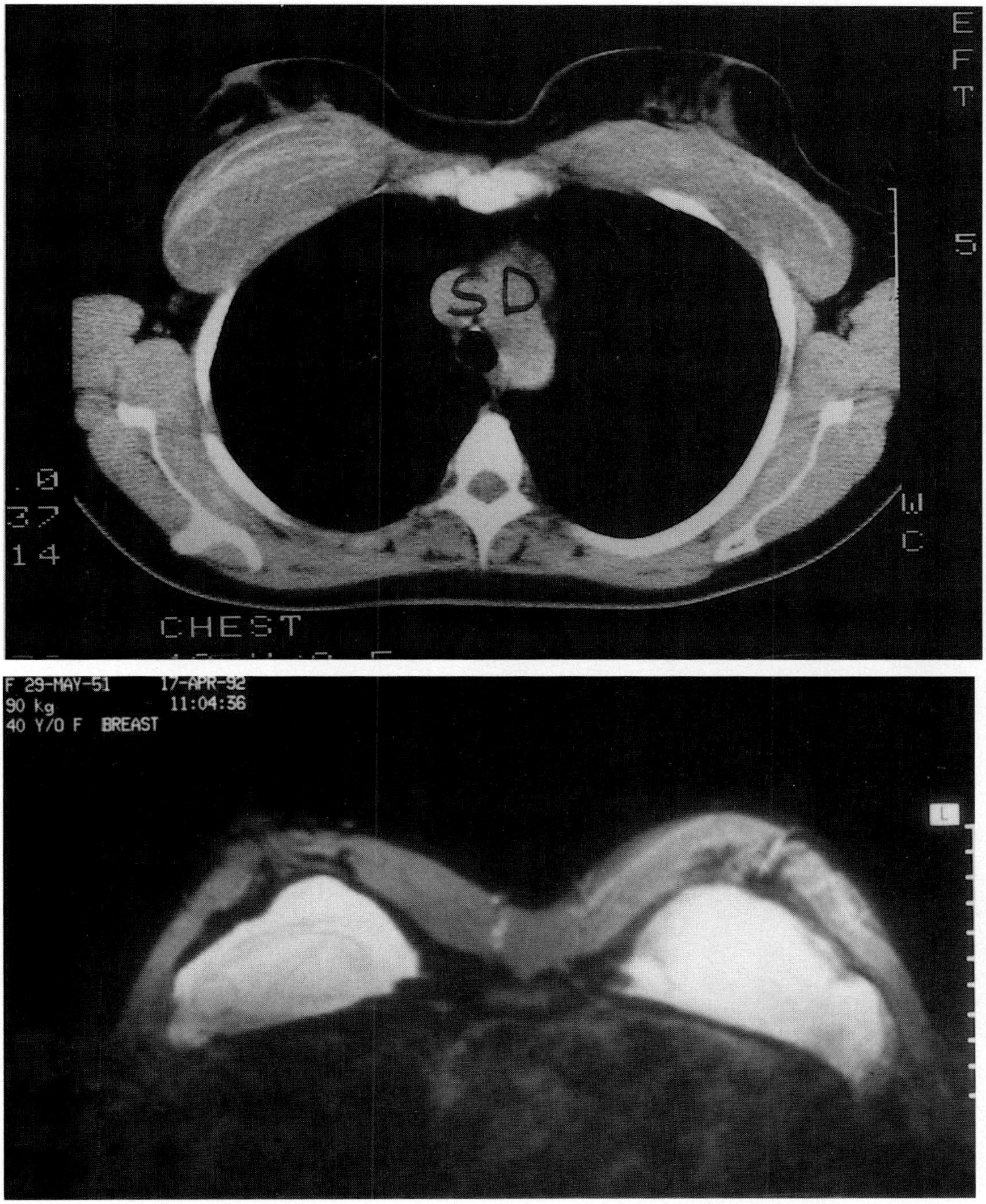

B

Figure 8–6. (**A**) CT scan of a patient with an intracapsular rupture on the right implant and extracapsular rupture on the left. (**B**) MR of the implants of the patient in **A**. Note that, on MR, the fibrous ring was more easily seen. The collapsed implant envelope, however, is more easily seen in CT.

implant rupture, but may also represent an advanced Baker's capsulitis.

Extracapsular rupture can be difficult to identify because of the poor soft tissue differentiation on CT imaging. It is not, however, impossible. The collapse of the white ring may or may not be present, but it is in the evaluation of the implant contour that the diagnosis can be made. Loss of the normal contour, especially in the region of the axilla, is the most reliable sign (Figs. 8–5 and 8–6). In these cases, searches in other areas of the chest are important also for migrating silicone (Fig. 8–7).

Double-lumen implants are very difficult to evaluate. CT can demonstrate the two lumens with the implant and, with a little history, it is possible to work out a correct diagnosis. In

A

B

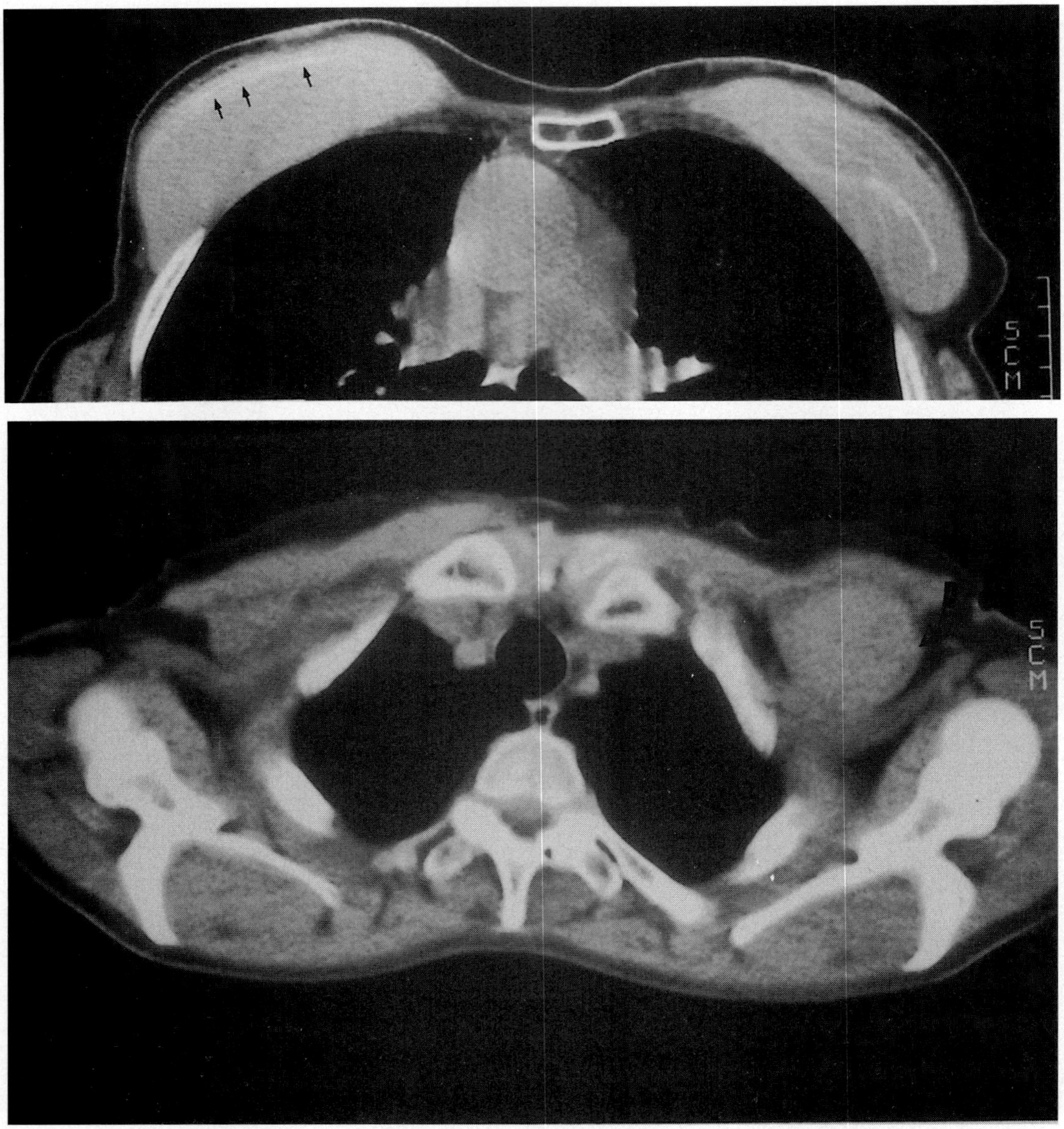

Figure 8–7. (**A**) CT scan of a patient with a noncollapsed rupture on the right and typical "linguine sign," or intracapsular rupture, on the left. The MR was not diagnostic because of the motion artifact. (**B**) A siliconoma seen on the CT scan in the left axilla was also identified only on CT in this examination.

Table 8–1. Efficacy of CT and MR in the Detection of Silicone Breast Implant Rupture

Imaging Study	*No. of Implants*	*True Positive*	*True Negative*	*False Negative*	*False Positive*	*Sensitivity*	*Specificity*
CT	141	40	77	11	13	78	86 Accuracy 83%
MR	141	46	77	5	13	90	86 Accuracy 87%

Note findings at surgery, which were used as the gold standard.

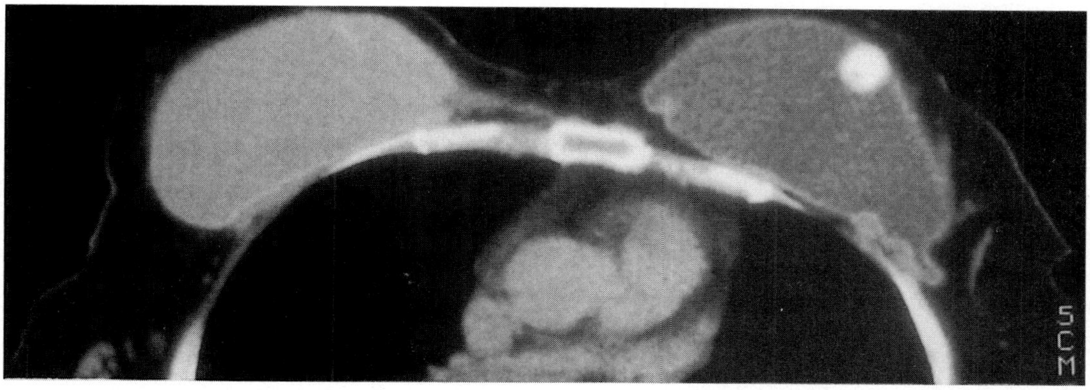

Figure 8–8. Example of intact silicone implant on the right and a saline implant, with its characteristic anterior valve, on the left.

the examples given, the first set of double-lumen implants shows the standard type, with a silicone lumen contained within a saline outer lumen (Fig. 8–8). When we were informed by the surgeon that there should be at least 20 to 30 cc of outer lumen saline, we felt that the image was inconsistent, and we surmised that this was a cause of outer-lumen rupture. Surgical explantation proved us right; however, this evaluation was based mostly on luck and not on the image.

Overall, CT evaluation of breast implant integrity proved to be quite good. Seventy-six patients had both MR and CT imaging of their implants prior to explantation. The results are summarized in Table 8–1.

■ DISCUSSION

The CT evaluation of silicone implants can be an alternative for patients who cannot have an MR evaluation of their implants. MR has its technical limitations, such as patient size, motion artifact, and chemical-shift artifacts. It is also limited by patients who are too claustrophobic to proceed with the examination. It is also important to note that except in major cities, dedicated breast coils for breast imaging are not readily available. Imaging without a dedicated breast coil yields information that is questionable at best.

The CT signs of implant collapse, such as collapse of the white ring into the gray density center in intracapsular rupture, or abnormal implant contours, such as in extracapsular rupture, mimic those seen on MR. Obviously CT does not have the degree of soft tissue differentiation or the ability to image in three planes with equal resolution that MR does, but in many cases this is not necessary. Furthermore, areas that cause difficulty on MR, such as capsule calcifications, are easily evaluated on CT (Fig. 8–9).

The fine detail imaging that is needed to visualize noncollapsed ruptures can also be detected on CT. The implant envelope represented by the fine white ring seen below the ho-

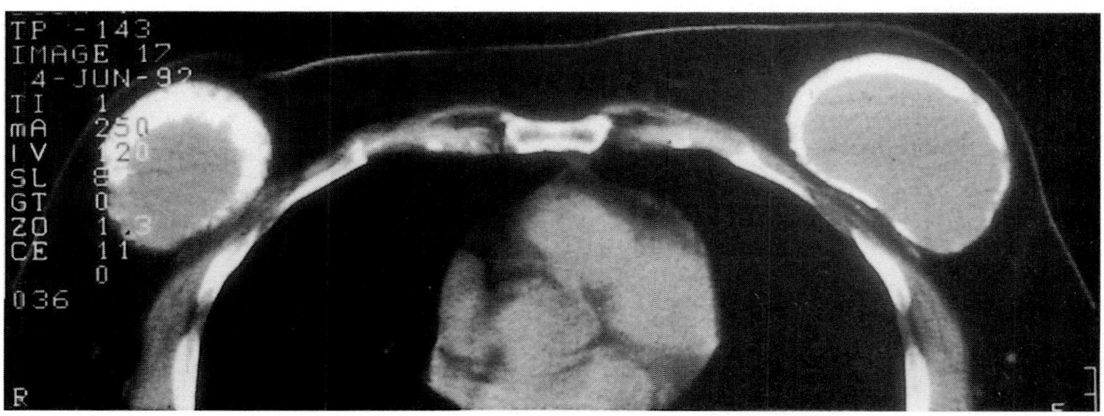

Figure 8–9. Example of heavily calcified implant envelopes in a patient who has had these implants for over 20 years.

mogeneous signal of the silicone gel and breast parenchyma is comparable to what is seen on an MR image. These types of ruptures cannot be detected on mammography and are difficult to see on sonography.

Radiation exposure from CT scanning, although less of a problem now than it was before, is still a drawback. For patients who have no alternative, however, the small radiation dose of a CT scan is felt to be acceptable. Compared with the risk of possibly not detecting a ruptured silicone implant, the radiation dosage should be considered a negligible risk. Cost is also a drawback, and many insurance companies refuse to cover the costs of either CT or MR imaging for evaluation of silicone breast implants. The patients are told that the insurance company will pay for the removal of the implants, but not for any associated imaging. The rationale here is not easily understood, and, in our viewpoint, a rupture should be verified prior to unnecessary surgery, especially if the patient is not experiencing any problems.

In conclusion, MR remains the best modality to evaluate breast implant integrity. CT scanning, however, remains a viable alternative and should be used in cases where MR is not possible or not advisable.

REFERENCES

1. Yoshida SH, Chang CC, Teuber SS, et al. Silicon and silicone: theoretical and clinical implications of breast implants. *Regul Toxicol Pharmacol.* 1993;17:3–18.
2. Silver RM, Sahn EE, Allen JA, et al. Demonstration of silicon in sites of connective-tissue disease in patients with silicone-gel breast implants. *Arch Dermatol.* 1993;129:63–68.
3. Varga J, Schumacher HR, Jimenez SA. Systemic sclerosis after augmentation mammoplasty with silicone implants. *Ann Intern Med.* 1989;111(5):377–383.
4. Weiner SR, Paulus HE. Chronic arthropathy occurring after augmentation mammaplasty. *Plast Reconstr Surg.* 1986;77(2): 185–187.
5. Sergott TJ, Limoli JP, Baldwin CM, et al. Human adjuvant disease, possible autoimmune disease after silicone implantation: a review of the literature, case studies, and speculation for the future. *Plast Reconstr Surg.* 1986;78:104–114.
6. Kaiser W, Biesenbach G, Stuby U, et al. Human adjuvant disease: remission of silicone induced autoimmune disease after explantation of breast augmentation. *Ann Rheum Dis.* 1990; 49:927–938.
7. Scott IR, Müller NL, Fitzpatrick DG, et al. Ruptured breast implant: computed tomographic and mammographic findings. *J Can Assoc Radiol.* 1988;39:152–154.
8. Andersen B, Hawtof D, Alani H, et al. The diagnosis of ruptured breast implants. *Plast Reconstr Surg.* 1989;84(6):903–907.
9. Silverstein MJ, Handel N, Gamagami P, et al. Breast cancer diagnosis and prognosis in women following augmentation with silicone gel-filled prostheses. *Eur J Cancer.* 1992;28(2,3): 635–640.
10. Leibman AJ, Kruse B. Breast cancer: mammographic and sonographic findings after augmentation mammoplasty. *Radiology.* 1990;174:195–198.
11. Everson LI, Parantainen H, Detlie T, et al. Diagnosis of breast implant rupture: imaging findings and relative efficacies of imaging techniques. *AJR.* 1994;163:57–60.
12. Gorczyca DP, DeBruhl ND, Ahn CY, et al. Silicone breast implant ruptures in an animal model: comparison of mammography, MR imaging, US, and CT. *Radiology.* 1994;190:227–232.
13. Chang CHJ, Sibala JL, Fritz SL, et al. Computed tomographic evaluation of the breast. *AJR.* 1978;131:459–464.
14. Chang CHJ, Nesbit DE, Fisher DR, et al. Computed tomographic mammography using a conventional body scanner. *AJR.* 1982;138:553–558.
15. Gisvold JJ, Reese DF, Karsell PR. Computed tomographic mammography (CTM). *AJR.* 1979;133:1143–1149.
16. Lindfors KK, Meyer JE, Busse PM, et al. CT evaluation of local and regional breast cancer recurrence. *AJR.* 1985;145: 833–837.

9

Magnetic Resonance Imaging of the Failing Implant

DAVID P. GORCZYCA

■ HISTORY OF BREAST MR IMAGING

Magnetic resonance (MR) imaging of silicone breast implants was first investigated in the early 1990s. As an increasing number of case reports of potential complications from silicone breast implants were made public, studies evaluating the ability of MR imaging to determine the integrity of silicone breast implants intensified. These complications included rupture and leakage, fibrous or calcific contracture, localized pain, paresthesias, and possibly even generalized autoimmune disorders.[1–3] The Plastic Surgery Department in conjunction with the Department of Radiological Sciences at UCLA were the first to systematically investigate the potential role of MR imaging in patients with silicone breast implants. Patients with silicone implants who were scheduled for implant explantation were enrolled in a study to determine if MR imaging of the breast could reliably determine if an implant was ruptured. The results of the MR imaging of the breast were not initially used in the decision of whether a patient should have her implants surgically removed.

In 1992 Gorczyca et al[4] published the first major prospective study on MR imaging of silicone breast implants, showing that MR imaging of silicone implants could detect implant ruptures with a sensitivity of 76% and specificity of 97%. Furthermore, this study showed that the majority of implant ruptures were intracapsular ruptures that were not detectable by mammography. The MR imaging finding of implant rupture described by Gorczyca et al as the "linguine sign," which represents the collapsed implant shell floating within the silicone gel, is commonly used today. Dedicated MR breast coils and optimized MR sequences have improved the sensitivity and specificity of MR imaging to detect silicone implant rupture to greater than 90%.[5–7] MR imaging of silicone breast implants is commonly used in clinical settings where it is important to determine if the silicone implant is ruptured prior to appropriate treatment.

Prior to the studies of MR imaging of silicone implants, MR imaging of the breast was investigated as a potential imaging modality to differentiate benign from malignant breast tumors. These studies were conducted in the mid-1980s.[8–13] The initial MR imaging studies were based primarily on breast tissue characterization using T1-weighted and T2-weighted images but failed to identify any useful role.[8–13] In 1986 Heywang et al[14] first applied the use of a MR contrast agent to determine if this would improve differentiating benign from malignant lesions. The results were encouraging, with most malignant tumors showing enhancement while most benign breast lesions did not enhance. Other investigators confirmed the initial experience with MR contrast agents in breast lesions and further contributed their experience and expertise to MR imaging of the breast.[15–21] However, more recent studies have shown that there is an overlap of enhancement patterns of benign and malignant tumors.[22]

Despite the inability of contrast-enhanced breast MR imaging to clearly differentiate benign from malignant tumors, there are several potential roles of MR imaging of breast tumors. MR imaging of the breast may detect lesions not imaged by mammography because of dense breast tissue, an indication that is particularly relevant for younger women. I include women who have had silicone oil injected

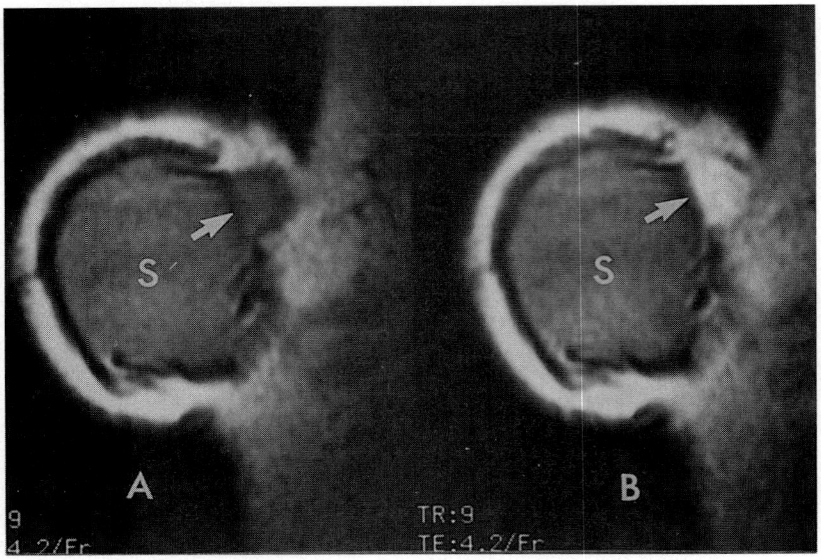

Figure 9–1. Dynamic contrast enhanced MR of infiltrating ductal carcinoma in patient with silicone implant (S); a 48-year-old woman with history of right mastectomy for breast carcinoma. Breast reconstruction was performed with a silicone implant (S). Patient presented with a palpable mass behind implant. Mammography showed no evidence of a mass. Sagittal T1-weighted dynamic MR image prior to (**A**) and 1 minute after (**B**) IV gadolinium shows rapid intense contrast uptake of lesion (arrows).

directly into their breasts for breast augmentation and women with silicone breast implants in the category of women with dense breasts (Fig. 9–1). By better depicting the abnormality, MR imaging could provide a better evaluation of the extent of lesions, including multiple foci of carcinoma in the same breast. Due to its high sensitivity, the fact that most postsurgical changes do not enhance after one year, and the limitations of mammography following lumpectomy, MR imaging will also probably have an important role in the surveillance of women who have had breast-conserving surgery for cancer. Large multicenter studies are under way to further define the role of MR imaging in evaluation of breast tumors.

The remainder of this chapter discusses the MR technique and MR findings of normal and failing silicone implants. Tumor detection is further discussed in Chapter 11.

■ EQUIPMENT

High field strength magnets of 1.0 to 1.5 T are preferred when imaging patients with silicone breast implants because of the ability to use MR sequences that can more readily suppress or emphasize the signal from water, fat, or silicone. In addition, the high field strength magnets produce additional signal allowing detection of more subtle signs of implant ruptures. Lower field strength magnets have been successfully used in imaging patients with silicone breasts; however, the number of different MR sequences available to suppress or emphasize the signal from water, fat, or silicone is limited.[23] In addition, the low field strength magnets may not produce sufficient signal to detect the more subtle signs of implant rupture.

The type of MR coil used in imaging patients with silicone breast implants is a very important component in obtaining optimal MR images.[7] A dedicated MR breast coil should be used when imaging patients with implants to obtain high-resolution images allowing detection of subtle signs of implant leakage or rupture. If a dedicated MR breast coil is not available, a general purpose 5-inch-round coil or a shoulder coil could be used with adequate results. The body coil should never be used to image patients with silicone breast implants. The resolution is not adequate to detect many breast ruptures. Ideally, the patient should be imaged prone. This will decrease respiratory motion and improve the image quality. The breast hangs freely in the dedicated breast coil or one can support the breast with soft pads. A claustrophobic patient can usually be imaged by placing her feet first into the bore of the magnet rather than the normal head-first position. It is important to shield the breast coil cable so no portion of the cable actually comes in contact with the patient. If the patient's body habitus is too large to fit in the bore of the magnet on a dedicated breast coil, consider placing the patient on her back while using a general purpose 5-inch-round coil or a shoulder coil. The image quality is usually not as optimal as the images from a dedicated breast coil, but are usually adequate for interpretation.

■ MR IMAGING TECHNIQUES

An understanding of the MR characteristics of silicone will be helpful to understand the different MR sequences that can be used to differentiate silicone from surrounding breast parenchyma. The chemical composition of most medical-grade silicones is dimethyl polysiloxane with varying degrees of polymerization (Fig. 9–2).[24] The MR signal is derived from the protons of the methyl groups. The implant shell (envelope) is also composed of silicone but differs from the gel because of the many additional cross-linkages between the methyl groups that result in an elastic solid. Al-

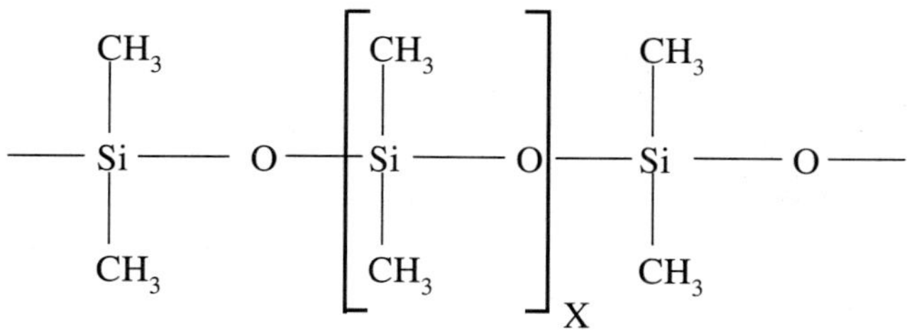

Figure 9–2. Chemical composition of silicone (dimethyl polysiloxane).

though the implant shell is composed of silicone, only minimal MR signal is produced from the silicone shell because of the many additional cross-linkages between the methyl groups.[25]

The selection of MR pulse sequences used to image breast implants is determined by the relative Larmor precessional frequencies, as well as the T1 and T2 properties of the tissues (fat, muscle, and silicone). The relative resonance frequency of silicone is approximately 100 Hz lower than fat and 320 Hz lower than water at 1.5 T (Fig. 9–3). Because the

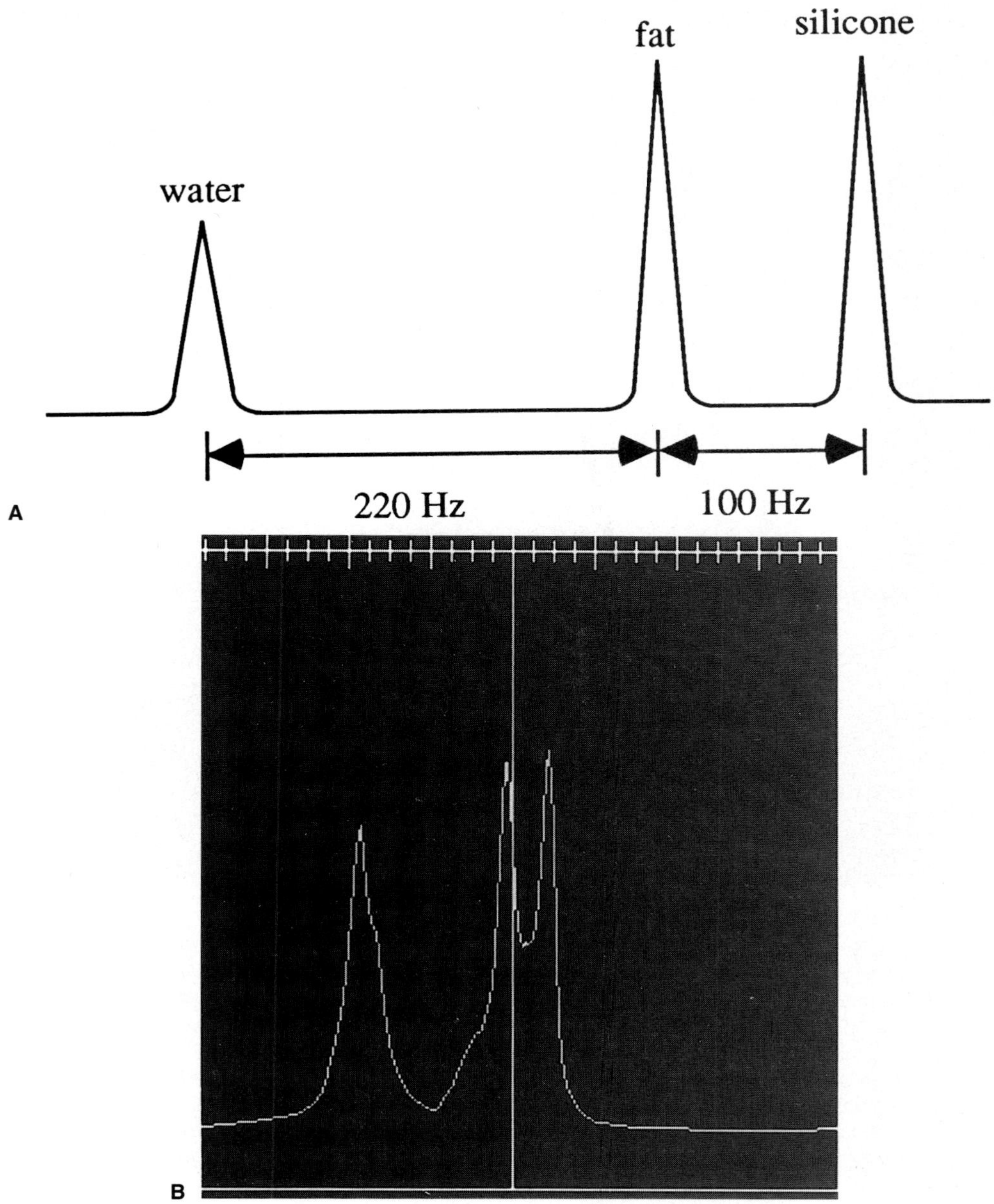

Figure 9–3. Relative resonance frequency differences between water, fat, and silicone at 1.5 T. (**A**) The resonance frequency of silicone is approximately 320 Hz lower than that of water and 100 Hz lower than that of fat. (**B**) Actual MR spectrum of patient with silicone implant.

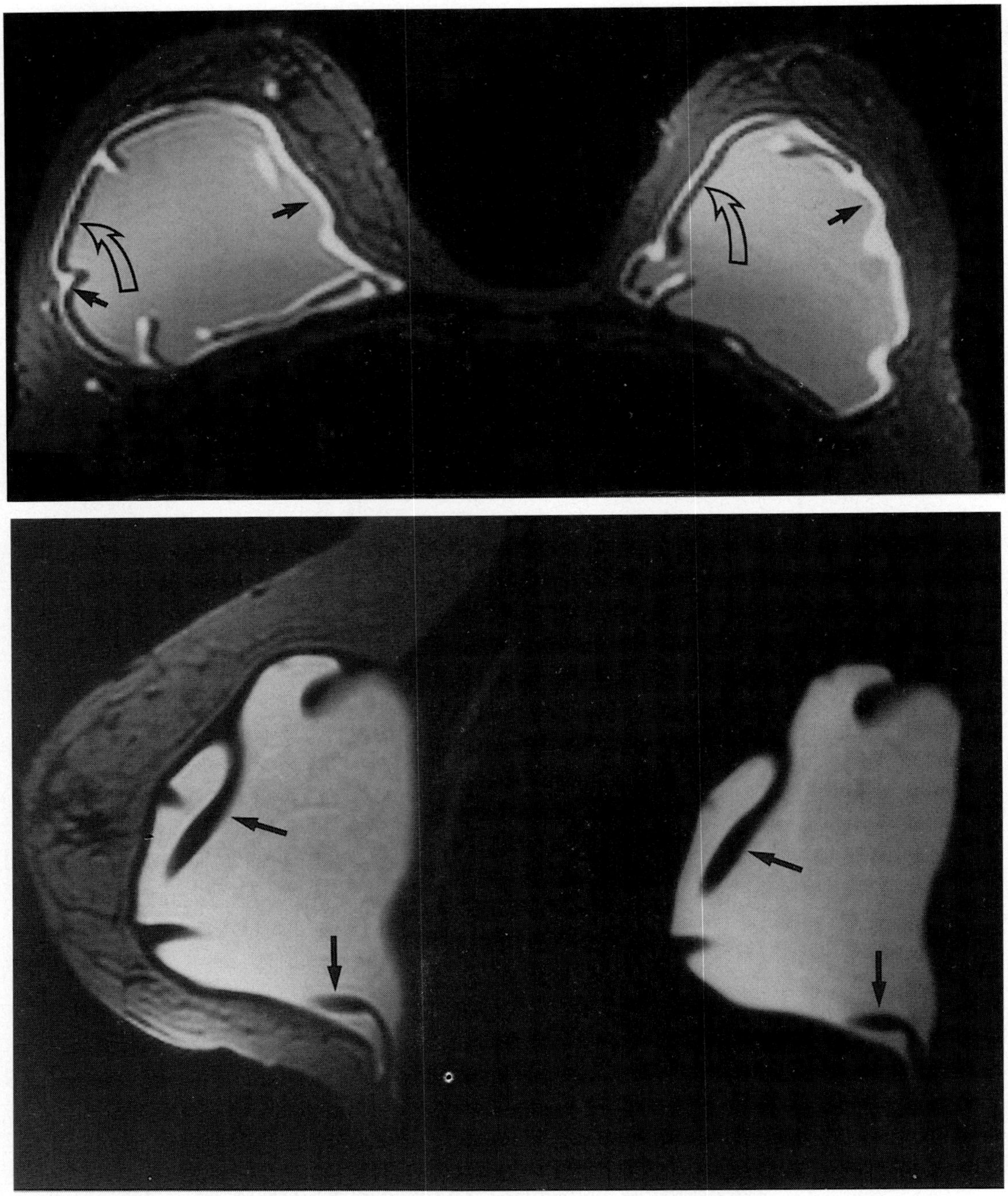

A

B

C

Figure 9–4. Normal double-lumen silicone implants. (**A**) Axial T2-weighted fast spin echo (FSE). The very high signal intensity (straight arrows) surrounding the lower signal silicone represents the saline filled outer lumen. The dark line (curved arrows) represents a chemical shift artifact caused by the different resonance frequencies of silicone, fat, and water. The chemical shift artifact is located only on one side of the implant and should not be mistaken for the fibrous capsule. (**B**) Sagittal T2-weighted FSE with water suppression. The saline outer lumen is of low signal intensity (straight arrows) on the sagittal T2-weighted FSE with water suppression. (**C**) Sagittal inversion recovery T2-weighted fast spin echo with chemical water suppression. This sequence has also been called a silicone selective sequence because the signal from fat is suppressed by the STIR and the signal from water is suppressed by the chemical water suppression pulse. Normal prominent radial folds (arrows).

Table 9–1. Signal Detection of MR Sequences

MR Sequence	Silicone	Fat	Water
Fast spin echo (FSE) T2-weighted (TR/TE 5000/200)	High	Medium	Very high
FSE with water suppression	High	Medium	Low
Inversion recovery FSE (IRFSE) (TR/TE 5000/90, TI = 150)	High	Low	Very high
IRFSE with water suppression	High	Low	Low
3-point Dixon (3PD) silicone only	High	None	None

resonance frequency of silicone is close to fat, when chemical suppression techniques (chemical fat or water suppression) are used the MR signal from silicone behaves similarly to fat. For chemical fat suppression at 1.5 T the MR imaging computer centers on the water resonance frequency and sends a radiofrequency (RF) pulse downfield approximately 220 Hz to suppress the fat resonance frequency peak. The water and fat resonance frequency peaks are approximately 220 Hz apart at 1.5 T. Because the silicone resonance frequency peak is close to the fat resonance frequency peak and the RF pulse produced has a broad peak, not only does the RF pulse suppress the MR signal from fat but it also suppresses the MR signal from silicone. Conversely, for chemical water suppression at 1.5 T, the MR imaging computer centers on the fat resonance frequency and sends an RF pulse upfield approximately 220 Hz to suppress the water resonance frequency peak. The chemical water suppression sequence will only suppress the MR signal from water and not from silicone. As a result, the silicone signal is high when chemical water suppression is used and the silicone signal is low when chemical fat suppression is used (Table 9–1).

The relative relaxation times of silicone, fat, and water can also be used to obtain MR sequences that selectively emphasize the signal from silicone. The relaxation times of fat are shorter than those of silicone. Therefore, one can use the relaxation time properties of silicone and fat to suppress the fat while maintaining a strong signal from silicone. The use of inversion recovery with a short TI (STIR) will suppress the signal from fat while maintaining signal from silicone.[26,27] To obtain a more selective silicone image, a chemical water suppression pulse can be used in conjunction with a STIR sequence to produce a silicone selective sequence (Fig. 9–4).

Chemical shift imaging (CSI) is another way to selectively image silicone.[5,28,29] This method uses the differences between the Larmor frequencies of silicone, fat, and water to separate the MR signal of silicone from the signal of fat and water. An example of a CSI MR sequence is the modified three-point Dixon technique.[5,29] This sequence produces a silicone only sequence and a simultaneous fat/water image with a single MR sequence (Fig. 9–5).

In our practice, MR imaging is performed with a dedicated breast coil with the patient prone. A 1.5-T superconducting magnet is used to acquire an axial scout image, fast gradient-recalled acquisition in the steady state (GRASS), followed by a sagittal T2-weighted fast spin echo (FSE) with water suppression and axial T2-weighted FSE sequences. A 256 × 256 matrix, 2 NEX with slice thickness between 3 and 5 mm to cover the entire implant are used to image the patients. Heavily T2-weighted FSE images, with TE approximately 200, are used to decrease the signal from the breast adipose tissue while keeping the signal from the silicone fairly high (Fig. 9–6). This examination requires between 20 and 30 minutes to complete. The relative signal intensities of silicone, fat, and water with various pulse sequences are summarized in Table 9–1.

■ APPEARANCE OF NORMAL IMPLANTS

Although hundreds of different types of silicone implants have been produced, single-lumen (Fig. 9–5) and double-lumen silicone implants (Fig. 9–4) are the most commonly encountered. A single-lumen silicone implant has an outer silicone Silastic shell containing homogeneous high signal intensity viscous silicone on T2-weighted images. A double-lumen silicone implant typically has an inner lumen of high signal intensity silicone surrounded by a smaller outer lumen that contains saline and has different signal intensities depending on the pulse sequence (Fig. 9–4). The implants are usually oval and have a smooth or textured surface. After

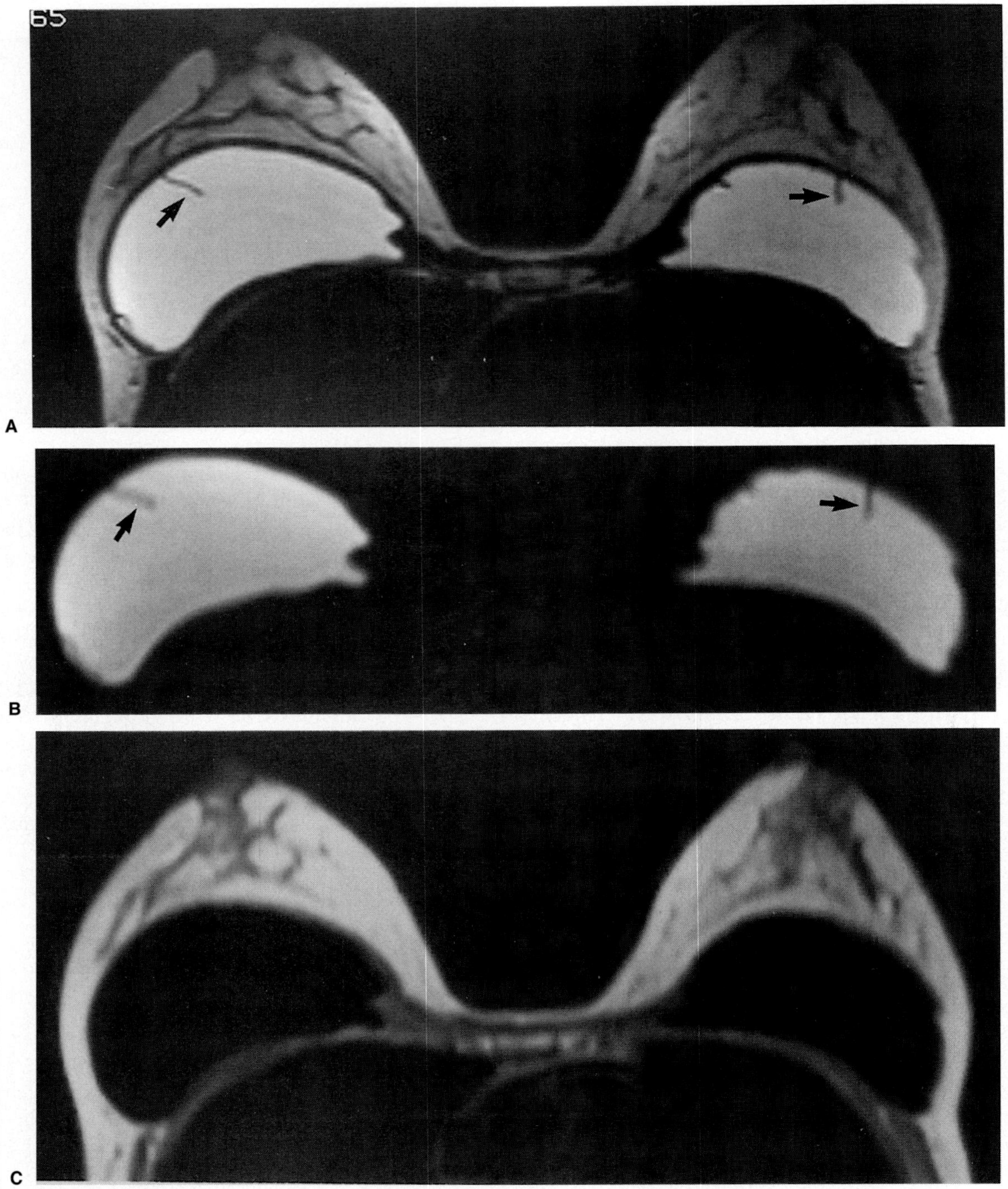

Figure 9–5. Normal single-lumen silicone gel implant. (**A**) Axial FSE T2-weighted image with water suppression. (**B**) Axial modified three-point Dixon (chemical shift imaging) silicone-only image. (**C**) Axial modified three-point Dixon fat/water image corresponding to image in **B**. Normal radial folds (arrows) of the silicone shell extending to the periphery of the implant. These folds are not indicative of rupture or leak.

surgical placement, a thin fibrous capsule (scar tissue) normally forms around the prosthesis. Breast implants may be surgically placed in a subglandular location, that is, anterior to the pectoralis major muscle, or subpectoral, posterior to the pectoralis major muscle (Fig. 9–7).

A variety of other types of implantable prostheses are occasionally encountered, including expander implants (reverse double lumens—saline in the inner lumen, silicone in the outer lumen), multicompartmental implants, foam implants, and single-lumen silicone implants with saline directly injected into the silicone at the time of surgery (Fig. 9–8). Occasionally, two or even more implants are placed in one breast, a configuration commonly known as stacked implants. Some implants have a coating of polyurethane covering the surface of the silicone envelope. These implants typically have a moderate to large amount of reactive fluid surrounding the implant (Fig. 9–8). The many different implantable prosthesis can be easily differentiated from direct silicone injections into the breast (Fig. 9–9). Saline implants, in which the lumen is filled with saline (Fig. 9–10), have become more popular since the Food and Drug Administration (FDA) limited the use of silicone gel implants in 1992.

MR imaging often shows radial folds, normal infoldings of the Silastic elastomer shell (Fig. 9–5). These folds may appear prominent (Fig. 9–11), but should not be confused with implant rupture or leak. Prominent radial folds are one of the major pitfalls in MR imaging of breast implants.

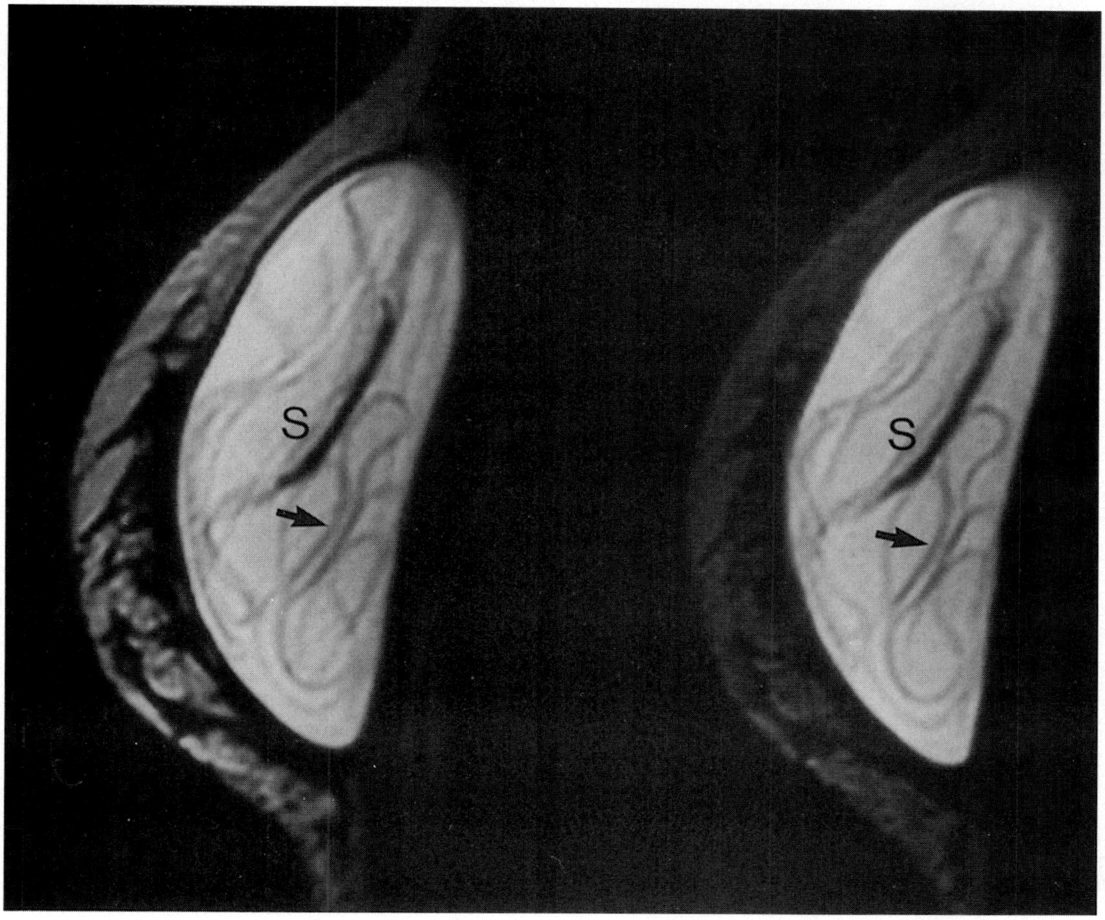

A B

Figure 9–6. Silicone-selective MR sequences using different MR parameters on an intracapsular rupture of a double-lumen implant. (**A**) FSE T2 sagittal image with TE = 130 (other MR parameters are equal), the fat signal is closer relative to the signal from silicone (S) when the TE is lower; linguine sign (arrow). (**B**) FSE T2 sagittal image with TE = 200 (other MR parameters are equal), the fat signal is much lower than the signal from silicone (S) when the TE is close to 200. *(continued)*

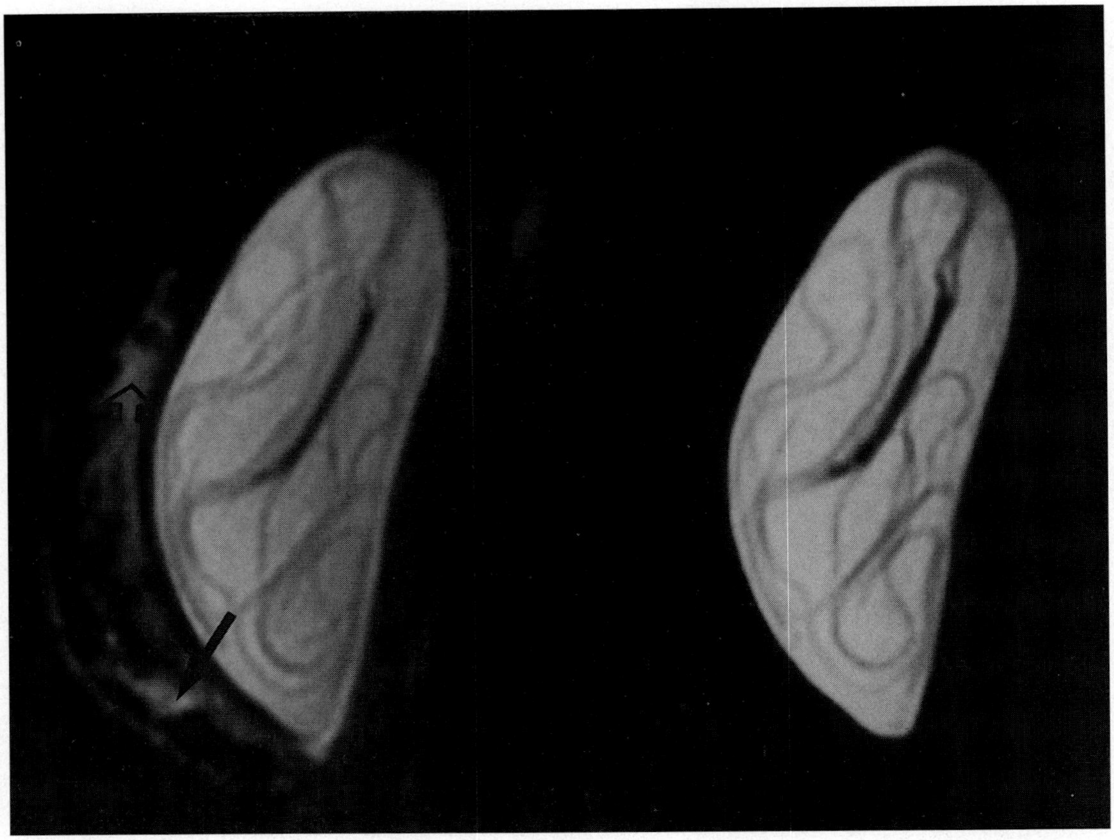

C D

9–6. ***(Continued)*** (**C**) FMPIR (STIR) sequence *without* chemical water suppression (other MR parameters are equal). The high signal area anterior to the implant (arrows) could represent either extracapsular silicone or normal fluid within the breast parenchyma. (**D**) FMPIR (STIR) sequence *with* chemical water suppression (silicone selective sequence) (other MR parameters are equal) shows that the high signal area within the breast parenchyma in **C** represented fluid and not extracapsular free silicone.

Some radiologists have confused prominent radial folds of intact silicone implants with the collapsed implant shell, "linguine sign," of a ruptured implant. The more experience one has in reviewing many different MR studies of silicone implants that have surgical correlation will help one avoid this major pitfall. Radial folds, even when prominent, extend to the periphery of the implant, and the folds are relatively few in number.

■ APPEARANCE OF RUPTURED BREAST IMPLANTS

Implant ruptures can be divided into two major categories, intracapsular and extracapsular rupture. Intracapsular implant rupture, the most common type of rupture, is defined as rupture of the implant shell (elastomer envelope) with silicone leakage that does not macroscopically extend beyond the fibrous capsule that commonly forms around silicone implants.[4,5] From 80 to 90% of all silicone implant ruptures are intracapsular ruptures.[4–6] The most reliable MR criterion for intracapsular rupture is the presence of multiple curvilinear low-signal-intensity lines seen within the high-signal-intensity silicone gel, the so-called linguine sign (Fig. 9–12).[4,25] These curvilinear lines represent the collapsed implant shell floating within the silicone gel. Rarely, intracapsular rupture will show multiple hyperintense foci on T2-weighted images or multiple hypointense foci on water-suppression images within the implant lumen (Fig. 9–8E). Without other MR evidence of implant rupture such as identifying the collapsed implant shell or free silicone within the breast parenchyma (with no previous history of implant rupture), water droplets or small amounts of air within a silicone implant are not reliable signs of implant rupture.

Extracapsular silicone implant rupture, the less common type of implant rupture, is defined as rupture of both the implant shell and the fibrous capsule with macroscopic silicone

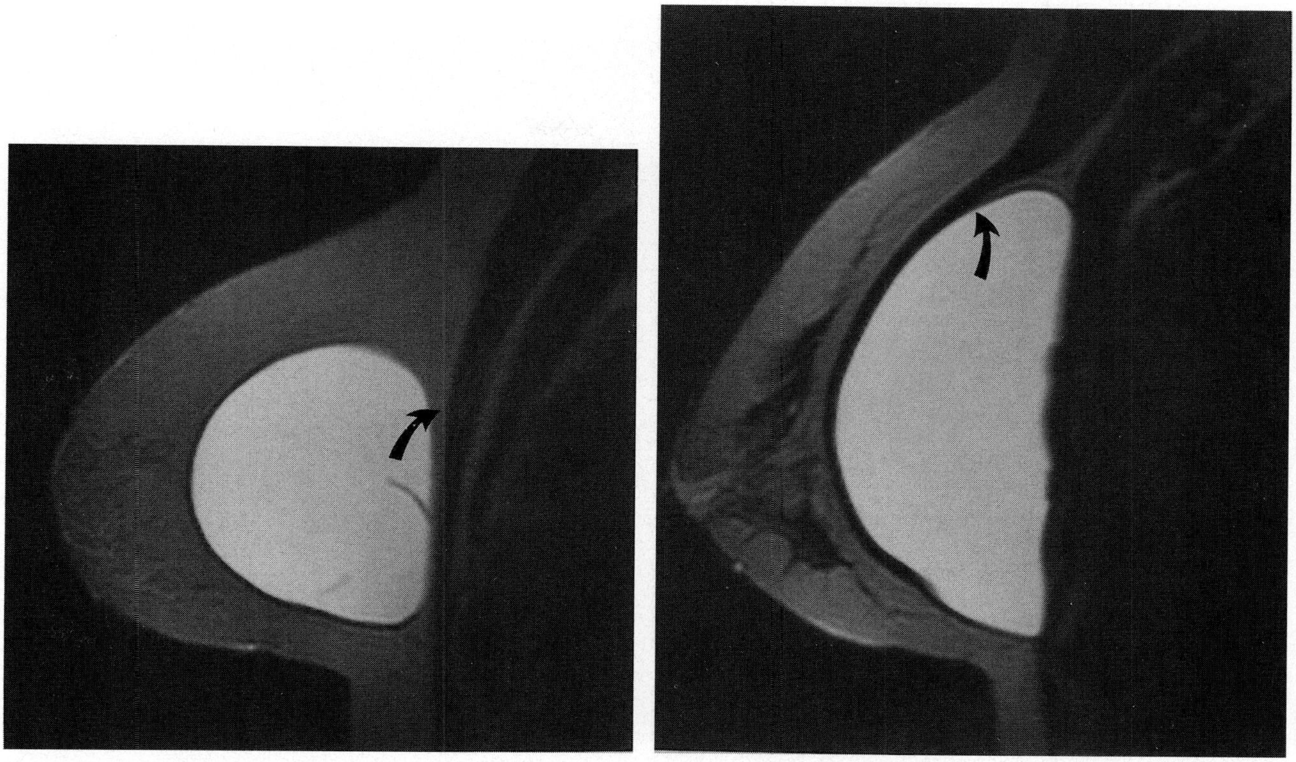

A B

Figure 9–7. (**A**) A woman with a subglandular single-lumen silicone implant. (**B**) A different woman with a subpectoral single lumen silicone implant. Pectoralis major muscle (arrow).

leakage that extends beyond the fibrous capsule into surrounding tissues. Focal areas of high signal intensity, representing free silicone, can be identified on MR images (Fig. 9–13).[4,6,30] In addition to free silicone in the surrounding breast parenchyma, the linguine sign is often present with extracapsular ruptures. The multiplanar capabilities of MR imaging allow precise localization of free silicone.

An uncollapsed silicone implant rupture is defined as a tear of the silicone implant shell; however, the implant shell does not collapse or only partially collapses. The linguine sign will not be present in an uncollapsed rupture. The reasons some ruptured implants do not completely collapse is unclear, but one theory is that some of the older implant shells are relatively stiff and some have fixation patches, making collapse less likely. The MR finding of an uncollapsed rupture is identifying free silicone outside the implant shell but still contained by the fibrous capsule. Commonly, free silicone can enter a radial fold and form the "inverted teardrop sign" (Fig. 9–14). An uncollapsed implant rupture is considered an intracapsular rupture because the free silicone is contained by the fibrous capsule. An uncollapsed silicone implant rupture can have a similar or identical MR appearance to a large gel bleed. However, when an inverted teardrop sign is identified on MR, the majority, greater than 90%, of implants will have a focal tear within the implant shell upon close examination. It is important for the surgeon to be aware of the possibility of an uncollapsed implant rupture, because a focal implant shell tear in an uncollapsed implant rupture can be easily overlooked if the silicone implant is not closely examined.

Unlike rupture, gel bleed is microscopic silicone leakage through an intact implant shell.[6,27,31] Most if not all implants will eventually have gel bleed; however, the majority of gel bleeds cannot be detected by MR imaging. Only when gel bleed is extensive can silicone gel be detected outside the silicone shell and form the inverted teardrop sign (Fig. 9–14).[6,27] A large amount of silicone gel oil can also be commonly identified outside the implant shell but contained by the fibrous capsule. The MR appearance of silicone gel oil and silicone gel bleed is identical. The difference can only be determined at surgery—silicone gel bleed is sticky and

(text continues on page 142)

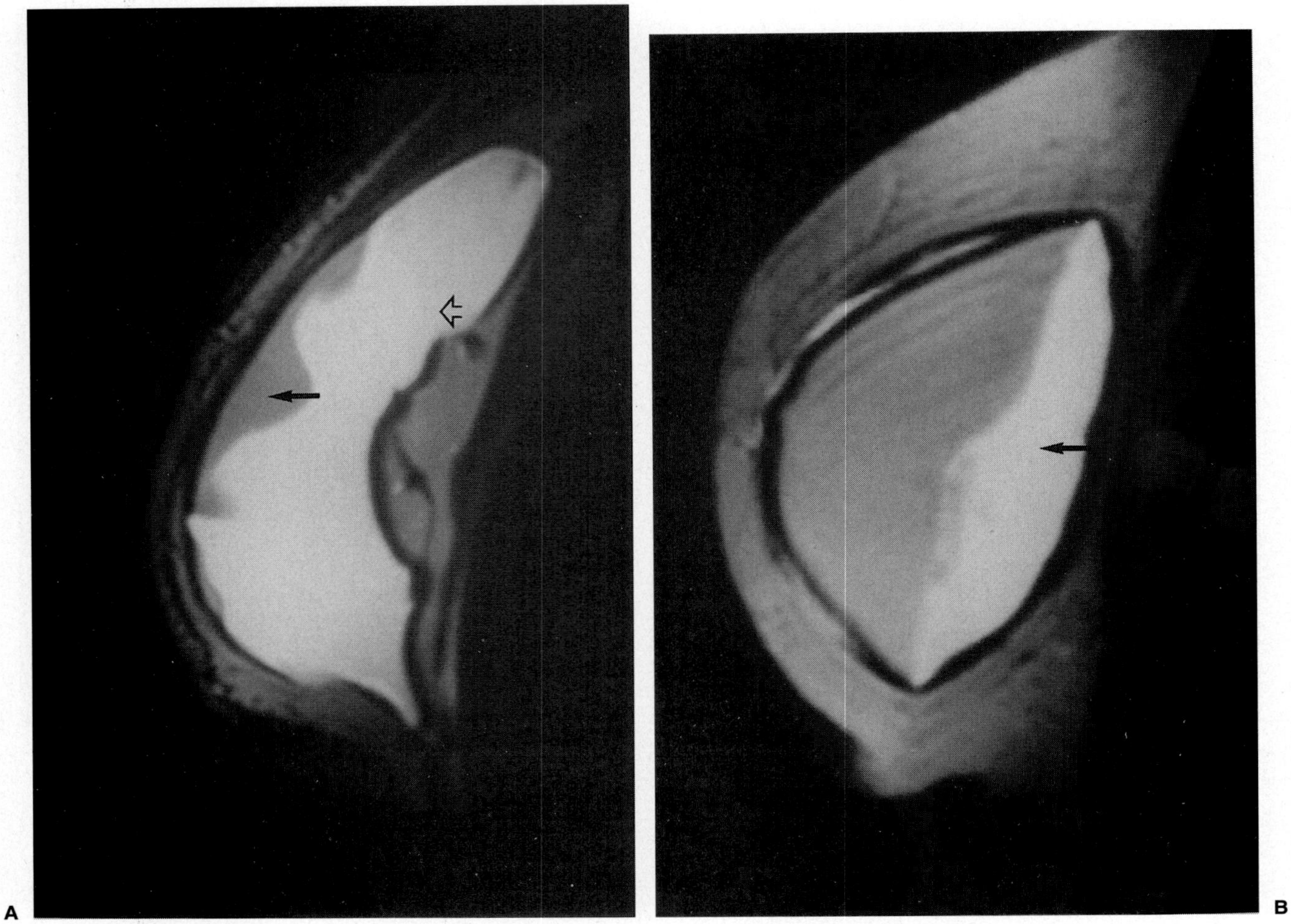

Figure 9–8. Different types of breast implants (all cases surgically confirmed). (**A**) A 46-year-old woman with reverse double-lumen or expander type implant. The silicone filled outer lumen (solid arrow) surrounds the inner saline-filled lesion (open arrow). (**B**) A 43-year-old woman with a single-lumen silicone-filled implant with a polyurethane-coated silicone envelope. A large amount of reactive fluid (arrow) is commonly associated with this type of implant. Reactive fluid is thought to result from an inflammatory response and is not indicative of implant rupture. *(continued)*

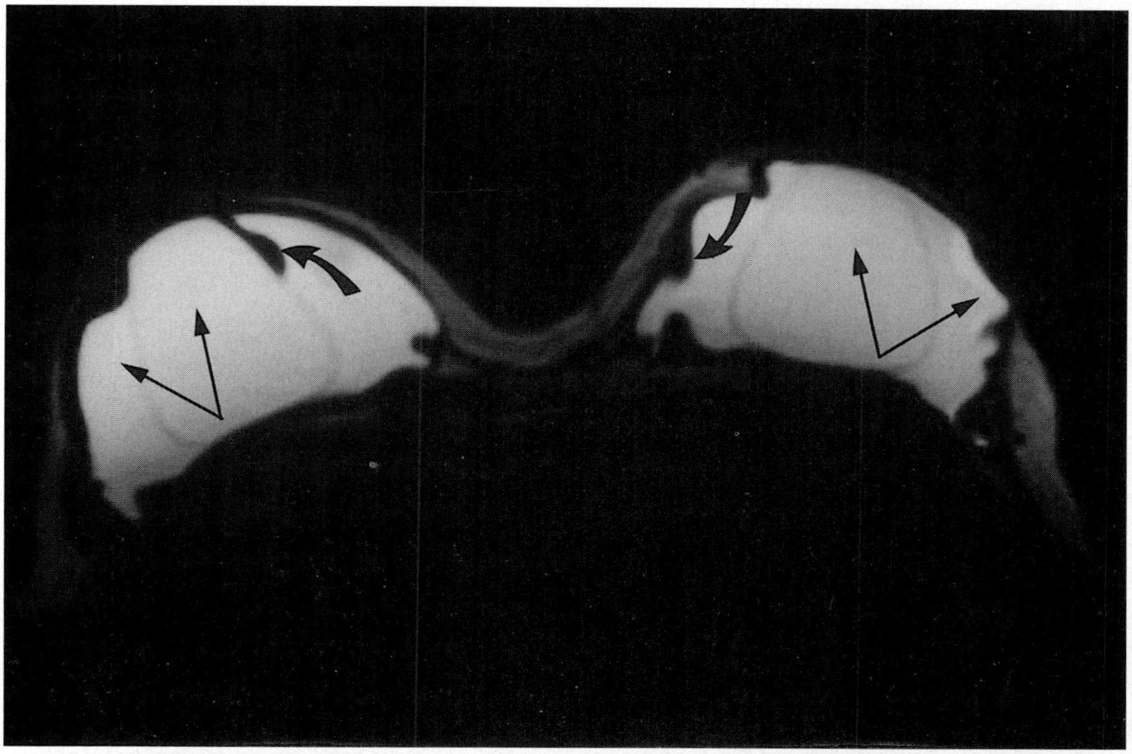

C

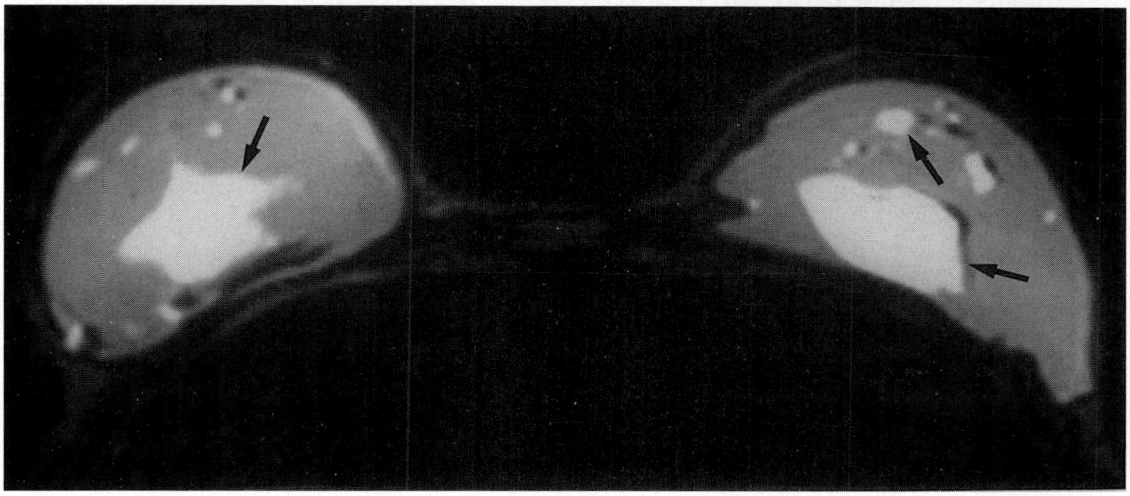

D

9–8. ***(Continued)*** (**C**) A 50-year-old woman with a multicompartmental implant composed of a outermost saline-filled lumen (curved arrow—saline suppressed by chemical water suppression) surrounding two inner silicone-filled compartments (straight arrows). (**D**) A 42-year-old woman with a single-lumen silicone implant with sa ine injected (arrows) into the silicone at the time of surgery to increase the volume of each prostheses. No rupture was found at surgery. *(continued)*

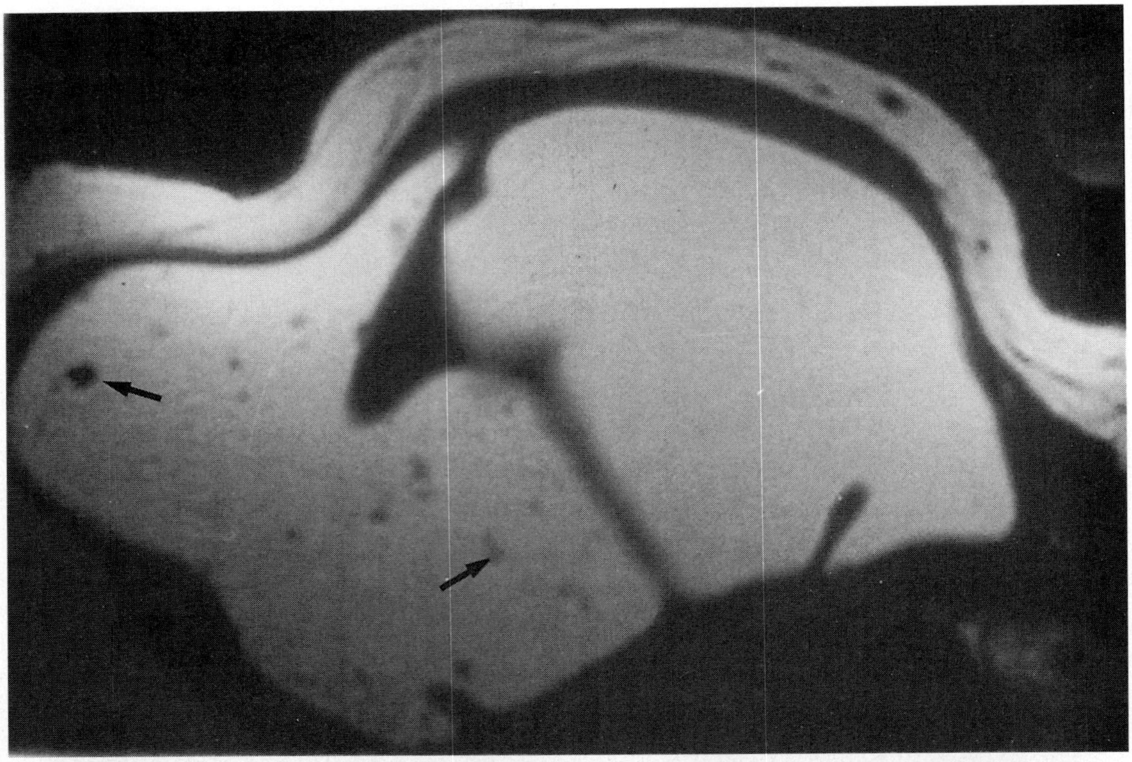

E

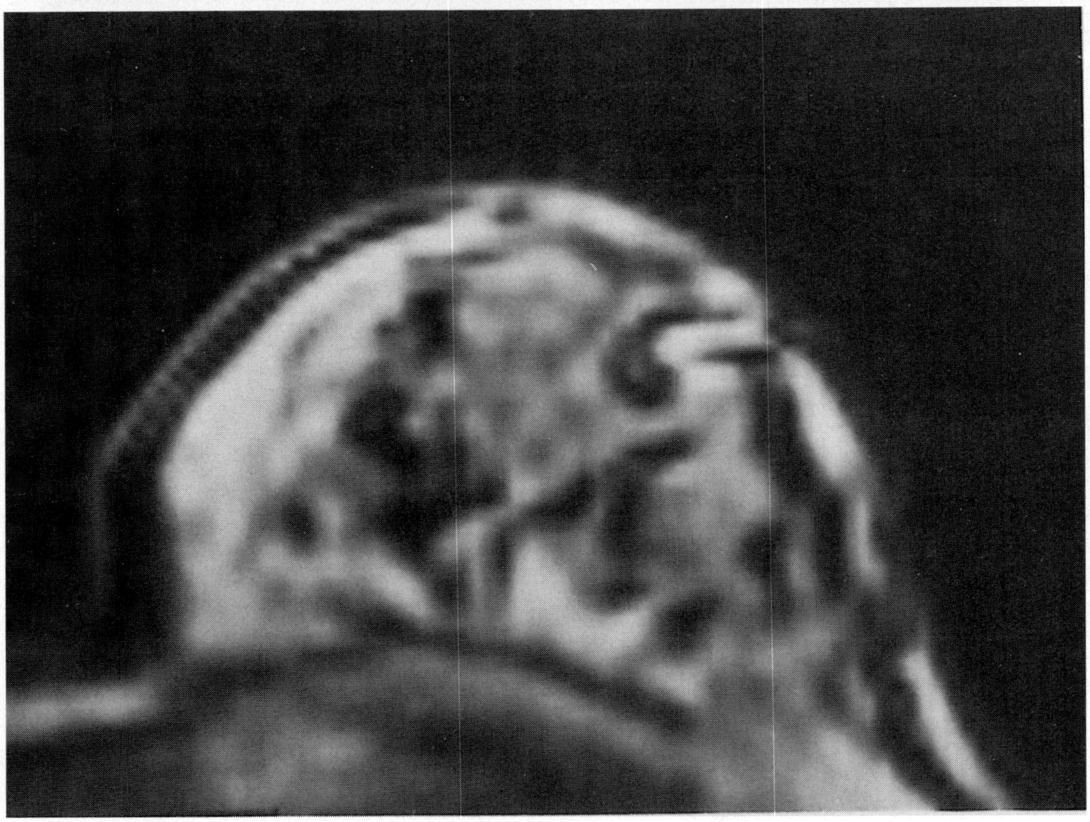

F

9–8. ***(Continued)*** (**E**) A 40-year-old woman with stacked breast implants. Axial T2-weighted FSE with water suppression shows stacked implants, which is composed of two or more implants placed in a single breast. Implant with multiple low-signal areas (arrow) shows an unusual appearance of an intracapsular rupture. The implant shell had not totally collapsed. However, several small fluid collections within an implant lumen can be normal, and this is not a reliable sign of implant rupture. (**F**) A 45-year-old woman with a foam implant that was placed in 1965 for Poland's syndrome. Sagittal T2-weighted FSE image shows low signal intensity foam mixed with high signal intensity reactive fluid. *(continued)*

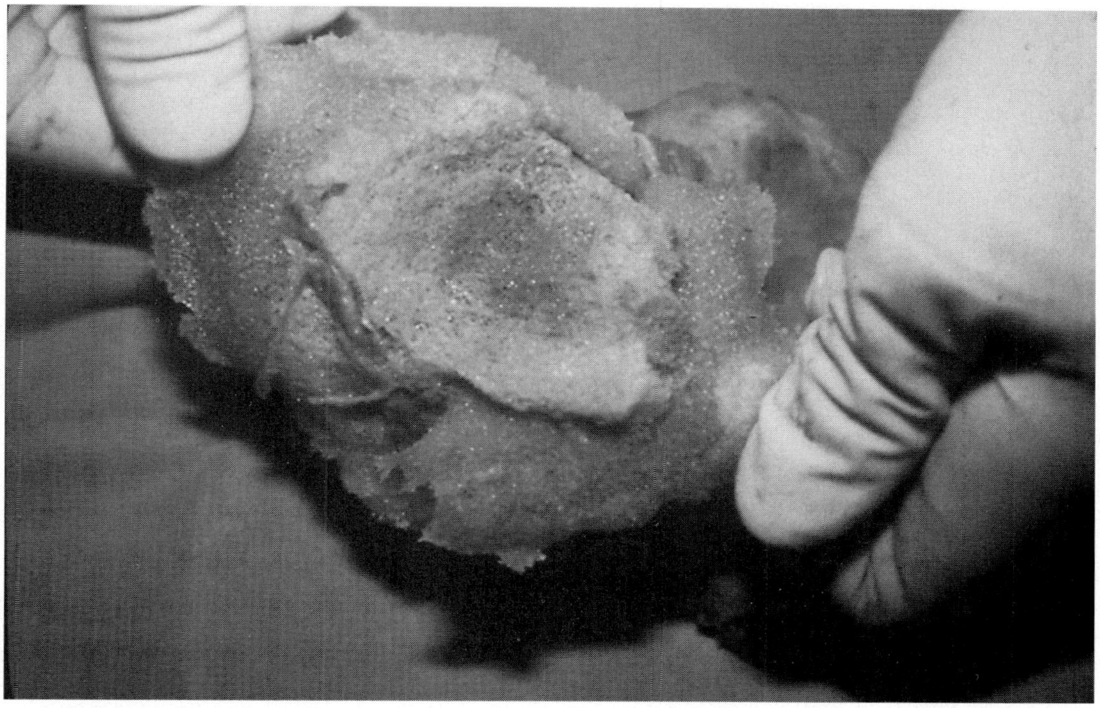

G

9–8. ***(Continued)*** (**G**) Surgical specimen of foam implant corresponding to MR image in **F**.

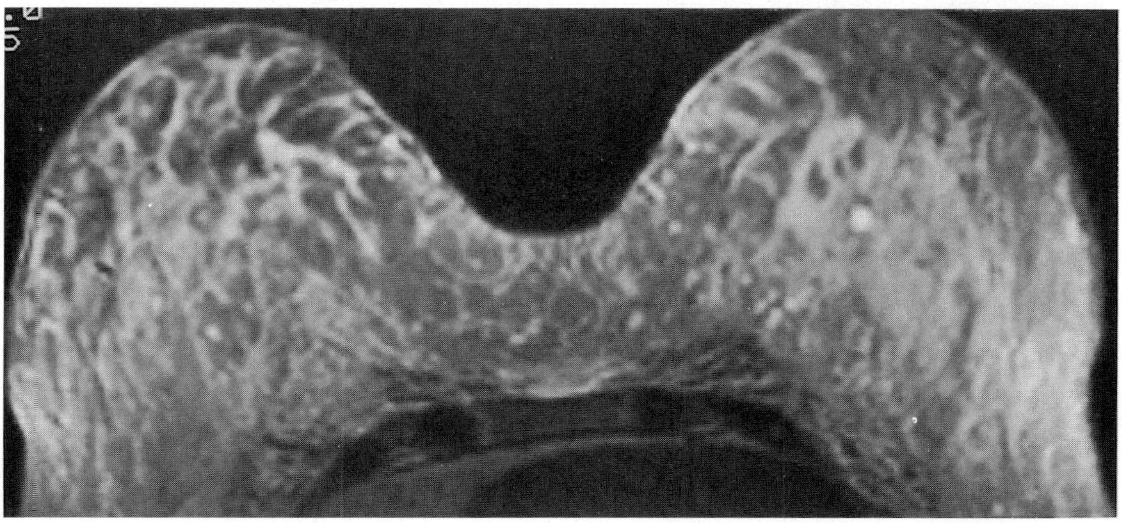

Figure 9–9. Silicone oil breast injections. Axial FSE T2-weighted image with water suppression demonstrating diffuse high signal throughout both breasts representing free silicone.

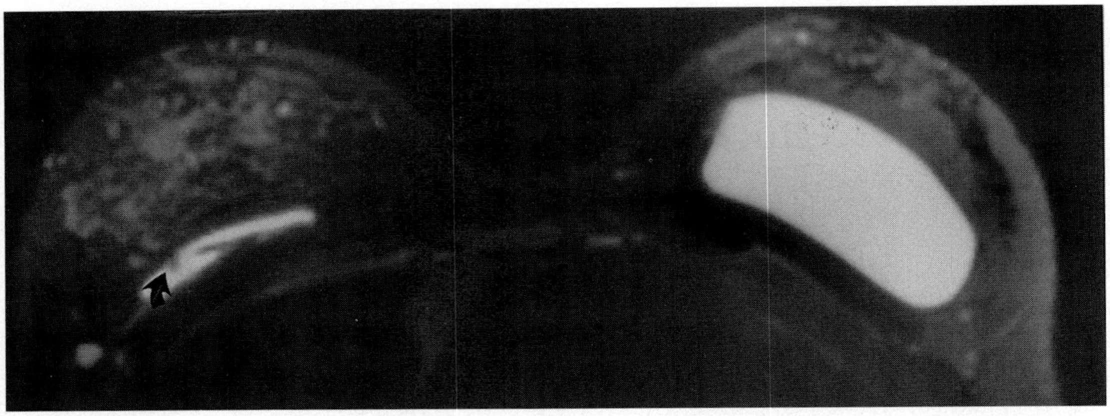

Figure 9–10. A 42-year-old woman with bilateral saline implants presented with loss of volume of right breast. Axial T2-FSE MR image shows a normal intact saline implant on the left and a collapsed saline implant on the right with only a small amount of residual saline (curved arrow). The saline is commonly reabsorbed when a saline implant ruptures or leaks. The linguine sign is not typically identified in a ruptured saline implant. Furthermore, a ruptured saline implant can easily be identified on mammography by identifying the collapsed implant shell. MR imaging is not indicated for the evaluation of ruptured saline breast implants.

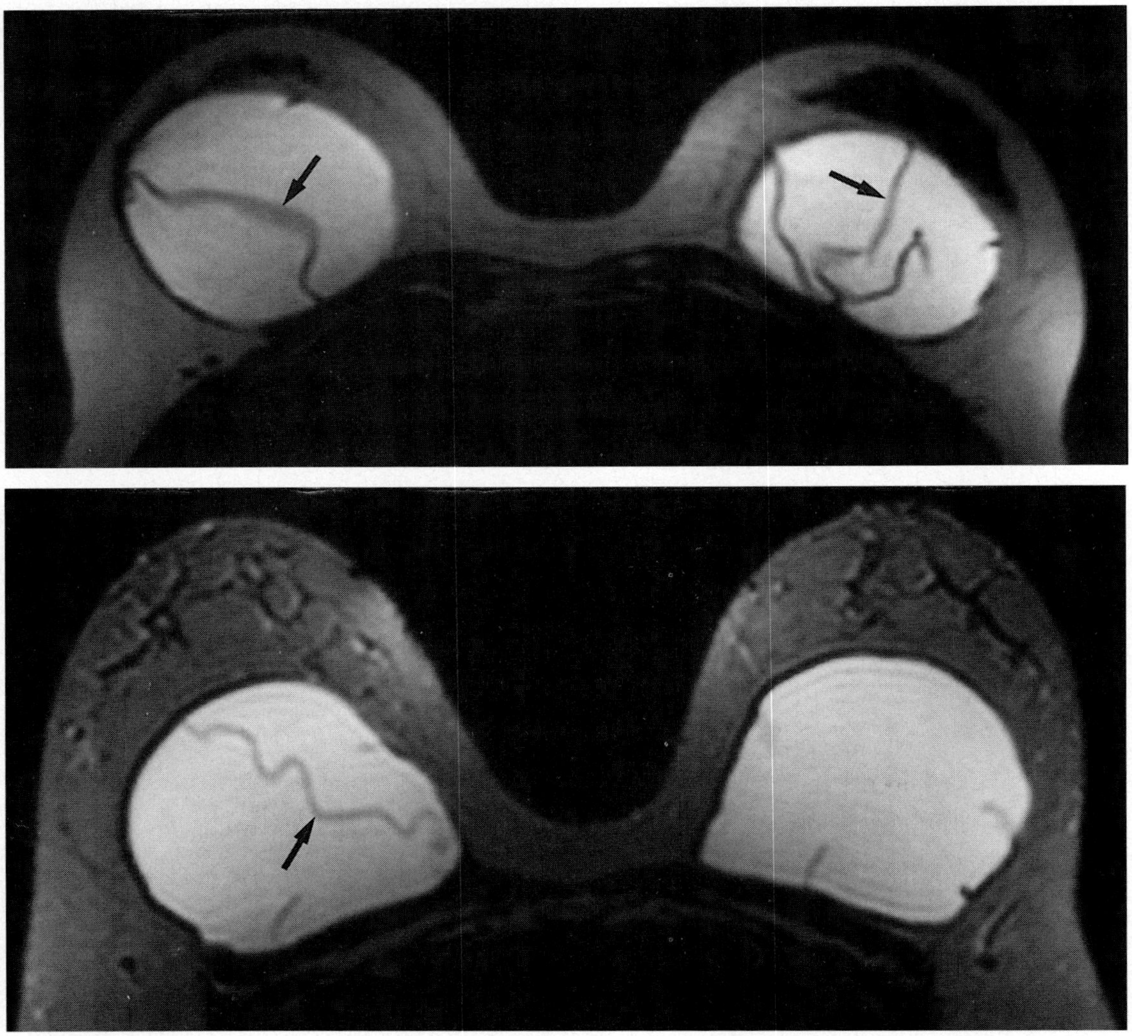

A

B

Figure 9–11. Prominent radial folds. (**A**) A 49-year-old woman with bilateral silicone implants for 20 years had pain in both breasts and implant "hardness." Axial T2-weighted FSE image with water suppression shows prominent radial folds (arrows) in single-lumen silicone implants in both breasts. All radial folds will extend to the periphery of the implant and are relatively few in number. These folds are not indicative of rupture or leak (surgically proven). (**B**) A 54-year-old woman with a prominent radial fold (arrow) in the right implant.

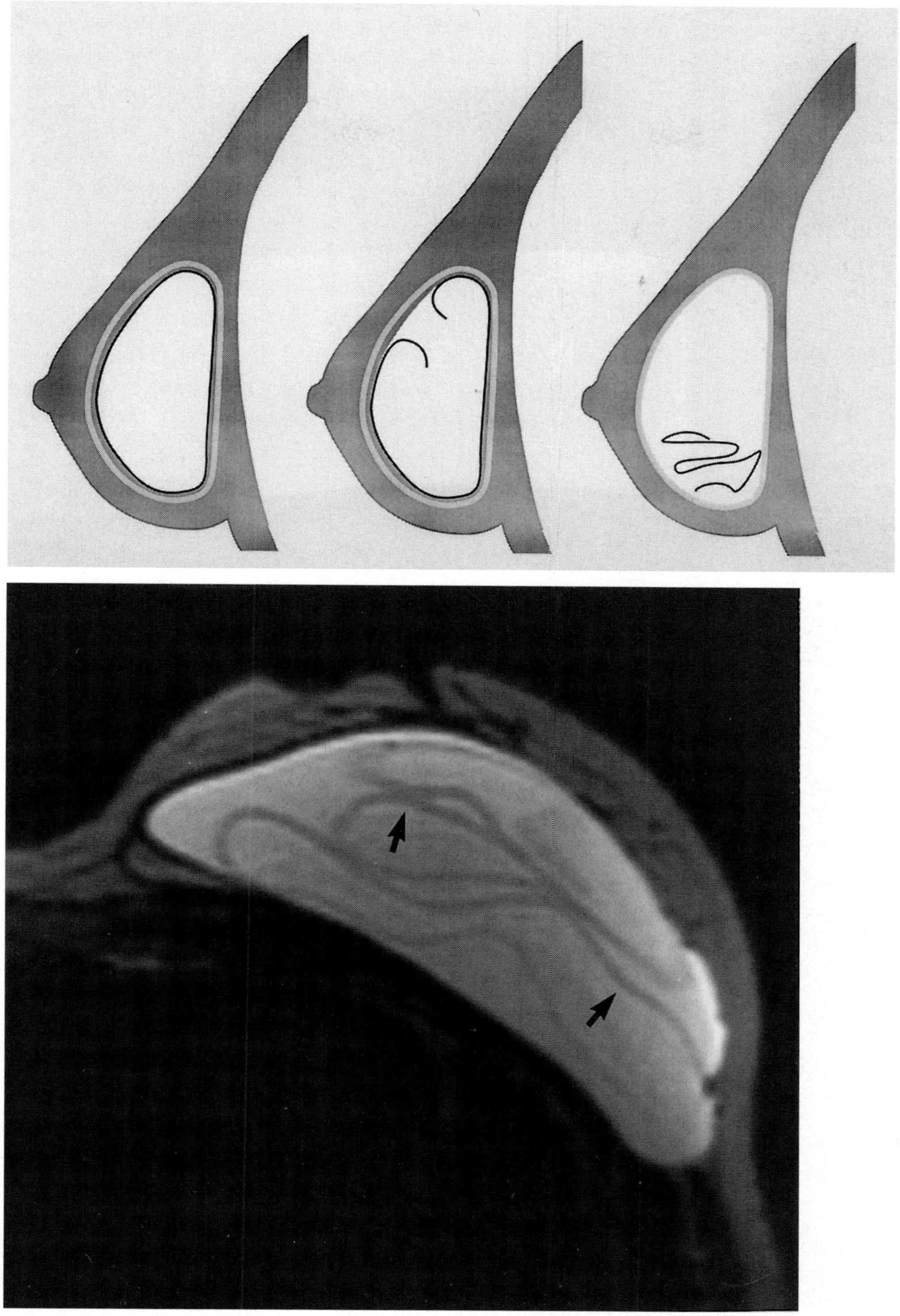

A

B

Figure 9–12. Intracapsular rupture. (**A**) Unlike an intact implant (left), in early intracapsular rupture (center) silicone gel surrounds implant shell, but is contained by the fibrous capsule. Later, the collapsed implant shell floats within the silicone gel (linguine sign, right). Light gray line, fibrous capsule; black line, implant shell; white, silicone gel. (**B**) Patient presented with pain in both breasts. Axial T2-weighted image shows multiple curvilinear low signal intensity lines within the left implant that represent the collapsed implant shell. The multiple curvilinear lines are known as the linguine sign (arrows). Intracapsular rupture of the left implant was found at surgery.

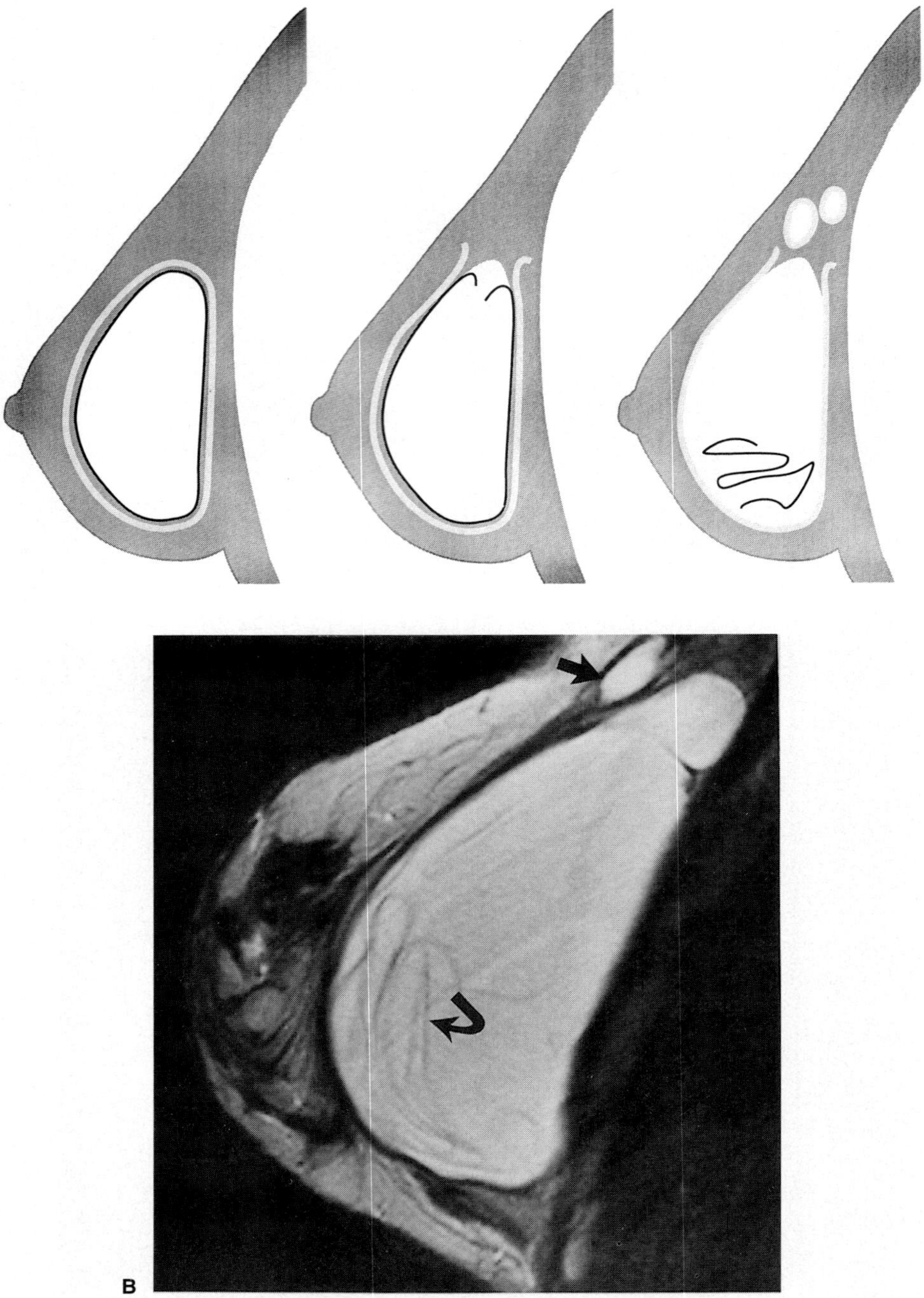

A

B

Figure 9–13. Extracapsular rupture. (**A**) Intact implant has uninterrupted shell and fibrous capsule (left). Disruption of shell and fibrous capsule (center) will allow silicone to extravasate into surrounding breast tissue (right). The collapsed implant shell (linguine sign) is commonly identified as extracapsular ruptures. Light gray line, fibrous capsule; black line, implant shell; white, silicone gel. (**B**) Patient presented with right breast pain following a closed capsulotomy, a procedure in which the surgeon attempts to manually break a rigid fibrous capsule. The sagittal T2-weighted image demonstrates extracapsular silicone (straight arrow) and collapse of the silicone shell (curved arrows).

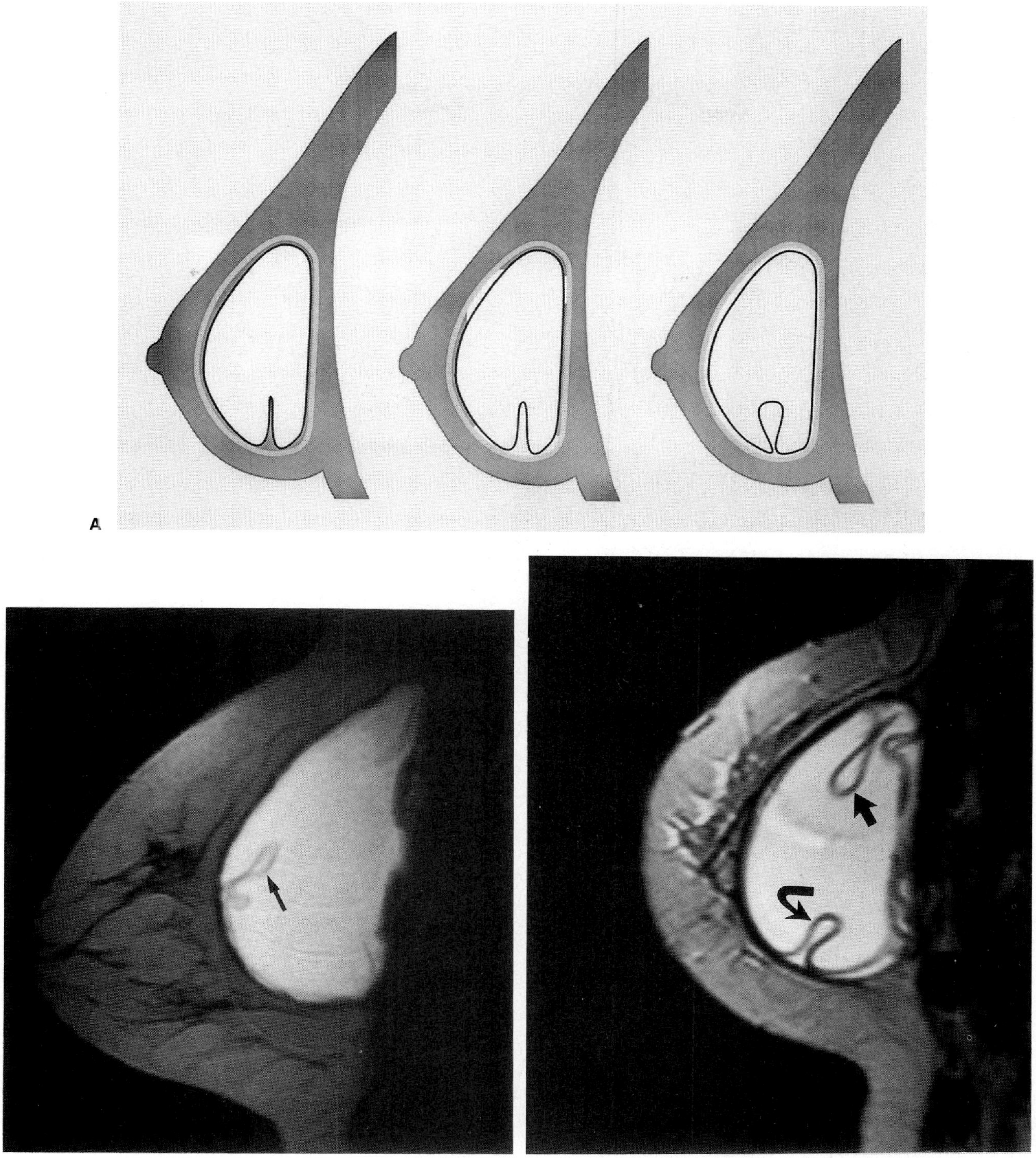

A B C

Figure 9–14. Extensive gel bleed or uncollapsed implant rupture (focal rupture without complete collapse of implant shell). (**A**) Normal infolding of implant shell causes radial folds (left). Gel bleed is microscopic silicone leakage through an intact implant shell (center). Silicone may enter a radial fold, resulting in an inverted teardrop sign (right). A focal tear in the implant shell without complete collapse of the implant shell can have an identical appearance. Light gray line, fibrous capsule; black line, implant shell; white, silicone gel. (**B**) Gel bleed. Sagittal T2-weighted FSE image shows the inverted teardrop sign (arrow) indicating silicone within a radial fold and outside of the implant lumen itself. At surgery, an extensive silicone-gel bleed and intact implant were found.(**C**) Uncollapsed implant. Sagittal T2-weighted FSE image shows inverted teardrop signs (straight arrow). A partial teardrop sign (curved arrow) has the same implication as the inverted teardrop sign. At surgery, a small tear within the implant shell was found. The inverted teardrop sign is not specific; we have seen this sign with both focal ruptures and extensive gel bleeds with intact implant shells. However, the majority of patients with the inverted teardrop sign will have a small focal implant rupture if the implant is closely examined.

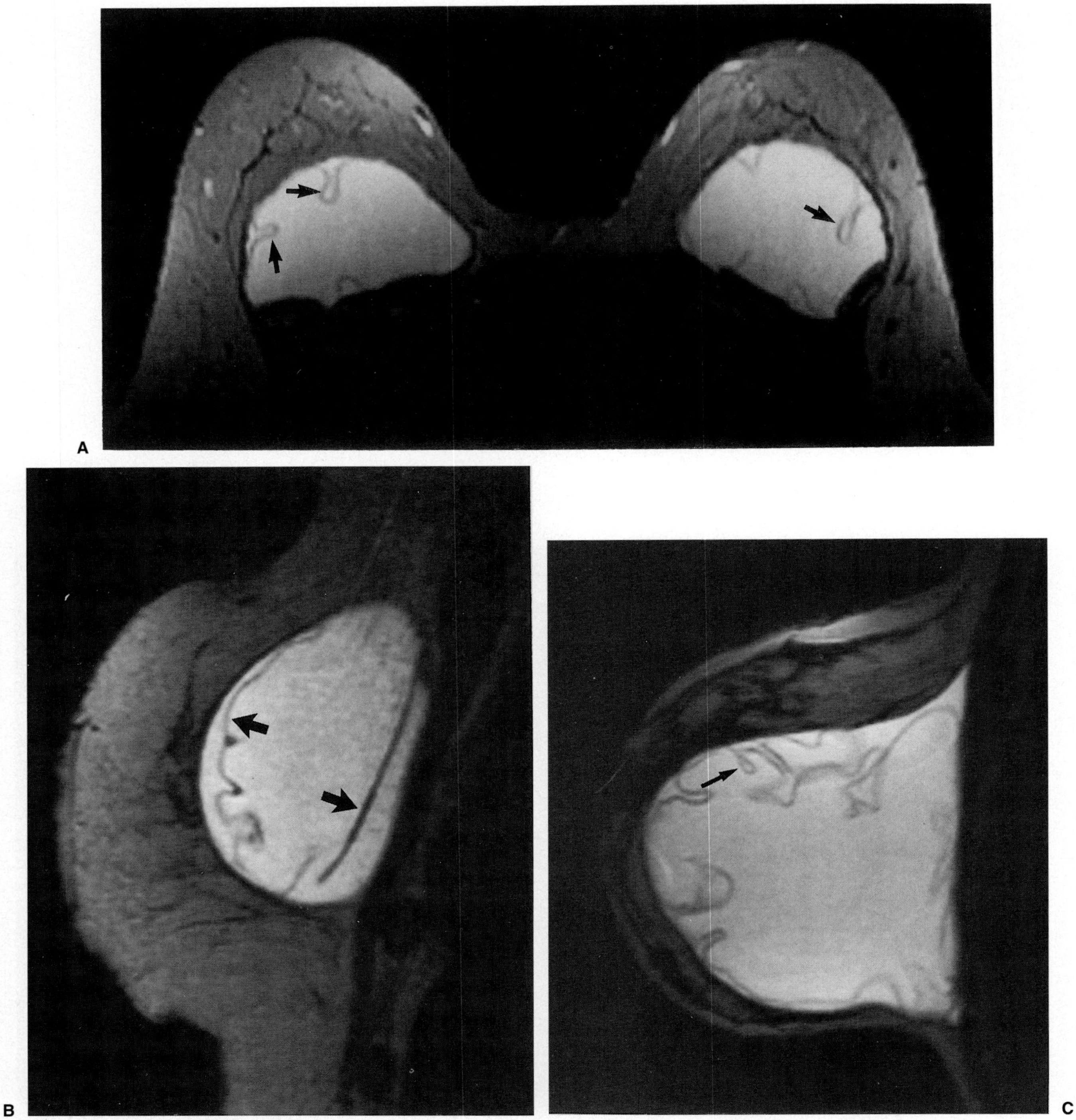

Figure 9–15. Different stages of intracapsular implant ruptures (all cases surgically proven). (**A**) Inverted teardrop and partial teardrop signs (arrows) are identified bilaterally in this patient with a surgically proven focal implant tear (uncollapsed implant rupture). (**B**) Uncollapsed implant rupture where the implant shell has pulled away from the fibrous capsule but has not totally collapsed. (**C**) Uncollapsed implant rupture in a different patient. The implant shell has not totally collapsed. Some inverted teardrop signs (arrow) are identified. *(continued)*

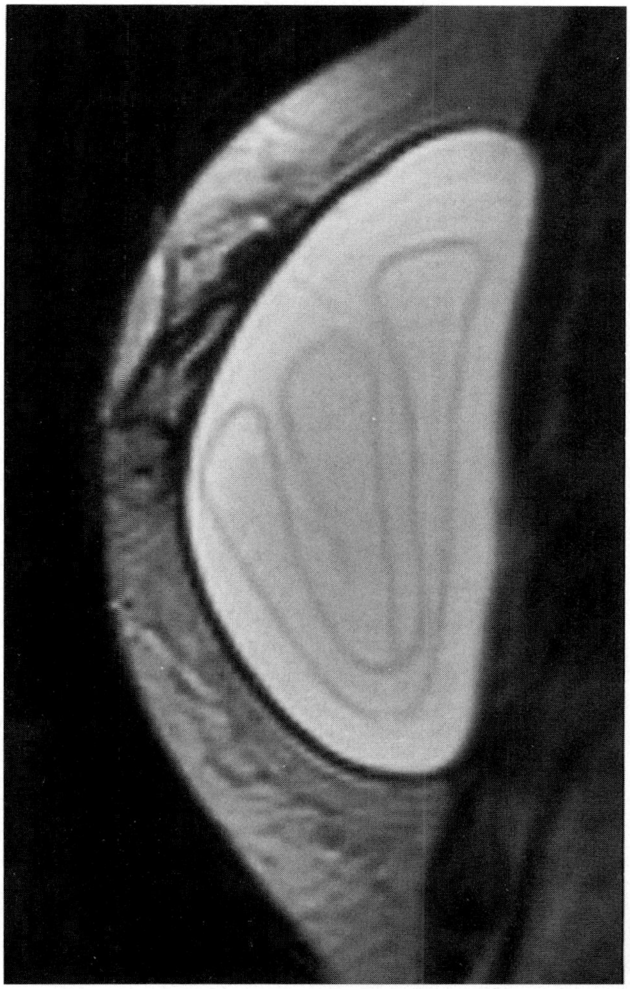

D

9–15. ***(Continued)*** (**D**) Totally collapsed implant shell (linguine sign) is identified in this patient with an intracapsular implant rupture.

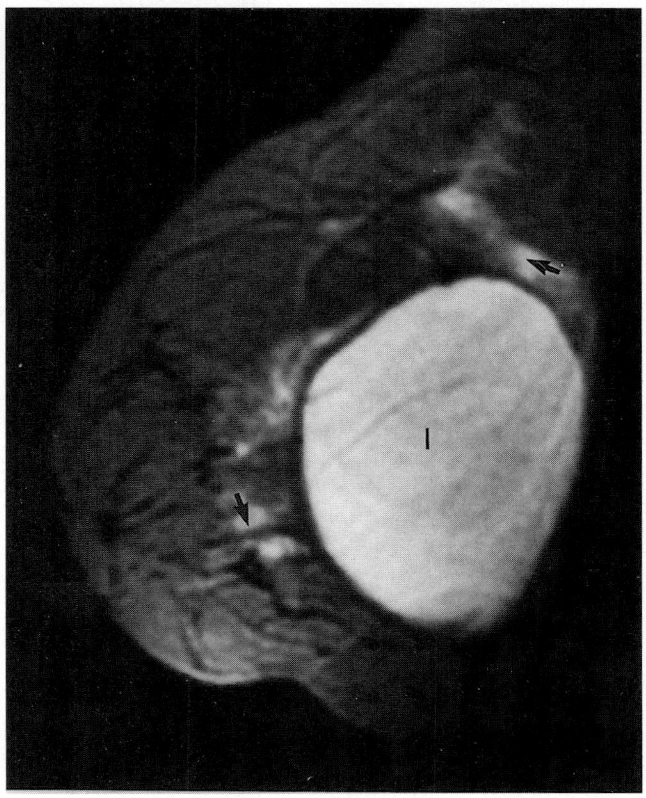

Figure 9–16. Patient with silicone breast injections (arrows) performed in the early 1960s and placement of a silicone breast implant (I) in the early 1970s.

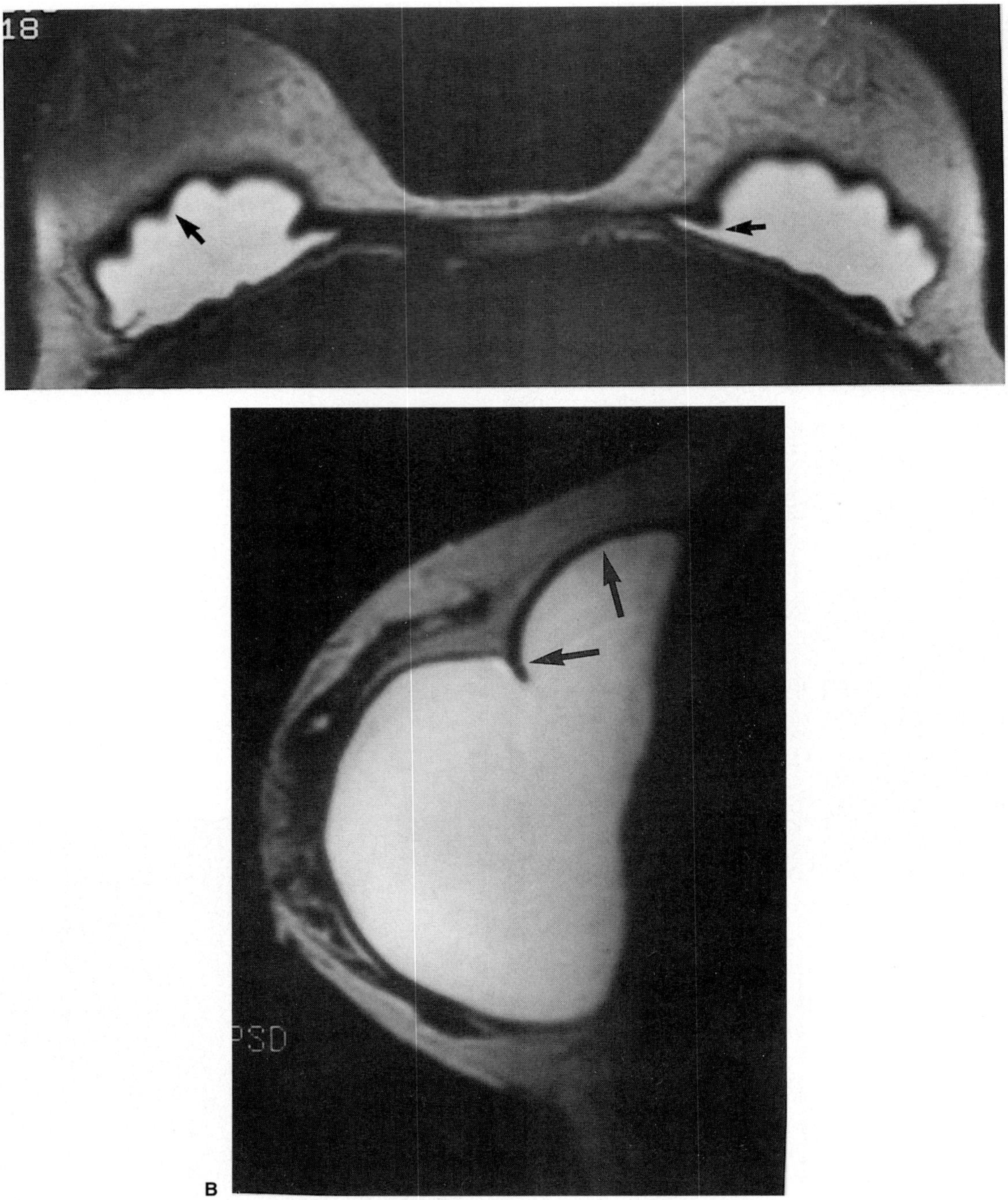

A

B

Figure 9–17. Contour irregularities of silicone implants. (**A**) Axial T2-weighted FSE shows diffuse irregularity of the contour (arrows) of the implant. Contour irregularities are not reliable signs of rupture. (**B**) Sagittal T2-weighted FSE shows herniation (arrow) of the silicone implant. Herniations of the implant are not reliable signs of rupture.

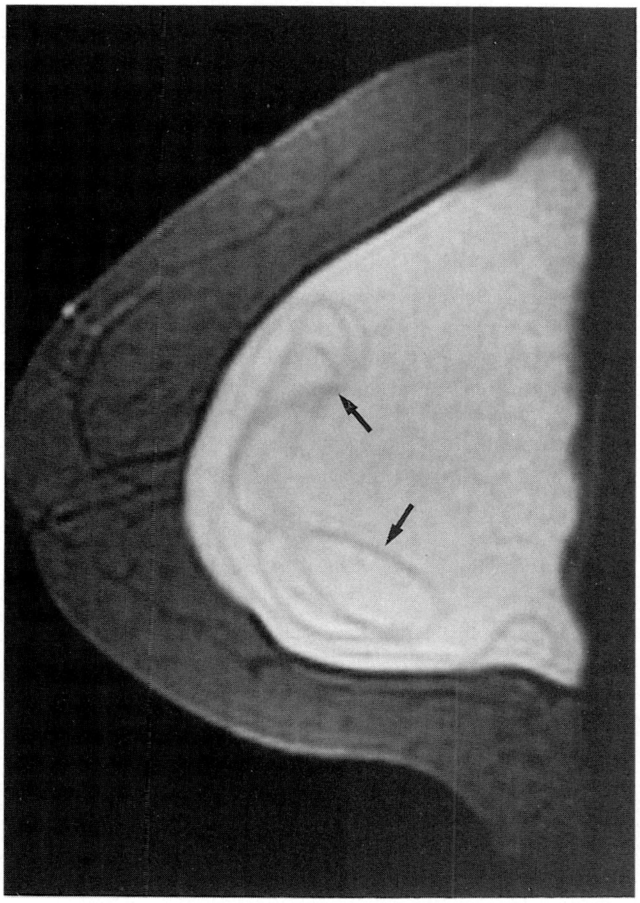

Figure 9–18. Patient with breast tenderness. Sagittal T2-weighted FSE MR image with water suppression shows intracapsular rupture of breast implant with curvilinear low signal intensity lines (linguine sign, arrow) representing the collapsed implant shell.

forms strands of silicone when touched; silicone oil has a slippery feel and does not form strands of silicone when touched. Silicone gel has many cross-linkages in the chemical composition of polydimethysiloxane while silicone oil has few or no cross-linkages. As previously stated, an uncollapsed implant rupture or early intracapsular rupture can have a similar or identical MR appearance to a large gel bleed or large collection of silicone oil and it can be difficult if not impossible to differentiate these two entities on MR images (Figs. 9–14 and 9–15).[6,27]

Direct silicone oil injections into the breast for breast augmentation started in the 1940s. There are many women in the United States and elsewhere who have had silicone oil breast injections. The MR imaging findings of direct silicone breast injections are high signal intensity areas scattered throughout the breast on T2-weighted images (Fig. 9–9). The free silicone can be easily identified and differentiated from multiple cysts on MR by performing a chemical water suppression MR sequence. The silicone will remain high signal intensity while any fluid within a breast cyst will be suppressed. There are a few women who have had both direct silicone breast injections and silicone breast implants (Fig. 9–16). It is difficult or impossible to differentiate the free silicone within the breast from prior direct silicone oil breast injections from extracapsular silicone implant ruptures. The main role of MR imaging in patients with direct silicone breast injections will probably be in the detection of breast tumors. MR imaging can easily suppress the signal from the silicone, and with the addition of MR contrast agents breast tumors can be identified by MR images. Ongoing research will eventually determine the role of MR imaging of the breast in patients with direct silicone breast injections.

In our experience, other signs, such as focal or diffuse irregularity of the contour of the implant, implant herniations (Fig. 9–17), or reactive fluid surrounding the implant, are not reliable indicators of silicone implant rupture. In approximately 20 to 25% of patients, a small amount of pleural fluid may be present of the image posterior to the breast. It is important not to confuse a normal small pleural effusion with an extracapsular rupture. Most patients are imaged in the prone position so any free pleural fluid will accumulate just posterior to the breast but within the thorax. Furthermore, this pleural fluid will not uniformly suppress with a chemical water-suppression sequence because of normal respiratory motion. If one is not convinced that the high signal posterior to the breast is a small pleural effusion, the patient can be imaged in the supine position using the body coil. Any free pleural fluid will accumulate along the posterior thorax. One must identify the multicurvilinear low signal intensity lines of an implant rupture (Fig. 9–18) or free silicone in the surrounding breast parenchyma, assuming no previous silicone implant rupture has occurred to diagnose an actual implant rupture.

■ SUMMARY

MR imaging has proven to be an excellent imaging modality in localizing free silicone and evaluating an implant for rupture with a sensitivity of approximately 94% and specificity of 97%. Silicone has a unique MR resonance frequency and long T1 and T2 relaxation times, which allows several MR sequences to provide excellent diagnostic images. The most commonly used sequences include T2-weighted, STIR, and chemical shift imaging. The T2-weighted and STIR sequences are commonly used in conjunction with chemical water suppression. The most reliable findings on MR imaging for detection of implant rupture include identification of the collapsed implant shell (linguine sign) and free silicone within the breast parenchyma.

REFERENCES

1. Marik PE, Kark AL, Zambakides A. Scleroderma after silicone augmentation mammoplasty: A report of two cases. *S Afr Med J.* 1990;77:212–213.
2. Weiner SR. Silicone augmentation mammoplasty and rheumatic disease. In: Stratmeyer ME, ed. *Silicone in Medical Devices: Proceedings of a Conference Held in Baltimore, MD, Feb 1–2, 1991.* Publication FDA 92-4249. Bethesda, MD: Department of Health and Human Services; 1991:81–102.
3. Bridges AJ, Vasey FB. Silicone breast implants: history, safety, and potential complications. *Arch Intern Med.* 1993;153: 2638–2644.
4. Gorczyca DP, Sinha S, Ahn CY, et al. Silicone breast implants in vivo: MR imaging. *Radiology.* 1992;185:407–410.
5. Gorczyca DP, Schneider E, DeBruhl ND, et al. Silicone breast implant rupture: comparison between three-point Dixon and fast spin-echo MR imaging. *AJR.* 1994;162:305–310.
6. Gorczyca DP. MR imaging of breast implants. *MRI Clin North Am.* 1994;2(4):659–672.
7. Sinha S, Gorczyca DP, DeBruhl ND, et al. MR imaging of silicone breast implants: comparison of different coil arrays. *Radiology.* 1993; 284–286.
8. Alcorn FS, Turner DA, Clark JW, et al. Magnetic resonance imaging in the study of the breast. *Radiographics.* 1985;5: 631–652.
9. Heywang SH, Fenzl G, Hahn D, et al. MR of the breast: histopathologic correlation. *Eur J Radiol.* 1987;3:175–183.
10. Murphy WA, Gohagan JK. Breast. In: Stark DD, Bradley WG Jr, eds. *Magnetic Resonance Imaging.* St. Louis: CV Mosby; 1987:861–886.
11. Partain CL, Kulkarni MV, Price RR, et al. Magnetic resonance imaging of the breast: functional T1 and three-dimensional imaging. *Cardiovasc Intervent Radiol.* 1986;8:292–299.
12. Stelling CB, Wang PC, Lieber A, Mattingly SS, Griffen WO, Powell DE. Prototype coil for magnetic resonance imaging of the female breast. *Radiology.* 1985;154:457–462.
13. Wiener JI, Chako AC, Merten CW, et al. Breast and axillary tissue MR imaging: correlations of signal intensities and relaxation times with pathologic findings. *Radiology.* 1986;160: 299–305.
14. Heywang SH, Hahn D, Schmid H, et al. MR imaging of the breast using gadolinium-DTPA. *J Comput Assist Tomogr.* 1986;10:199–204.

15. Harms SE, Flamig DP, Hesley KL, et al. Fat-suppressed three-dimensional MR imaging of the breast. *Radiographics.* 1993; 13(2):247–267.
16. Harms SE, Flamig DP, Hesley KL, et al. MR imaging of the breast with rotating delivery of excitation off resonance: clinical experience with pathologic correlation. *Radiology.* 1993; 186:493–501.
17. Heywang SH, Wolf A, Pruss E, et al. MR imaging of the breast with Gd-DTPA: use and limitations. *Radiology.* 1989;171:9.
18. Heywang-Kobrunner SH. Nonmammographic breast imaging techniques. *Curr Opinion Radiol.* 1992;4:146–154.
19. Heywang-Kobrunner SH. Contrast-enhanced MRI of the breast—overview after 1250 patient examinations. *Electromedica.* 1993;2:43–52.
20. Heywang-Kobrunner SH. Contrast-enhanced magnetic resonance imaging of the breast. *Invest Radiol.* 1994;29:94–104.
21. Kaiser WA. MRM promises earlier breast cancer diagnosis. *Diagn Imaging Int.* 1992;11:44–50.
22. Orel S, Schnall MD, LiVolsi VA, Troupin RH. Suspicious breast lesions: MR imaging with radiologic-pathologic correlation. *Radiology.* 1994;190:485–493.
23. Derby KA, Frankel SD, Kaufman L, et al. Differentiation of silicone gel from water and fat in MR phase imaging of protons at 0.064 T. *Radiology.* 1993;189(2):617–620.
24. Habal MB. The biologic basis for the clinical application of the silicones. *Arch Surg.* 1984;119:843–848.
25. Gorczyca DP, DeBruhl ND, Mund D, Bassett LW. Linguine sign at MR imaging: Does it represent the collapsed silicone implant shell? *Radiology.* 1994;191:576–577.
26. Mukundan S, Dixon WT, Kruse BD, et al. MR imaging of silicone gel-filled breast implants in vivo with a method that visualizes silicone selectively. *J Magn Reson Imaging.* 1993;3: 713–717.
27. Mund DF, Farria DM, Gorczyca DP, et al. MR imaging of the breast in patients with silicone-gel implants: spectrum of findings. *AJR.* 1993;161:773–778.
28. Garrido L, Kwong KK, Pfleiderer B, et al. Echo-planar chemical shift imaging of silicone gel prostheses. *Magn Reson Imaging.* 1993;11(5):625–634.
29. Schneider E, Chan TW. Selective MR imaging of silicone with the 3-point Dixon technique. *Radiology.* 1993;187:89–93.
30. Ahn CY, Shaw WW, Narayanan K, et al. Definitive diagnosis of breast implant rupture using magnetic resonance imaging. *Plast Reconstr Surg.* 1993;94(4):681–691.
31. Brody GS. Fact and fiction about breast implant "bleed." *Plast Reconstr Surg.* 1977;60:615–616.

10

Comparison of Imaging Modalities for the Failing Implant

DAVID P. GORCZYCA, NANETTE D. DEBRUHL, R. JAMES BRENNER, AND LAWRENCE W. BASSETT

Different methods for identifying the integrity of the silicone implant and extent of possible leakage have been described in detail in previous chapters of this text. The discussion by necessity has often included incidental references to other imaging modalities. In this chapter, we review all of these methods with the specific intent of comparing and contrasting their applications in clinical practice.

Mammography, ultrasonography (US), computed tomography (CT), and magnetic resonance imaging (MRI) have all been used to evaluate the integrity of silicone breast implants.[1–27] Each modality has specific strengths and weaknesses that may make a particular modality the study of choice for an individual patient. One of the first parameters that is commonly evaluated when comparing imaging modalities is the sensitivity and specificity. If all other factors are equal, the imaging modality with the highest sensitivity and specificity would be the imaging modality of choice; however, other important factors can influence which imaging modality should be used to evaluate the integrity of silicone breast implants. These factors include the cost of the examination, the availability of an imaging modality in the community, the expertise of the radiologist performing and interpreting the study, and potential contraindications or limitations that would prevent the utilization of a specific imaging modality.

For example, MR imaging of silicone breast implants has the highest sensitivity and specificity for detection of silicone implant rupture; however, contraindications such as cardiac pacemakers, aneurysm clips, or severe claustrophobia prevent some patients from having an MRI examination.[24,25,27] Ultrasonography has a respectable sensitivity and specificity for detection of silicone implant rupture, but is very operator dependent. The experience and expertise of a radiologist performing the examination, especially an ultrasound study, can have a significant impact on the ability to diagnose a silicone implant failure.[9–13,24,25,27] Computed tomography has a high sensitivity and specificity for detection of intracapsular silicone implant ruptures; however, extracapsular silicone implant ruptures are not as easily detected.[25,27] Furthermore, ionizing radiation used in CT imaging is a relative contraindication in younger women. Mammography is widely available, relatively inexpensive, and can easily detect extracapsular silicone implant ruptures.[1,27] Unfortunately, 80 to 90% of all silicone implant ruptures are intracapsular ruptures that cannot be identified by mammography.[14,18]

Several studies have been designed to directly compare the different imaging modalities in their ability to detect implant failure. One of the studies comparing the different imaging modalities was in an animal model designed to determine the most accurate imaging modality for detection of silicone implant ruptures.[25] In this study, 40 single-lumen silicone implants were surgically placed in 20 rabbits. Each received one intact and one ruptured implant and was examined with mammography, ultrasonography, computed tomography, and MR imaging. Five radiologists reviewed all images in a random fashion and graded each for rupture. MR imaging and CT were the most accurate modalities in detec-

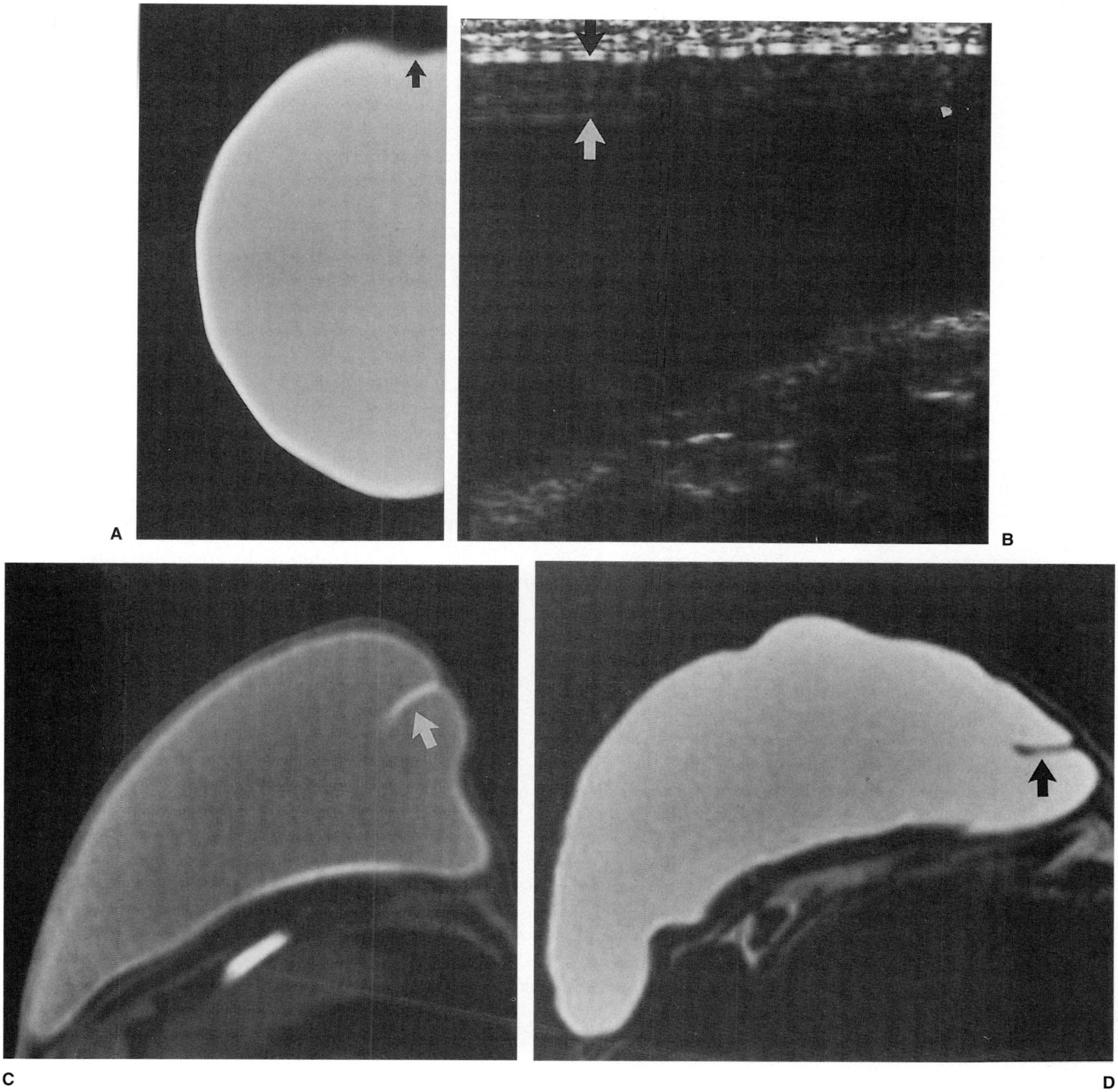

Figure 10–1. Normal intact silicone implant with a radial fold. (**A**) Mammogram shows slight contour deformity (arrow). (**B**) US image shows an anechoic interior with minimal reverberation artifact (between arrows) in anterior region of implant. (**C**) CT image shows the normal radial fold (arrow). (**D**) MR image shows a low signal intensity line that extends to the periphery (arrow), which represents a normal radial fold.

(text continues on page 148)

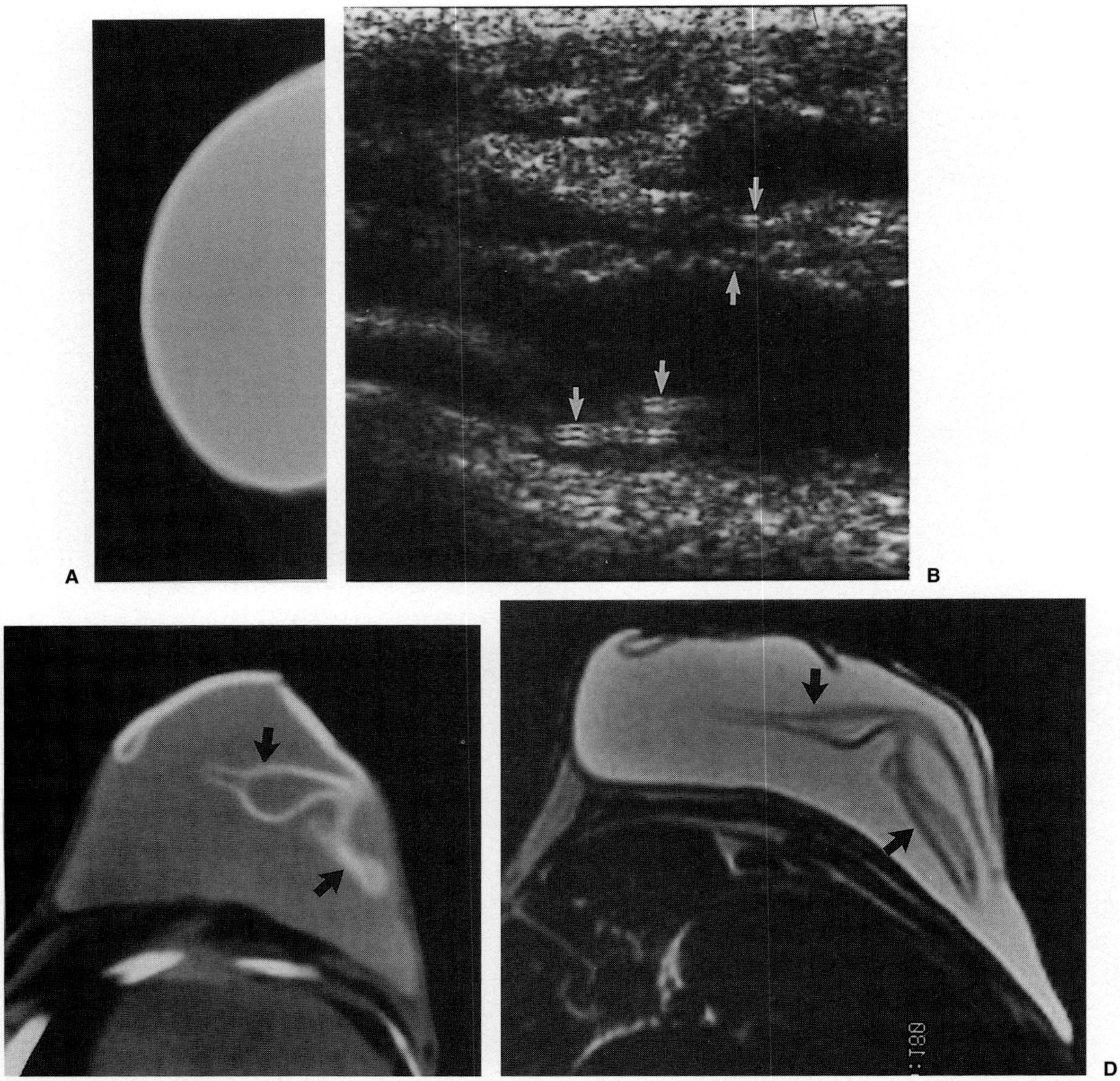

Figure 10–2. Intracapsular rupture of silicone implant. (**A**) Mammogram shows no abnormalities. (**B**) US image shows the collapsed implant shell as multiple echogenic lines (arrows—the stepladder sign). (**C**) CT image shows multiple curvilinear lines (arrows), which correspond to the linguine sign in **D**. (**D**) MR image shows multiple curvilinear lines (arrows) with low signal intensity (the linguine sign), which represents the collapsed implant shell.

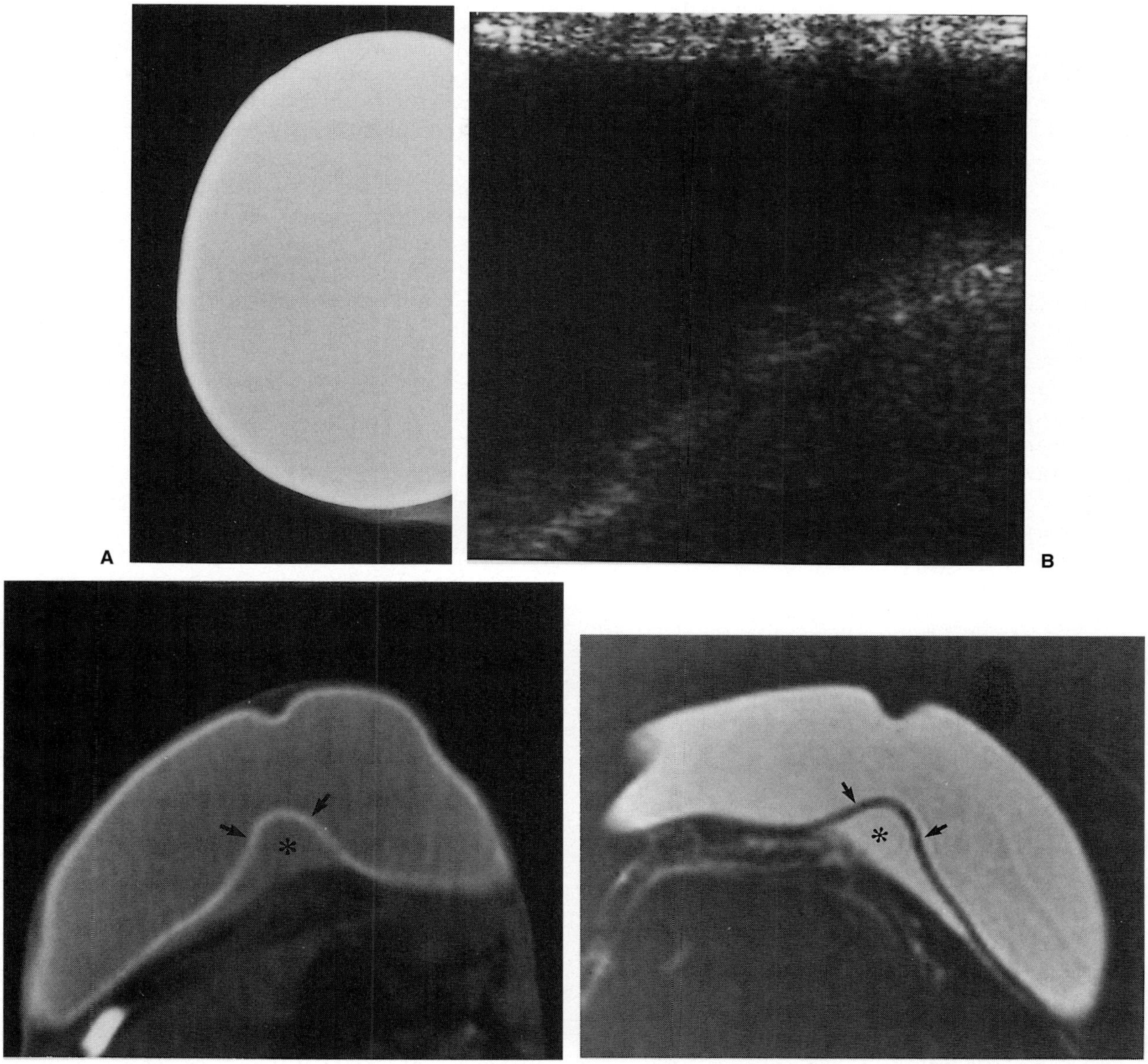

Figure 10–3. Uncollapsed rupture of silicone implant. (**A**) Mammogram shows no abnormalities. (**B**) US image shows an anechoic interior without evidence of rupture. (**C**) CT image shows silicone (asterisk), which has low attenuation, outside the implant shell. (**D**) MR image shows high signal intensity silicone (asterisk) outside the low signal intensity implant shell.

tion of intracapsular implant ruptures with receiver operating characteristic (ROC) values of .95 and .91 respectively; mammography and US were statistically significantly inferior with ROC values of .77 for each (p <.05). However, Gorczyca and DeBruhl found no statistical difference between the detectability of intracapsular rupture between MRI, CT, or US as long as the experienced radiologist performing the US examination interpreted the study at the time of scanning (Figs. 10–1 through 10–3). In a separate study comparing MR imaging and US, Berg et al[24] found the accuracy of MR imaging to be 84% compared with an accuracy of US of 49% in evaluation of intracapsular leaks. Additional comparative studies are under way to evaluate and directly compare the different imaging modalities. Most experts would agree that if all factors were equal between the different imaging modalities, MR imaging would be the study of choice because it has the highest sensitivity and specificity and has the ability to image the entire implant without the use of ionizing radiation. However, MR imaging of the breast is the most expensive imaging modality, and some patients are unable to have an MRI examination. Therefore, mammography, ultrasonography, and computed tomography will have roles in the evaluation of silicone breast implants. This chapter summarizes the advantages and limitations of each imaging modality and describes the key findings in detection of silicone implant failure.°

■ MAMMOGRAPHIC EVALUATION OF SILICONE BREAST IMPLANTS

Advantages

Mammography is relatively inexpensive and many women over 50 years of age, including women with silicone implants, receive yearly screening examinations. Therefore, the radiologist is able to evaluate the silicone implant on a yearly basis and detect any change in configuration or identify any new free silicone within the breast parenchyma. Because mammography can easily detect free silicone within the breast parenchyma, extracapsular silicone implant ruptures can be identified. Unfortunately, only 10 to 20% of silicone implant ruptures are of the extracapsular variety. Therefore, most of implant ruptures will not be detectable by mammography.

Limitations

Mammography is limited in its ability to depict silicone rupture and leakage, particularly of intracapsular ruptures, which account for approximately 80 to 90% of implant failures (Figs. 10–2A, 10–3A, and 10–4A).[1,24,25,27] The dense silicone is not easily penetrated by the x-ray energies used for typical screening mammography. Therefore, the classic finding of intracapsular rupture, the "linguine sign," cannot be identified. Even when one can penetrate the implant such as when using xeromammography which is no longer commercially available, it is difficult if not impossible to differentiate the collapsed implant shell from prominent radial folds on two-dimensional images.

Although, there are no documented cases of implant rupture due to mammography compression, we are aware of several unsubstantiated cases of rupture attributed to mammography. While new, nonimplanted silicone gel bags can withstand considerable mammographic compression, it is suspected that over time implanted silicone gel bags may be subject to fatigue and trauma, making them vulnerable. Therefore, radiologists should at least be aware of the potential for implant rupture during mammography and should have a protocol within their facilities to deal with any complications that may arise. Clinical signs of implant rupture include palpable silicone nodules, decreased breast size, asymmetry, tenderness, and a change in texture of the implant. Breakage of the fibrous capsule around the implant may occur with compression, and may be accompanied by an audible "pop." Thus, mammographic compression can potentially convert an intracapsular rupture to an extracapsular rupture. This same process may occur when a clinician performs "closed capsulotomy" to relieve capsular contracture causing deformity of the implant.

The possibility of implant rupture from mammography compression has led some professional liability carriers to suggest that a signed consent form be obtained prior to the performance of mammography on women with breast implants. Radiologists have voiced concern over the need of such informed consents in the absence of any documented evidence of a relationship between mammography and implant rupture. Radiologists are also concerned that informed consents might alarm women and prevent them from having mammograms done. The American College of Radiology does not recommend that routine consent forms be obtained for mammography of women with breast implants, but educational information for these women is encouraged.

Findings

Mammographic features that are not specific to implant rupture include a measurable periprosthetic dense band or rim of tissue that might correlate with a fibrous capsule around the implant, periprosthetic calcification, asymmetry of implant size or shape, and focal herniation of the implant. Specific mammographic evidence of implant rupture is extravasation of silicone outside the implant shell.[1,5,8] Before diagnosing an extracapsular implant rupture by mammography, obtain a good clinical history to make sure that the patient has not had a previous implant rupture that

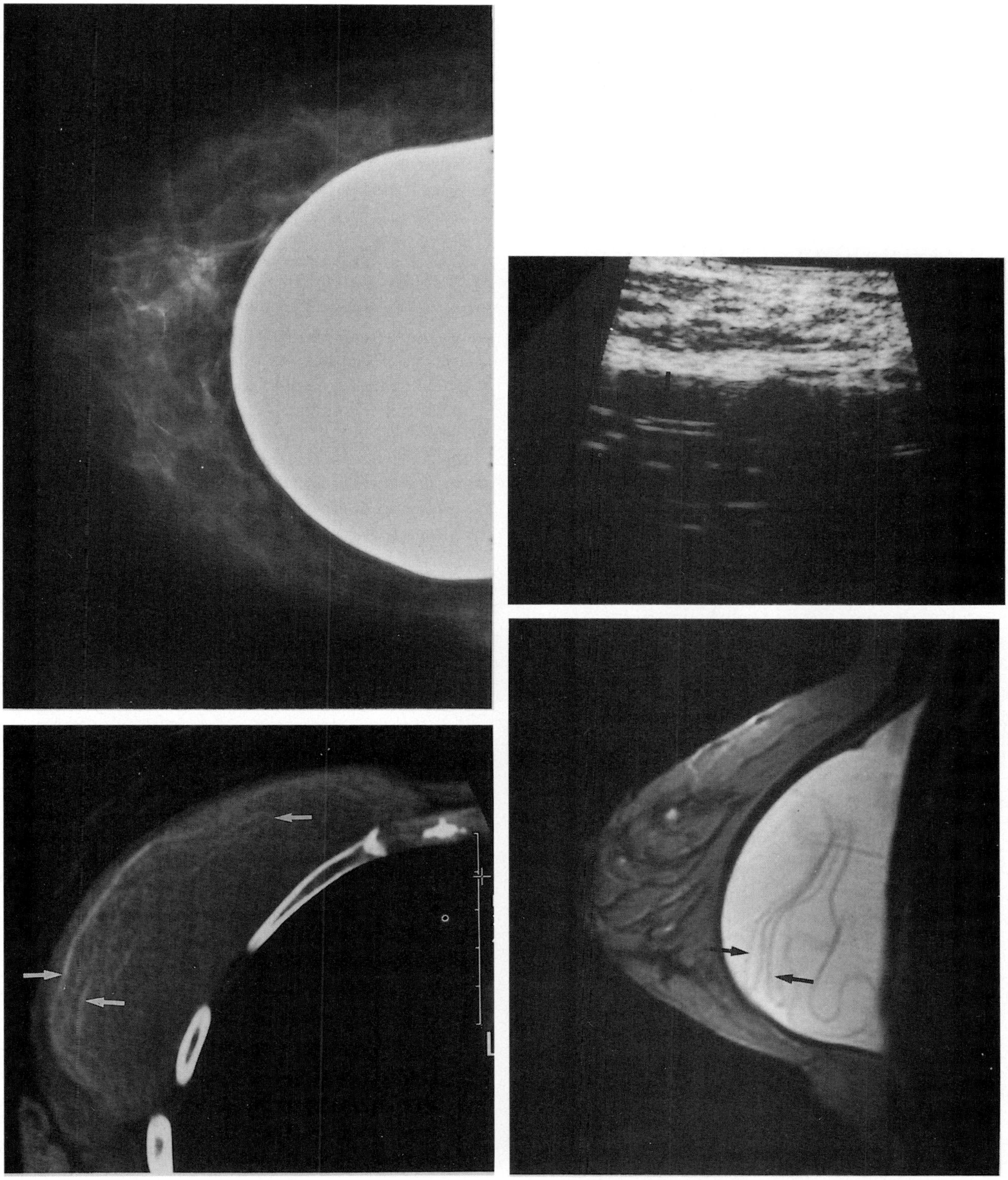

Figure 10–4. Intracapsular silicone implant rupture in a 40-year-old woman with bilateral silicone gel implants who presented with pain in the right breast for one year. (**A**) Mammogram shows no abnormalities. (**B**) US scan shows the collapsed implant shell as multiple echogenic lines (arrows), which represents the stepladder sign. (**C**) Axial CT scan shows high-density curvilinear lines (linguine sign, arrows) representing the collapsed implant shell. (**D**) Sagittal MR image shows the collapsed implant shell (arrow) indicating an intracapsular rupture.

was replaced with another silicone implant, or verify that the patient has not had direct silicone injections prior to silicone implant augmentation. Free silicone in the breast may be manifested by dense mass, linear streaks, or lymph node opacification. Silicone may be seen in lymph nodes beyond the fibrous capsule secondary to excessive gel bleed without implant rupture.

■ ULTRASONOGRAPHIC EVALUATION OF SILICONE BREAST IMPLANTS

Advantages

Ultrasonography is relatively inexpensive when compared with MRI or CT and no ionizing radiation is used. In the hands of an experienced operator, the entire sonographic examination of both silicone breast implants can be performed in less than 15 minutes. Furthermore, ultrasonography can detect small amounts of free silicone mixed within the surrounding breast tissues by the characteristic echogenic "snowstorm."[11] Ultrasonography can also detect intracapsular rupture by identifying a series of horizontal echogenic straight or curvilinear lines, somewhat parallel, traversing the interior of the implant commonly known as the "stepladder sign" (Figs. 10–2B and 10–4B).[12] It is important not to confuse the stepladder sign with normal prominent radial folds. Ultrasonography is very useful in patients who are claustrophobic or have a contraindication for MR imaging such as cardiac pacemakers or aneurysm clips.

Limitations

We have encountered some important limitations in the sonographic evaluation of implants. Due to marked attenuation of the ultrasound beam by silicone, sonography is limited in the evaluation of the back wall of an implant and the tissue posterior to it (Fig. 10–3B).[12] Prominent reverberation artifact can be confused with abnormalities of the implant. Previous silicone injections make it impossible to rule out extracapsular rupture in patients who have subsequent placement of silicone prostheses. In addition, extensive silicone injections can make it extremely difficult to evaluate the interior of a subsequently placed silicone implant due to attenuation of the ultrasound beam by the injected silicone and granuloma formation. In the same way, residual silicone granulomas from extracapsular rupture of explanted silicone implants compromise the evaluation of a new implant.

Findings

There are conflicting reports on the usefulness of ultrasonography for detecting implant ruptures.[9–13,24,25,27] The varying results in the literature may reflect the experience of the operator, type of equipment used, and technical factors. Ultrasonography is operator dependent and requires on site evaluation to accomplish the best results. A steep learning curve is needed to be proficient in US evaluation of implants. A high-resolution transducer (7.5 to 10 MHz) is required to evaluate the integrity of the silicone implant. However, a 5-MHz transducer may be required to depict the posterior aspects of the implant or better visualize a subpectoral implant. The implant should be examined systematically, to ensure evaluation of all areas of the implant, surrounding breast, and axilla. Clockwise scanning of the breast is used in our practice to be sure that the examination is complete. Selected hard-copy images are obtained for documentation.

The most reliable sign of an intact implant is an anechoic interior. However, reverberation artifacts are commonly encountered in the anterior aspect of the implant and should not be confused with abnormalities (Fig. 10–1B). The reverberation artifact is usually no thicker than the breast tissue anterior to the implant. The implant membrane, sometimes visualized as a thin echogenic line at the parenchymal tissue–implant interface, should be continuous and intact. Radial folds present as echogenic lines that extend from the periphery to the interior of the implant. These folds are normal infoldings of the implant membrane into the silicone gel. Radial folds are commonly found in normal implants but are frequently seen and may be more prominent in the presence of capsular contracture.

Sonographic Signs of Implant Rupture

The reported signs of implant rupture include hyperechoic or hypoechoic masses, dispersion of the sonographic beam ("snowstorm"), discontinuity of the implant membrane, multiple parallel echogenic lines within the implant interior (stepladder sign), and heterogeneous aggregates of medium to low-level echoes within the interior of the implant.[9–13] In our experience, the stepladder sign is the most reliable sonographic evidence of an intracapsular rupture (Figs. 10–2B and 10–4B.[12] The stepladder sign is a series of horizontal echogenic straight or curvilinear lines, somewhat parallel, traversing the interior of the implant. This sign represents the collapsed implant membrane floating within the silicone gel, and is analogous to the linguine sign seen on MR imaging. The continuity of these echogenic lines is usually not obvious on sonography because of the narrow field of view.

The most reliable sign of an extracapsular rupture is a focal nodule of generalized increase in echogenicity of the breast tissue and loss of normal parenchymal interfaces due to dispersion of the ultrasound beam, referred to as the "snowstorm sign." The nodules represent silicone granulomas, composed of free silicone and surrounding fibrous tissue reaction, lying outside the confines of the fibrous capsule. The granulomas have been associated with an echodense posterior band, sometimes referred to as "echodense noise." The granulomas are differentiated from breast tumors through correlation of clinical, mammographic, and sonographic findings.

As would be expected, sonographic signs of intracapsular rupture can be expected to accompany extracapsular rupture. Therefore, when sonographic signs of intracapsular rupture are present, a careful search for extracapsular rupture should be made, including a search for silicone nodules in the axilla.

■ COMPUTED TOMOGRAPHY EVALUATION OF SILICONE BREAST IMPLANTS

Advantages

Computed tomography is widely available and can be used in the evaluation of silicone breast implant failure. CT is accurate in detecting intracapsular silicone breast implant ruptures, and is capable of depicting the linguine sign (Figs. 10–2C and 10–4C).[4,25,27] Even in communities where MRI and US are commonly used for evaluation of silicone implants, it would be useful for radiologists to be familiar with the CT findings of implant rupture because silicone implants are commonly imaged during CT examination of the chest and upper abdomen. Many patients who have had mastectomies for breast cancer have had breast reconstruction with silicone implants. Furthermore, many of these patients will have CT scans of their chests and abdomens for staging of their breast cancer, and this is an ideal opportunity to evaluate the integrity of the silicone breast implants. Some patients who are unable to complete an MR examination because of claustrophobia can complete a CT examination. Furthermore, some patients who are not able to undergo an MRI because of size or weight restrictions may qualify for a CT scan. Most CT scanners have higher weight limits and larger bores than most MRI units.

Limitations

Computed tomography uses ionizing radiation to obtain images; therefore, this modality should not be the study of choice, especially in young women in the evaluation of silicone breast implants. The ability of computed tomography to detect extracapsular silicone is also limited because of the similar hounsfield units between silicone and soft tissues. However, in most cases of extracapsular silicone implant ruptures, one can identify the collapsed implant shell, so a ruptured silicone implant will usually not be missed by CT. In most communities CT is more expensive than US and mammography but is typically less expensive than MR imaging.

Findings

Computed tomography of an intact silicone implant is characterized by a homogeneous, gray density with a surrounding high-density ring (Fig. 10–1C). The intact silicone implant is usually oval in shape but can commonly have contour deformities or implant bulges or hernias. The CT findings of intracapsular silicone implant rupture are similar to MRI findings. The collapsed implant shell can usually be easily identified on the CT images (Figs. 10–2C and 10–4C). Signs of intracapsular implant rupture on CT consist of collapse of the white ring into the silicone gel center to form the linguine sign. Extracapsular rupture can be difficult to identify because of the poor soft tissue differentiation on CT imaging. As with MRI, it is important to differentiate normal prominent radial folds from an actual collapsed implant shell.

■ MRI EVALUATION OF SILICONE BREAST IMPLANTS

Advantages

MR imaging is the most accurate method for the detection of silicone breast implant ruptures and in determining if the silicone implant is intact. Other advantages of MR imaging are that no ionizing radiation is used, and many different MR pulse sequences can be used to optimize the silicone image, allowing optimal visualization of the silicone implants. Furthermore, MR imaging has multiplanar capability, allowing visualization of the silicone implant in any plane.

Limitation

MR imaging is the most expensive imaging modality for the evaluation of silicone breast implants. Furthermore, to obtain high-quality images, a dedicated breast coil is required. If a dedicated breast coil is not used, the image quality suffers and the ability to detect subtle implant ruptures will be compromised. Not all patients are able to undergo MR imaging because of cardiac pacemakers, aneurysm clips, or metallic foreign bodies with the orbits, which are not compatible with MR imaging. Some patients are very claustrophobic and are unable to complete an MRI examination. Size and weight restrictions also prevent some patients from having an MRI examination of the breast.

Findings

MR images of an intact single-lumen silicone implant show an outer silicone Silastic shell containing homogeneous high signal intensity silicone on T2-weighted images (Fig. 11–1D). A double-lumen silicone implant typically has an inner lumen of high signal intensity silicone surrounded by a smaller outer lumen that contains saline and has different signal intensities depending on the pulse sequence. The silicone implants are usually oval or round in shape.

The most reliable MR criterion for intracapsular rupture is the presence of the multiple curvilinear low signal intensity lines seen within the high signal intensity silicone gel, the so-called linguine sign (Figs. 10–2D and 10–4D).[14,19] These curvilinear lines represent the collapsed implant membrane floating within the silicone gel.[19] In early stages the curvilinear lines may be located near the periphery of the implant (Fig. 10–3D). The teardrop sign is sometimes the only indication of implant rupture.[18] This sign represents silicone that has leaked out of the ruptured silicone implant and entered one of the radial folds on the exterior of the implant. This finding is not definitive for an implant rupture, because it has also been attributed to extensive gel bleed.

The definitive sign of extracapsular rupture is the presence of free silicone in the breast parenchyma. On MR imaging free silicone presents as focal areas of high signal intensity. The multiplanar capabilities of MR imaging allow precise localization of free silicone. Other causes of silicone in the parenchyma are previous silicone oil injections or silicone remaining from previous rupture of a silicone implant that has been removed. Because extracapsular rupture is an extension of intracapsular rupture, all of the signs of intracapsular rupture can be present as well. For example, the linguine sign, the most reliable sign of intracapsular rupture, is almost always seen in cases of extracapsular rupture.

■ SELECTION OF IMAGING MODALITY

The imaging protocol for a patient with breast implants depends on many factors. If the woman is referred for screening or diagnostic evaluation for possible breast cancer, then mammography should include implant displaced views whenever possible. Mammography may detect extracapsular silicone implant rupture. If the patient is referred for evaluation of a possible implant rupture, and explantation is being contemplated, ultrasonography or MR imaging may be required. Ultrasonography should be limited to practices where the radiologist has sufficient experience to identify both intracapsular and extracapsular ruptures with confidence. Even in the latter situation, MR imaging may be required to resolve questionable ultrasonographic findings. MR imaging is the modality of choice for the evaluation of silicone implants prior to surgical explantation in most practices. CT is reserved for patients in whom MR imaging is contraindicated due to severe claustrophobia or indwelling metallic devices that are not compatible with magnetic resonance. It is important to emphasize that if there is no expectation that a detected rupture would lead to surgery, then there is no reason to perform expensive and time-consuming imaging procedures.

REFERENCES

1. Destouet JM, Monsees BS, Oser RF, Nemecek JR, Young VL, Pilgram TK. Screening mammography in 350 women with breast implants: prevalence and findings of implant complications. *AJR.* 1992; 973–978.
2. Eklund GW, Busby RC, Miller SH, et al. Improved imaging of the augmented breast. *AJR.* 1988;151:469–473.
3. Dershaw DD, Chaglassian TA. Mammography after prosthesis placement for augmentation or reconstructive mammoplasty. *Radiology.* 1989;170:69–74.
4. Scott IR, Muller NL, Fitzpatrick DG, et al. Ruptured breast implant: computed tomographic and mammographic findings. *J Canad Assoc Radiol.* 1988;39:152–154.
5. Young VL, Bartell T, Destouet JM, Monsees B, Logan SE. Calcification of breast implant capsule. *South Med J.* 1989;82: 1171–1173.
6. Bassett LW, Brenner RJ. Considerations when imaging women with breast implants. *AJR.* 1992;159:979–981.
7. Bassett LW, Hendrick RE, Bassford TL, et al. *Quality Determinants of Mammography.* Clinical Practice Guideline, no. 13. AHCPR Publication No. 95-0632. Rockville, MD: Agency for Health Care Policy and Research, Public Health Service, U.S. Department of Health and Human Services; 1994.
8. Leibman AJ, Kruse B. Breast cancer: mammographic and sonographic findings after augmentation mammoplasty. *Radiology.* 1990;174:195–198.
9. Levine RA, Collins TL. Definitive diagnosis of breast implant rupture by ultrasonography. *Plast Reconstr Surg.* 1991;87: 1126–1128.
10. Rosculet KA, Ikeda DM, Forrest ME, et al. Ruptured gel-filled silicone breast implants: sonographic findings in 19 cases. *AJR.* 1992;159:711–716.
11. Harris KM, Ganott MA, Shestak KC, et al. Silicone implant rupture: detection with US. *Radiology.* 1993;187:761–768.
12. DeBruhl ND, Gorczyca DP, Ahn CY, Shaw WW, Bassett LW. Silicone breast implants: US evaluation. *Radiology.* 1993; 189:95–98.
13. Ganott MA, Harris KM, Ilkhanipour ZS, Costa-Creco MA. Augmentation mammoplasty: normal and abnormal findings with mammography and US. *RadioGraphics.* 1992;12:281–295.
14. Gorczyca DP, Sinha S, Ahn C, et al. Silicone breast implants in vivo: MR imaging. *Radiology.* 1992;185:407–410.
15. Ahn CY, Shaw WW, Narayanan K, et al. Definitive diagnosis of breast implant rupture using magnetic resonance imaging. *Plast Reconstr Surg.* 1993;94(4):681–691.
16. Gorczyca DP, Schneider E, DeBruhl ND, et al. Silicone breast implant rupture: comparison between three-point Dixon and fast spin-echo MR imaging. *AJR.* 1994;162:305–310.
17. Schneider E, Chan TW. Selective MR imaging of silicone with the 3-point Dixon technique. *Radiology.* 1993;187:89–93.
18. Gorczyca DP. MR imaging of breast implants. *MRI Clin North Am.* 1994;2(4):659–672.
19. Gorczyca DP, DeBruhl ND, Mund DF, Bassett LW. Linguine sign at MR imaging: Does it represent the collapsed silicone implant shell? *Radiology.* 1994;191:576–577.
20. Garrido L, Kwong KK, Pfleiderer B, et al. Echo-planar chemical shift imaging of silicone gel prostheses. *Magn Reson Imaging.* 1993;11(5):625–634.
21. Mukundan S, Dixon WT, Kruse BD, et al. MR imaging of silicone gel-filled breast implants in vivo with a method that visualizes silicone selectively. *JMRI.* 1993;3:713–717.
22. Mund DF, Farria DM, Gorczyca DP, et al. MR imaging of the breast in patients with silicone-gel implants: spectrum of findings. *AJR.* 1993;161:773–778.

23. Derby KA, Frankel SD, Kaufman L, et al. Differentiation of silicone gel from water and fat in MR phase imaging of protons at 0.064 T. *Radiology.* 1993;189(2):617–620.
24. Berg WA, Caskey CI, Hamper UM. Diagnosing breast implant rupture with MR imaging, US, and mammography. *RadioGraphics.* 1993;13:1323.
25. Gorczyca DP, DeBruhl ND, Ahn CY, et al. Silicone breast implant ruptures in an animal model: comparison of mammography, MR imaging, US, and CT. *Radiology.* 1994;190:227–232.
26. Steinbach BG, Hardt NS, Abbitt PL, et al. Breast implants, common complications, and concurrent breast disease. *Radiographics.* 1993;13:95–118.
27. Everson LI, Parantainen H, Detlie T, et al. Diagnosis of breast implant rupture: imaging findings and relative efficacies of imaging techniques. *AJR.* 1994;163:57–60.

11

Tumor Detection in the Augmented Breast

R. JAMES BRENNER

Although imaging is an important aspect in evaluating the breast for potential implant failure, its paramount role remains the detection of breast cancer. The incidence of breast cancer in the United States is approximately 180,000 per year and is neither better nor worse for women with breast implants or injected silicone.[1] Such projections, however, need to be modified for this population of nearly 2 million women.

First, at least 20% of women who currently have breast implants have undergone augmentation because of prior breast cancer surgery. Implants are usually placed following mastectomy but may be placed for cosmetic symmetry in patients who have undergone conservation therapy (eg, lumpectomy). The incidence of cancer in patients who have undergone mastectomy would be expected to be lower than in the general population, but it is not. On the other hand, these women are at increased risk for the development of breast cancer in the other (contralateral) breast. Women who have undergone conservation surgery are at higher risk for the development of either recurrent breast cancer in the same area or another breast cancer in a different area of the breast. Indeed, the possibility of recurrent cancer on the operated side persists even in a patient who has undergone modified radical mastectomy because even aggressive current techniques make it virtually impossible to remove absolutely all breast tissue. Furthermore, the possibility of recurrent local disease that has already spread microscopically to the chest wall or internal mammary nodes remains a challenge for detection in the woman who has undergone mastectomy.

Second, although the presence of an implant or injected silicone has no known direct causative relationship to the induction of breast cancer, [notwithstanding the theoretical carcinogenic risk of 2,4-toluenediamine (TDA), a breakdown product of polyurethane that coats perhaps 10% of implanted prostheses], the presence of implants is associated with delayed stages of detection and consequently poorer prognosis at time of diagnosis. Although most breast cancers currently detected are by size stage 0 (confined to the mammary duct without penetration or infiltration) or stage I (less than 2 cm in maximum diameter), especially in women undergoing regular screening, this is not the situation in women who have undergone augmentation mammoplasty.

The delay in diagnosis of breast cancer in women undergoing breast implants has been observed in several studies. Silverstein et al[2] reported on a series of 42 women with prior augmentation in which 95% of the tumors were detected by clinical examination an average of 8.4 years following implantation surgery, most of which were not visible on mammogram. Among this population, 90% had infiltrating carcinomas, 45% had metastases to axillary nodes, seven have had recurrence, and five have died.

French investigators Ouimet-Oliva and Hebert[3] reported their results of women who had undergone silicone implant placement for either augmentation or reconstruction over a 6-year period. They found 22 cancers, all palpable at time of detection, among a population of 230 women with mammography failing to demonstrate an abnormality in 41% of cases. This was compared with 920 patients with mammograms showing cancer in which a little over one third of the lesions were not palpable during physical examination.

Leibman and Kruse[4] reported on 11 patients with augmentation implants and breast cancer. Fifty-five percent of the cancers were palpable, 73% were infiltrating carcinomas, and 36% had spread to the lymph nodes.

Fajardo et al[5] retrospectively reviewed a large clinic population, most of whom were being followed asymptomatically, and reported on 18 patients with cancer who had had a mammogram within 8 months of diagnosis. Eighty-nine percent of these patients had palpable abnormalities at diagnosis, 89% had invasive carcinomas, and 39% had spread to the axillary lymph nodes.

Destouet et al[6] reported on a series of screening mammograms in 350 asymptomatic women, incidentally finding two cancers in the population, one stage 0 and one stage II.

The finding of a breast cancer with less favorable prognostic features in populations of studied patients who have breast implants, compared with large-scale screening studies in which a majority of lesions are found at stage 0 or stage 1 and often by mammography alone, implies that implants interfere with both the clinical and mammographic detection of cancer. Fajardo et al[5] indicated that among the 18 patients studied with palpable cancers, standard mammographic views were negative in 17 of them (94%), and implant displacement views showed abnormalities in 12 patients (67%). As discussed above, such delayed detection reported for small groups of patients needs to be reconciled with a woman's other reasons for deciding to undergo prosthetic implantation.

It is difficult to know precise reasons for delay. Imaging of the augmented breast requires special techniques and attention to detail that have been discussed elsewhere (see Chapter 10). An interesting phenomenon was reported by Morgenstern et al,[7] who reviewed the histopathology surrounding 12 patients who had undergone direct silicone injections, the majority of which were subject to mastectomy. They found that those patients with tumor demonstrated little desmoplastic (fibrotic) reaction to the tumor when it was admixed with silicone, whereas tumors distal to areas of free silicone showed normal reactive fibrosis. The absence of any inflammatory reaction to the tumor not only makes detection more difficult, but may affect overall prognosis.[8] Furthermore, Morgenstern and colleagues observed a relationship between silicone nodal involvement and tumor spread; namely, the greater the involvement of the node with free silicone, the greater the propensity for tumor invasion, implying an enhancing effect of free silicone on tumor spread.

Postoperative scarring involved in both reconstructed and augmented procedures may produce features that mimic malignancy. Although controversial, it is suspected that the placement of implants into the subpectoral location rather than the subglandular location—a more difficult procedure—may induce fewer mammographic features of scarring and permit better demonstration of breast tissue. The difficulties of tumor detection in the postoperative breast for any reason have been discussed elsewhere.[5,9,10]

The mammographic (and sonographic) features of malignancy in the patient with a breast implant are no different from those in a patient without an implant, and have been reviewed extensively in other publications and general texts to which the reader is referred. In particular, masses with irregular margins, with or without calcifications, and clustered pleomorphic microcalcifications, especially in an identifiable ductal distribution, are the most common radiographic signs of breast cancer. Other signs may be more or less specific than in a woman who has not undergone surgery or silicone injection. For example, the presence of architectural distortion, which may indicate a malignant process and/or tissue response to malignancy (eg, desmoplasia), is also a common mammographic feature of postoperative scarring. In like manner asymmetries of the breast following surgery may be more difficult to distinguish with respect to benign or malignant etiology. Finally, image-defined or clinical palpated masses need to be distinguished with respect to parenchymal disturbances such as cancer and findings associated with implantation such as silicone granuloma or prosthetic valve. Finally, sequelae following explantation may also mimic mammographic or sonographic features of malignancy.

The evaluation of a patient with a palpable mass frequently involves imaging of the mass as well as any other nonpalpable abnormalities (eg, screening the remainder of the ipsilateral and entire contralateral breast). Evaluation is facilitated by direct tissue sampling. In a patient with an implant, needle biopsy may be more difficult and thus restricted, and imaging assumes greater importance for two reasons. First, the possibility of implant puncture during blind needle biopsy of a palpable abnormality exists when the position of the implant is not easily defined on physical examination. Second, the area of palpation may be related to the implant rather than the breast, or inseparable from the implant and its fibrous capsule. Imaging under such circumstances provides not only an anatomical evaluation of the area of palpable findings and its relationship to the implant, but also the opportunity for an image-guided approach to the lesion in question. On the other hand, the latter procedure is not always indicated and in fact is less feasible when an area of clinical suspicion has no correlative imaging features to help guide needle placement.

A variety of clinical situations emerge in the image evaluation of a woman who has undergone augmentation mammoplasty when she is either being screened for breast cancer or evaluated for signs or symptoms of breast cancer following physical examination. At times, evaluation is direct and at other times so complicated as to involve sophisticated technology. The essential decision regarding biopsy for an area of clinical or imaging concern, which is determined by the woman in consultation with her physician, may be more influenced by cosmetic considerations in women who have undergone augmentation for cosmesis than in the general population. Nonetheless, the importance of identifying breast cancer, and especially early breast cancer, remains the pri-

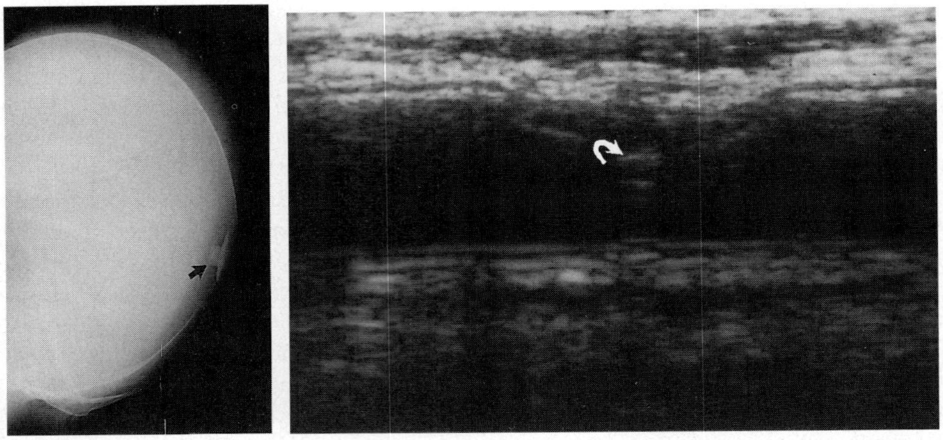

A B

Figure 11–1. (**A**) Cranial-caudal view of breast with saline implant. Arrow points to valve that was the cause of the palpable mass. (**B**) Ultrasound image of implant over the palpable area. Arrow indicates position of "palpable" valve.

mary concern. Thus recommendations for biopsy require, as always, due deliberation and critical analysis. As in much of medicine, the particular techniques and subjective interpretations of both clinical and imaging examinations are not entirely standardized, and vary among institutions. Successful management decisions are frequently dependent on judgment founded in both expertise and experience.

Consider the situation of a 39-year-old woman who presented with a sharp-feeling lump near her nipple. The physician requested both a mammogram and ultrasound examination (Fig. 11–1). Both imaging studies identified the implant valve as corresponding to and accounting for the clinical finding, obviating further intervention and anxiety.

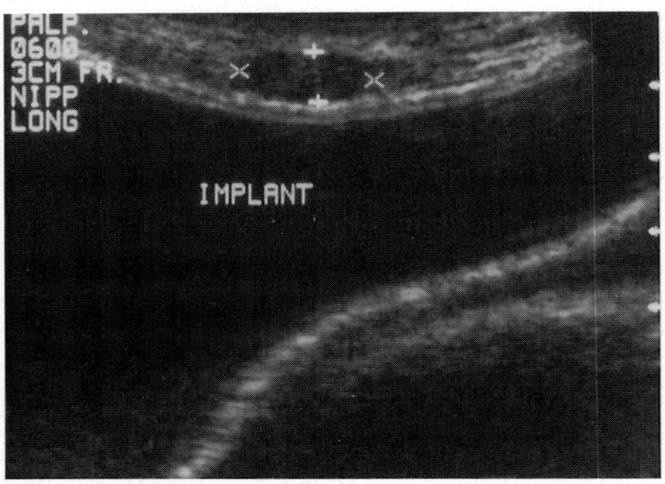

Figure 11–2. Ultrasound image of a palpable solid mass anterior to intact implant. The mass is well circumscribed with low-amplitude internal echoes. Acoustic enhancement or shadowing is difficult to ascertain because sound waves encounter interference from both the fibrous capsule and the implant posterior to the mass. Diagnosis: fibroadenoma.

In contrast to the above case, a 46-year-old woman with breast implants presented with a palpable mass in the 6 o'-clock position of the right breast. Mammography showed no evidence of a mass but ultrasound examination over the mass demonstrates a well-circumscribed solid mass anterior to the implant (Fig. 11–2). Both the preoperative and final surgical diagnoses was benign fibroadenoma. Had the mass shown irregular margins by sonography it would have been considered suspicious for malignancy in a manner similar to evaluation of a patient without implantation. It is sometimes difficult to distinguish by imaging or physical examination or both a focal collection of silicone, either eventrated or herniated through a weakened portion of the fibrous capsule, or free silicone (especially with surrounding granulation tissue) from a breast parenchymal mass. In the case of this patient, there were no other signs of intracapsular leak (eg, stepladder sign, snowstorm appearance, see Chapter X), and the normal unaltered contour of the implant was easily defined. Free silicone is sometimes defined mammographically by its density, or sonographically by its highly echogenic characteristics, a feature usually inconsistent with both fibroadenoma or carcinoma, the two most common lesions that need to be considered in a differential diagnosis. At times, coexistent signs of silicone leak and a true breast mass may make evaluation even more difficult. In such cases, mammographic and sonographic features together with clinical presentation should help distinguish such processes, but further and more sophisticated imaging may be required.

Such is the case of a 45-year-old woman who had undergone a mastectomy and silicone implant reconstruction and presented with a new palpable mass in the inner aspect of

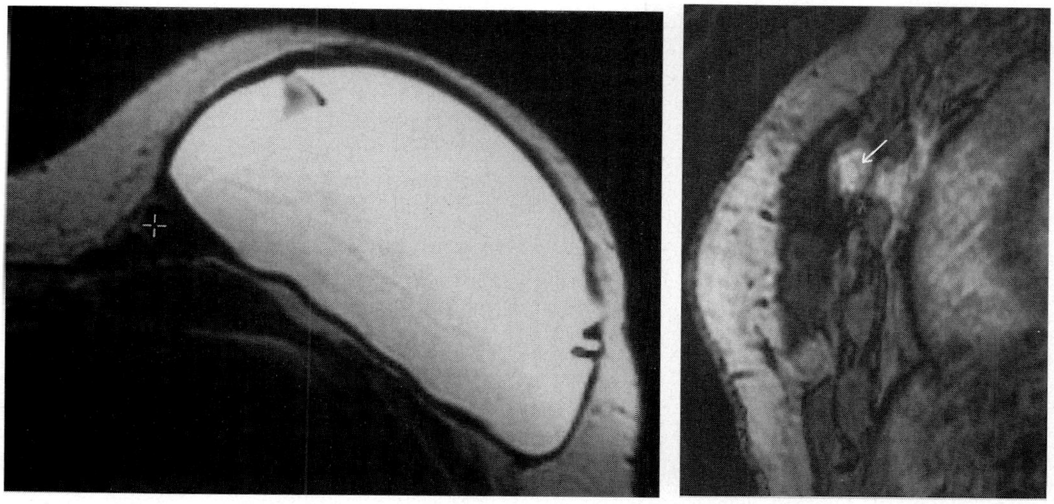

Figure 11–3. (**A**) MRI with T2-weighted axial image. Area of the mass is indicated by crosshatches, which are electronically linked to position shown in **B**, in the area of the palpable mass. The mass is displacing the implant, but there is no bright (silicone) signal associated with the mass. Based on this image alone, the mass could represent simple fibrous tissue, but not silicone. (**B**) MRI study without subtraction, T1-weighted sagittal image, following injection of gadolinium contrast agent. Arrow indicates precise location of a palpable mass, corresponding to that seen in axial image in **A**. The dumbbell-shaped lesion enhances rapidly in the first minute and is shown extending through the chest wall, infiltrating both anteriorly and posteriorly. Diagnosis: recurrent cancer involving internal mammary lymph node.

her breast. The anatomic area of the mass was impossible to image mammographically and difficult to image sonographically because the mass was posterior to the implant (Fig. 11–3A). In this case, magnetic resonance imaging (MRI) was performed. The first MRI study (Fig. 11–3B) confirmed an intact implant with no silicone signal beyond the fibrous capsule in the area of palpable findings, indicating that the mass did not represent a silicone leak. The second MRI study (Fig. 11–3C) showed a contrast-enhancing mass with a dumbbell shape, suspicious for recurrent malignancy within an internal mammary lymph node, which was confirmed by surgery.

A similar presentation in a different clinical setting illustrates both the limitations and potentials of sophisticated imaging techniques in complicated cases of palpable abnormalities that are not sufficiently imaged with more conventional techniques such as mammography and ultrasound. A 39-year-old woman with silicone implants had been studied elsewhere and told that her palpable mass was not associated with silicone as evidenced on MRI examination (Fig. 11–4A). Reevaluation of the patient with ultrasound examination showed an echogenic mass in the area of palpable concern, suggesting either a focus of free silicone or a lymph node infiltrated with silicone (see Fig. 11–7 for the sonographic appearance of a lymph node infiltrated with silicone). Because of the prior reported results, however, a tumor-seeking gadolinium-contrast MRI was performed showing an enhancing mass in the area of palpable and sonographic findings with a suggestion of silicone signal corresponding to the inferior aspect of the mass (Fig. 11–4B,C). The combination of features suggested a preoperative diagnosis of inflamed lymph node secondary to silicone, either from gel bleed or leak. Review of the prior MRI study performed at another institution faintly shows the lymph node (mass) but not extracapsular silicone because the entire area is obscured by technique artifact. The patient declined needle biopsy because of the fear of implant penetration. The nodule decreased in size and was eventually removed during implant revision several months later. At surgery a lymph node was found that included silicone.

That clinical and imaging results are best considered in tandem is illustrated by the case of a 58-year-old woman who had undergone modified radical mastectomy for cancer several years earlier and now presented because she had developed a palpable mass. Conventional mammography showed minimal residual tissue and no evidence of silicone leak (Fig. 11–5A). Special spot compression magnification mammographic views demonstrated an ill-defined soft tissue mass at the site of the palpable mass (Fig. 11–5B), possibly representing the implant bulging through a weakened area of the fibrous capsule. Ultrasound demonstrated a solid mass distinct from and anterior to the silicone implant (Fig. 11–5C). The mass was not associated with a valve, and was unlikely to be related to free silicone for the same reasons as

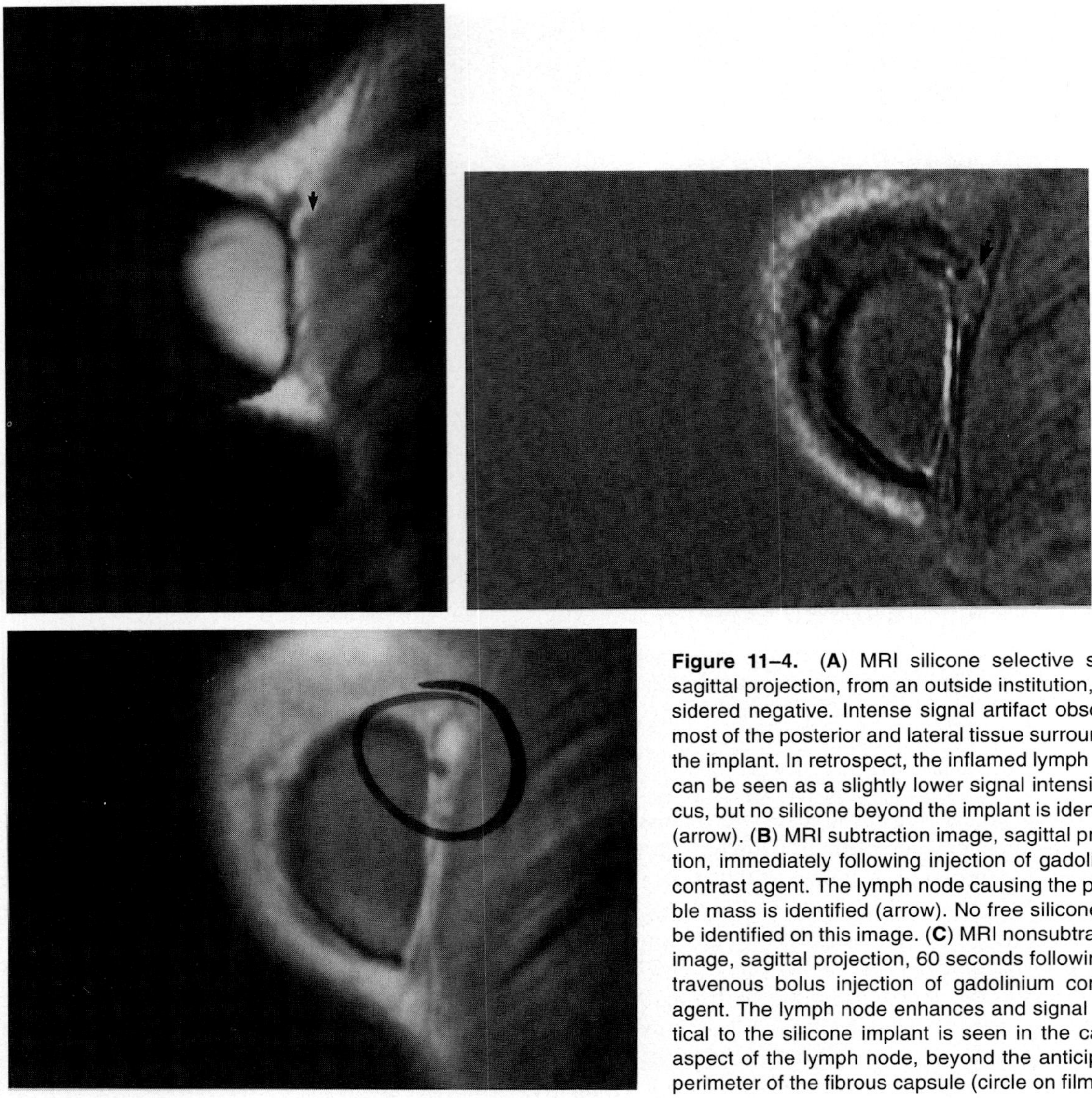

Figure 11–4. (A) MRI silicone selective study, sagittal projection, from an outside institution, considered negative. Intense signal artifact obscures most of the posterior and lateral tissue surrounding the implant. In retrospect, the inflamed lymph node can be seen as a slightly lower signal intensity focus, but no silicone beyond the implant is identified (arrow). (B) MRI subtraction image, sagittal projection, immediately following injection of gadolinium contrast agent. The lymph node causing the palpable mass is identified (arrow). No free silicone can be identified on this image. (C) MRI nonsubtraction image, sagittal projection, 60 seconds following intravenous bolus injection of gadolinium contrast agent. The lymph node enhances and signal identical to the silicone implant is seen in the caudal aspect of the lymph node, beyond the anticipated perimeter of the fibrous capsule (circle on film).

discussed in Figure 11–2. Therefore, in a postmenopausal patient who had undergone mastectomy, a new solid mass was by definition highly suggestive of recurrent malignancy, which was found at surgery.

Masses that cannot be palpated at physical examination (clinically occult) but are detected mammographically need to be managed in a manner independent of whether or not a woman has breast implants. When detected in patients who have undergone mastectomy, a very high index of suspicion must be raised, as in the above case (Fig. 11–5). Masses must also be distinguished from silicone, which, as described, may be difficult.

In Figure 11–6 a soft tissue mass was identified on mammography in the lower outer quadrant of a 43-year-old patient's right breast and not felt during clinical examination. The mass was distinguishable from extensive silicone mastopathy, including silicone cyst formation; the patient had undergone free silicone injections many years earlier. The margins of the mass as defined on the mammogram were microlobulated with a density sufficiently different from silicone to indicate a parenchymal origin. Surgical removal of the mass was performed, revealing a benign "clump" of tissue without silicone ("fibrocystic mass").

Contrast the patient in Figure 11–6 with the one illustrated in Figure 11–7. Two nonpalpable soft tissue–appearing masses were detected during routine mammography (Fig. 11–7A). When subjected to mammographic spot compression magnification examination, silicone-dense material can be seen infiltrating the two masses, the morphology of which indicated probable lymph nodes (Fig. 11–7B). Ultra-

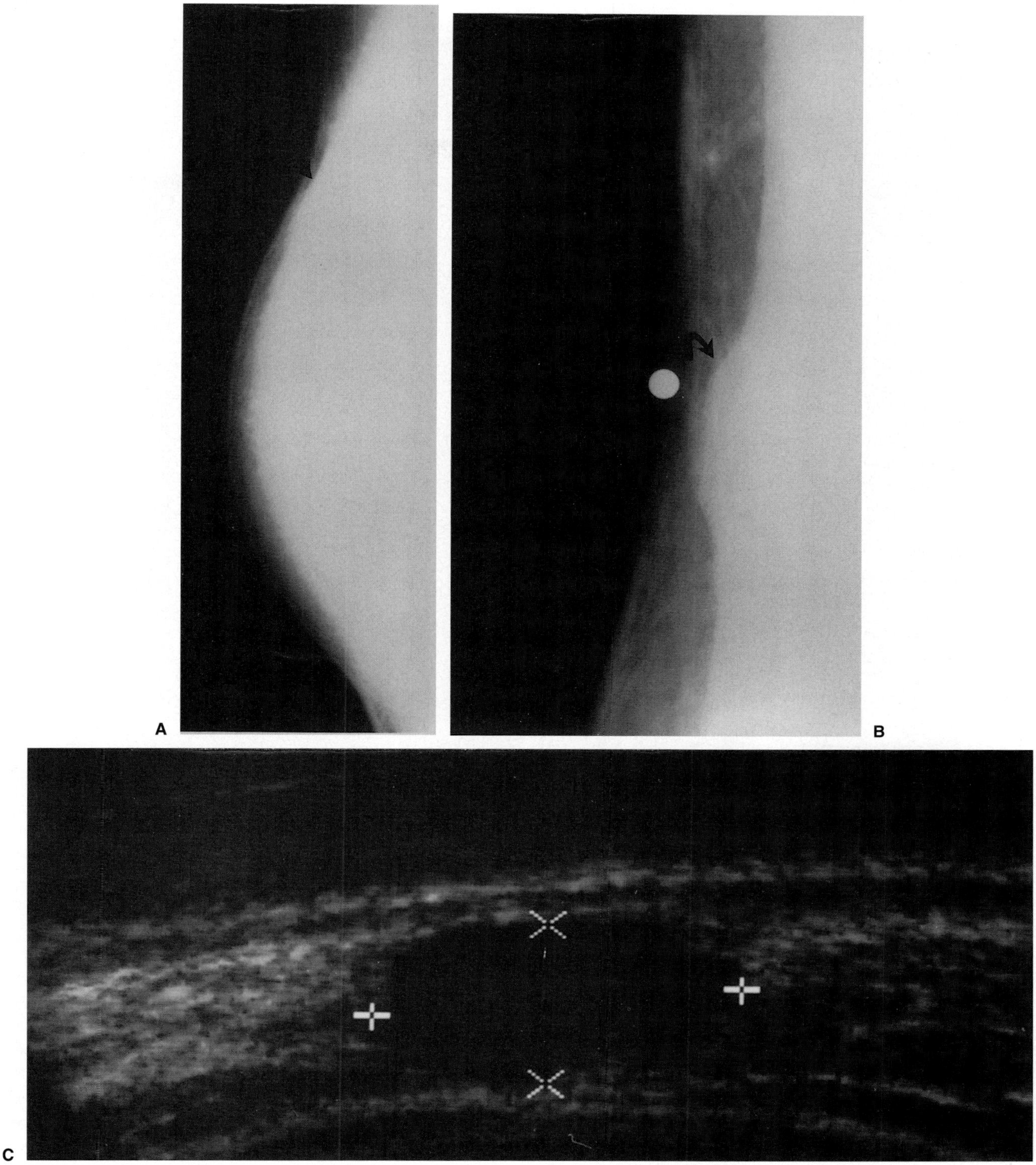

Figure 11–5 (**A**) Postmastectomy lateral mammographic view showing silicone implant (arrow) and minimal residual fibroglandular tissue. (**B**) Coned compression spot mammographic view over area of palpable concern. Soft tissue density is seen, which was not identified on the conventional full breast projection and may represent eventration or herniation of a focal area of the implant or parenchymal mass (arrow). (**C**) Ultrasound image of a palpable mass, distinctly hypoechoic with respect to the remaining breast tissue (callipers). Low-amplitude echoes are difficult to appreciate on this reproduced image. Note the acute angles of the mass with respect to fibrous capsule, which is intact, inconsistent with a herniated or eventrated implant, the sonographic appearance of which might otherwise be similar. Masses abutting fibrous capsules and implants may not easily demonstrate acoustical enhancement or shadowing because of the interference with sound waves posterior to the mass. Diagnosis: recurrent carcinoma.

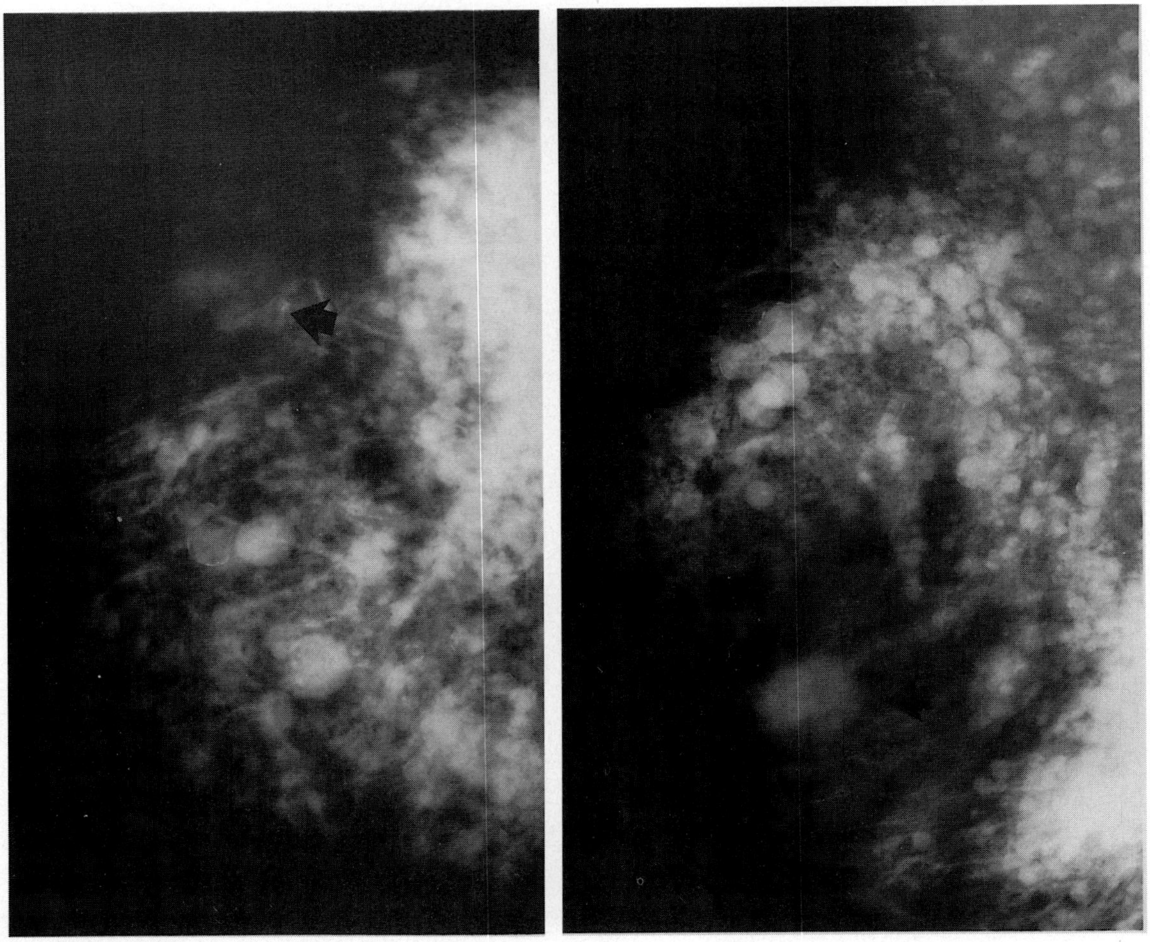

Figure 11–6. Cranial-caudal (**A**) and mediolateral oblique (**B**) views of a breast with a history of silicone injections. Much of the silicone has migrated inferolaterally and is "clumped" together. Elsewhere, multiple silicone cysts are seen. A soft tissue mass, the density of which is distinguished from silicone, with microlobulated borders is identified in the lower outer quadrant of the breast (arrow). Diagnosis: fibrocystic mass.

sound examination showed the masses to be echogenic with an associated posterior snowstorm appearance, corroborating the mammographic features indicating silicone within lymph nodes (Fig. 11–7C) (see Chapter X). MRI was performed showing no evidence of either intracapsular or extracapsular silicone leak. The patient declined surgery and remains asymptomatic 3 years following initial evaluation.

Mammographic evaluation of calcifications employs a logic similar to that of masses; namely, those features that are suspicious in a patient without implants remain suspicious in patients with implants. As with masses, certain mammographic features associated with implants may make evaluation of calcifications more difficult. In addition to a higher incidence of dystrophic calcifications and calcifications associated with fat necrosis in the postoperative breast, calcifications associated with the fibrous capsule surrounding the implant may be at times mammographically indistinguishable from malignant calcifications, as illustrated in Figure 11–8. Although capsular calcifications were suspected in this 42-year-old woman who had undergone explantation several years prior to the mammogram, they were not sufficiently identifiable as within the fibrous capsule remnant to exclude the possibility of malignancy, which was entertained because of their anatomically clustered appearance (Fig. 11–8A). MRI was not performed because the absence of any soft tissue mass and the relative insensitivity of MRI to cancers detected by mammography as clustered calcifications would only render a "negative" study as inconclusive. Preoperative localization followed by surgical excision showed the dystrophic nature of the calcifications in a

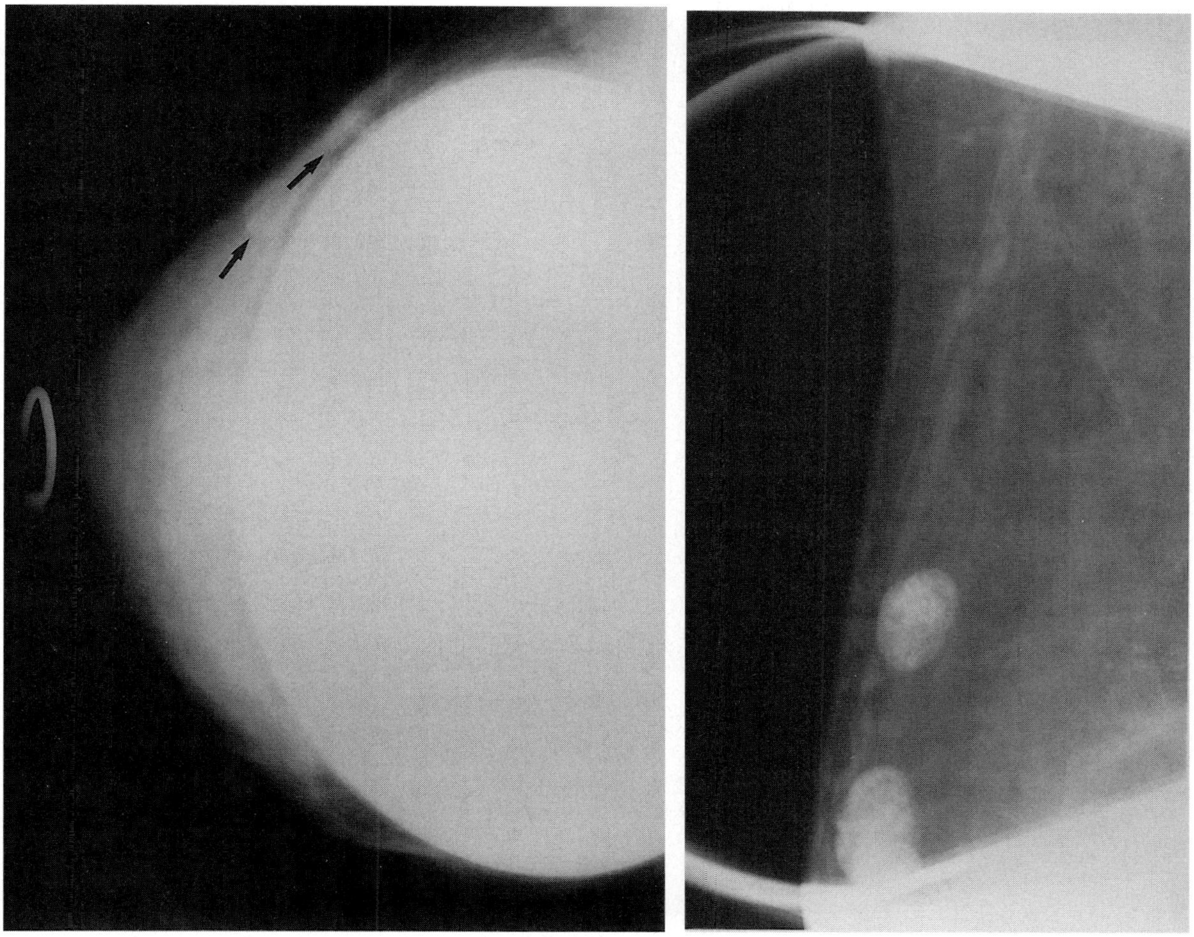

A B

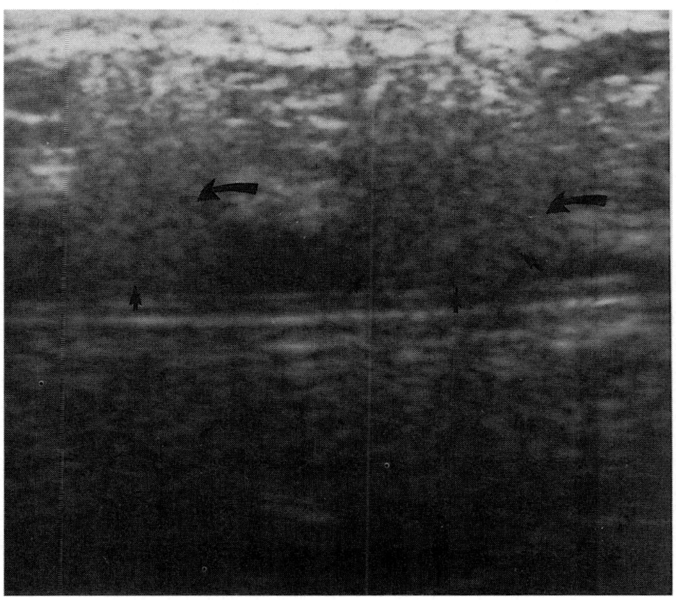

C

Figure 11–7. (**A**) Mediolateral mammogram of breast. Two small masses are identified in the superior aspect (arrows). (**B**) Coned compression spot mammographic magnification view of these masses shows a lentiform shape with silicone infiltrating the apparent cortical aspects of these presumed intramammary lymph nodes. (**C**) Ultrasound of these masses (curved arrows) shows internal consistency more echogenic than surrounding breast tissue, with posterior echoes resembling "snowstorm" appearance (straight arrowhead). Presumptive diagnosis: intramammary lymph nodes with silicone, presumably from gel bleed.

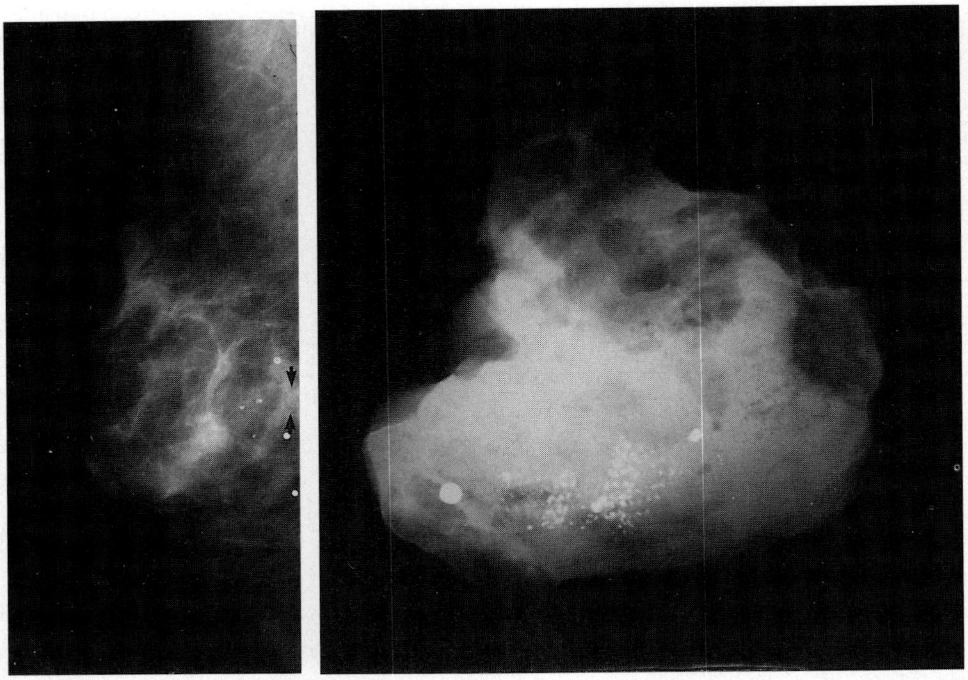

A B

Figure 11–8. (**A**) Mediolateral mammographic view of explanted breast. Large dystrophic calcifications are easily seen. Small cluster of microcalcifications are noted posteriorly and could not be adequately analyzed by a spot compression magnification view because of fibrosis and the inability to position them under the compression device (arrows). These were localized preoperatively for surgical excision (see Figure 11–15). (**B**) Specimen radiograph demonstrates the calcifications to be arranged in a "sheet" along the remnant fibrous capsule.

bandlike appearance conforming to probable silicone implant coating remaining on the fibrous capsule. Imaging techniques of material in vivo (outside the patient) may be applied (during specimen radiography) that do not lend themselves to the patient's existing breast tissue (Fig. 11–8B).

Compare the similarity of many of the calcifications in Figure 11–8 to those seen overlying the fibrous capsule in Figure 11–9, the case of a 45-year-old asymptomatic woman with saline implants who was found to have an abnormal mammogram. While the extent of the calcifications seen in this case is inconsistent with an origin exclusive to the fibrous capsule surrounding the implant, those calcifications that are near or abutting the capsule are difficult to distinguish from the calcifications associated with the capsule remnant of Figure 11–8. Needle localized biopsy of these latter calcifications demonstrated evidence of infiltrative ductal carcinoma.

A more typical case of detected clustered microcalcifications in the lower outer quadrant of an asymptomatic patient with breast implants is shown in Figure 11–10A and B. A spot compression magnification mammographic view demonstrates characteristics of the calcifications of pleomorphism (polymorphism), a ductal and lobular distribution, particles of differing density per unit size and multiple clustered foci within the breast (Fig. 11–10C). These features constitute criteria for clustered microcalcifications which are highly suggestive of malignancy and indicate extensive involvement. Biopsy showed infiltrating comedocarcinoma with extensive intraductal component.

The importance of preoperative mammography for patients with silicone implants is emphasized by the patient illustrated in Figure 11–11. Following the biopsy of a palpable mass that was shown to be malignant, a mammogram was obtained prior to wider excision. A spot compression magnified mammographic view indicates the presence of multiple small clusters of microcalcifications, two clusters of which proved to be other sites of intraductal carcinoma. This case also indicates, as in the prior case, that high-detail mammography can be successfully performed on patients with implants, even in the postoperative setting.

Explantation may also result in occasional difficulties in mammographic evaluation. Polyethylene foam, which covers many of the silicone envelopes, may dissolve within the breast, inciting dystrophic calcific deposits, which are usually not difficult to define. Further increase in calcification

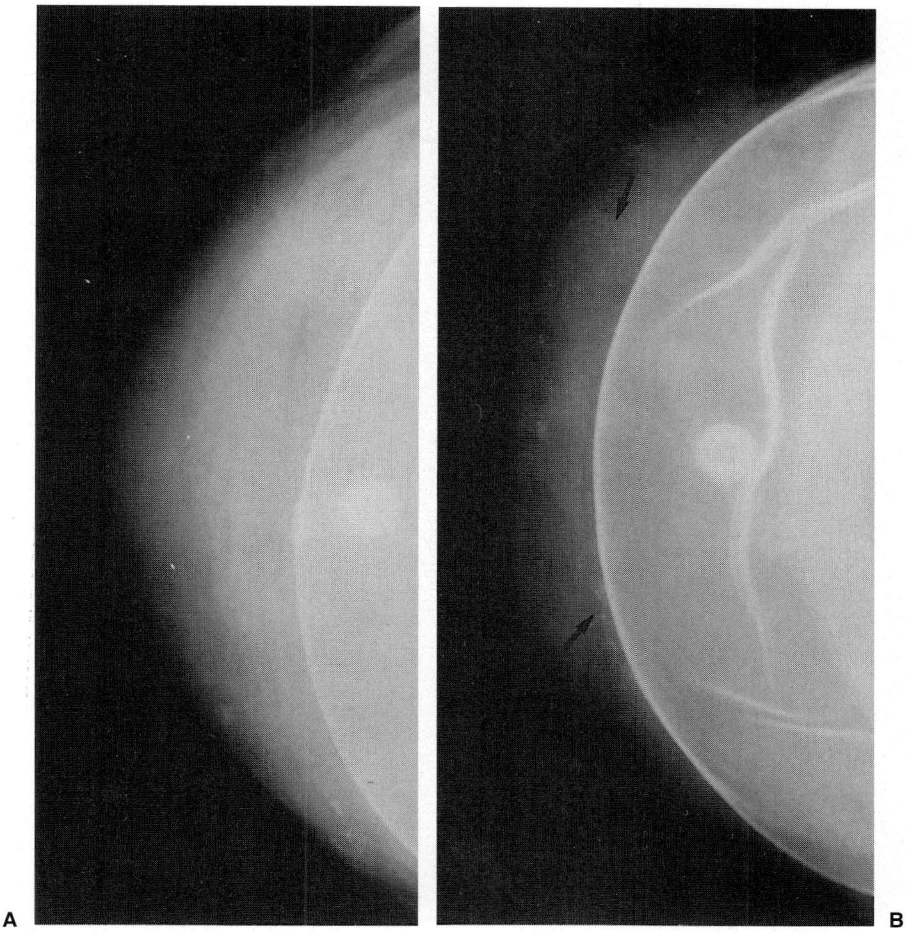

Figure 11–9. Cranial-caudal (**A**) and mediolateral (**B**) mammographic views of a breast with saline implants. Note radial folds and valve. Clusters of microcalcifications are identified in multiple areas of the breast (arrows). Note, especially on lateral projection, how the calcifications abutting the fibrous capsule are similar to those seen in Figure 11–8. Diagnosis: infiltrating ductal carcinoma.

deposition may occur over time. When the calcifications are large and benign in appearance, such serial changes are not a diagnostic problem (Fig. 11–12). However, portions of the fibrous capsule coated with foam or other foreign material may induce the deposition of dystrophic calcifications that may not be readily identifiable as benign and lead to biopsy (Fig. 11–13).

Many clusters of microcalcifications and clinically occult masses may lack sufficient benign characteristics to permit reasonable management recommendations other than biopsy. Preoperative localization is performed in a manner consistent with those of patients without implants, taking special care to avoid puncturing the implant. This possibility, however, should be included in the informed consent obtained during the procedure. Many commentators suggest extending the needle through the lesion, a practice that may need modification when a lesion is found in a breast with implants. Successful accomplishment requires that the lesion be seen in two orthogonal views, similar to requirements for diagnosis. More than 40 lesions in this author's experience have been successfully localized with such parameters (Fig. 11–14).

Routine imagine of a breast that has undergone autogenous flap reconstruction for purposes of tumor detection is an undecided issue. There is one case reported in the medical literature in which malignancy was identified in the reconstructed breast, presumably caused by tissue remaining on the chest wall and growing into the flap (recall that surgery cannot remove 100% of breast tissue).[12] More frequently imaging is performed on such patients to evaluate complications of flap reconstruction, especially when they present as clinical problems. For example, fat necrosis may present as

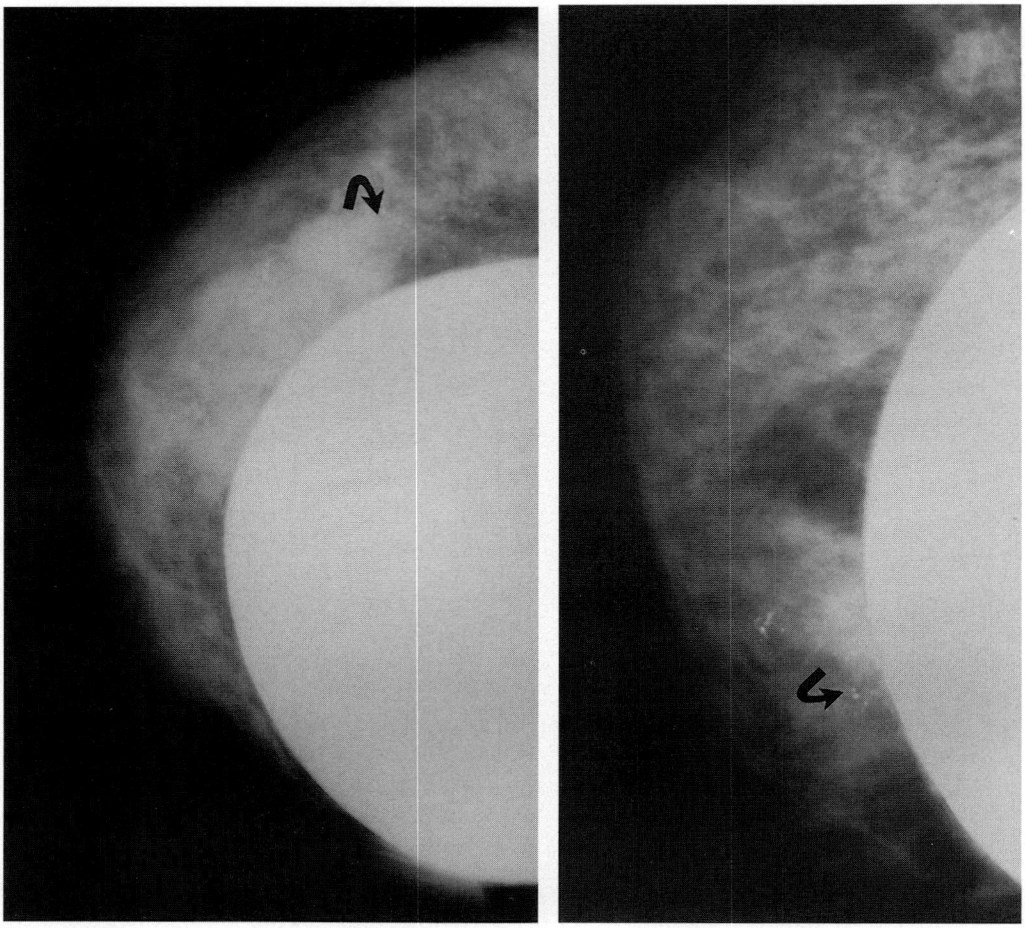

A B

Figure 11–10. Cranial-caudal (**A**) and mediolateral (**B**) mammographic views of a breast with silicone implants. Multiple suspicious clusters are readily identified in the lower outer quadrant. *(continued)*

a palpable mass and can often be specifically diagnosed on the mammographic examination. Imaging of the mastectomy remnant of patients who have not undergone reconstruction of any kind has not shown convincing efficacy.[13] Cancers detected by imaging alone and not by palpation in such patients have either not been reported or are exceedingly rare. This is similar to the situation shown in Figure 11–3. However, in the case shown in Figure 11–3, a patient who had undergone implant reconstruction, the issue of a palpable abnormality being related to the implant as opposed to the remnant breast tissue distinguishes the efficacy of imaging the former and not the latter.

Finally, the detection of tumors, as in all of radiology, should be sought beyond the specific indication for the study, where such features are demonstrated incidentally. Figure 11–16 demonstrates the detection of an incidental lesion in the liver during a localizing sequence on MR examination in the evaluation of implants. The lesion was subject to ultrasound evaluation, showing an echogenic mass, with the presumptive diagnosis of hemangioma.[14]

The evaluation of patients with implants requires attention to detail, both in technique and image evaluation. Assessment of the implant, as has been discussed in a separate chapter, is now an integral part of the radiology report. Evaluation of such breast for malignancy remains the primary directive for the radiologist who must combine experience and knowledge of mammographic features of both malignancy and scarring in forming a deliberate assessment. Be-

(text continues on page 169)

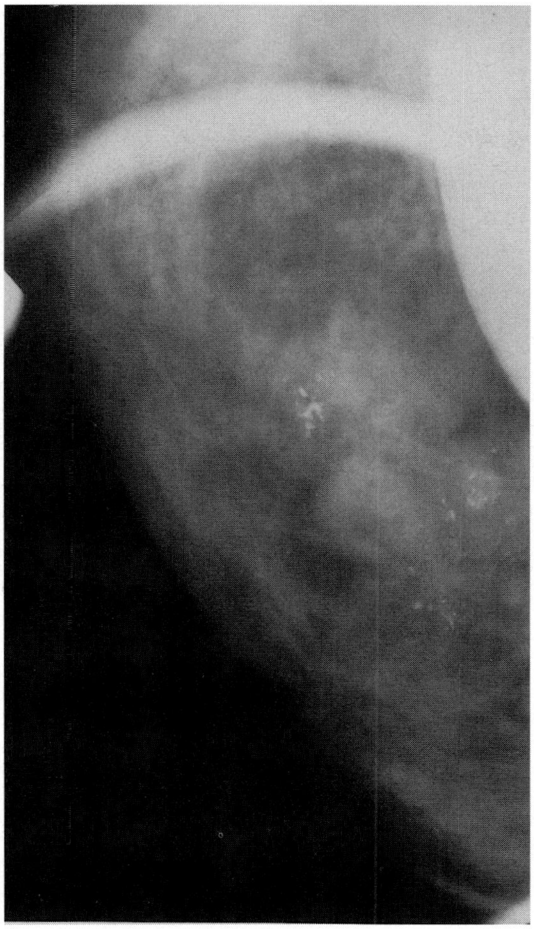

C

11–10. ***(Continued)*** (**C**) Coned compression spot magnification mammogram demonstrates highly suspicious features of the calcifications (arrows). Diagnosis: infiltrating comedocarcinoma with extensive intraductal involvement.

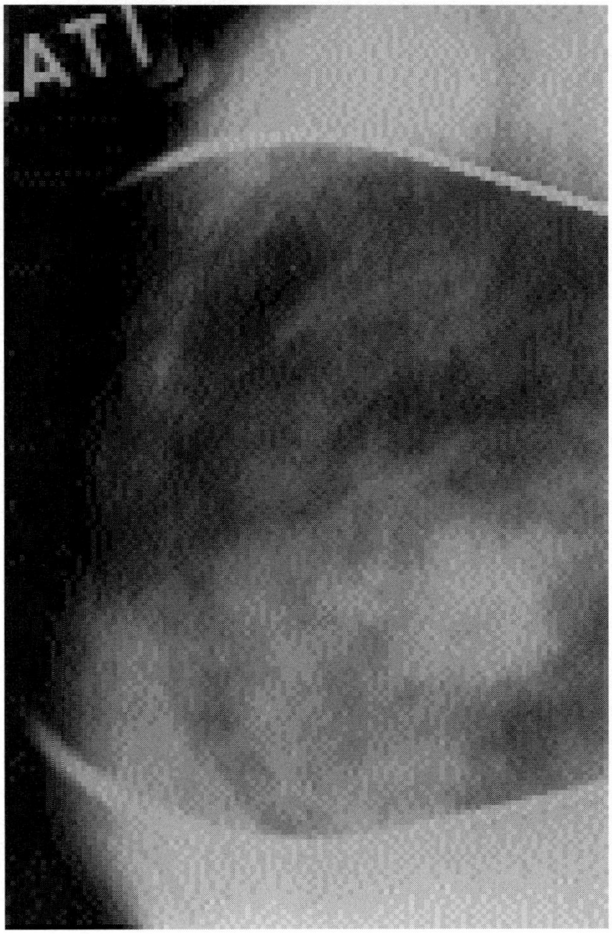

Figure 11–11. Coned compression spot magnification mammographic view following excisional biopsy of a palpable carcinoma shows high detailed views of other areas of clustered microcalcifications representing intraductal carcinoma.

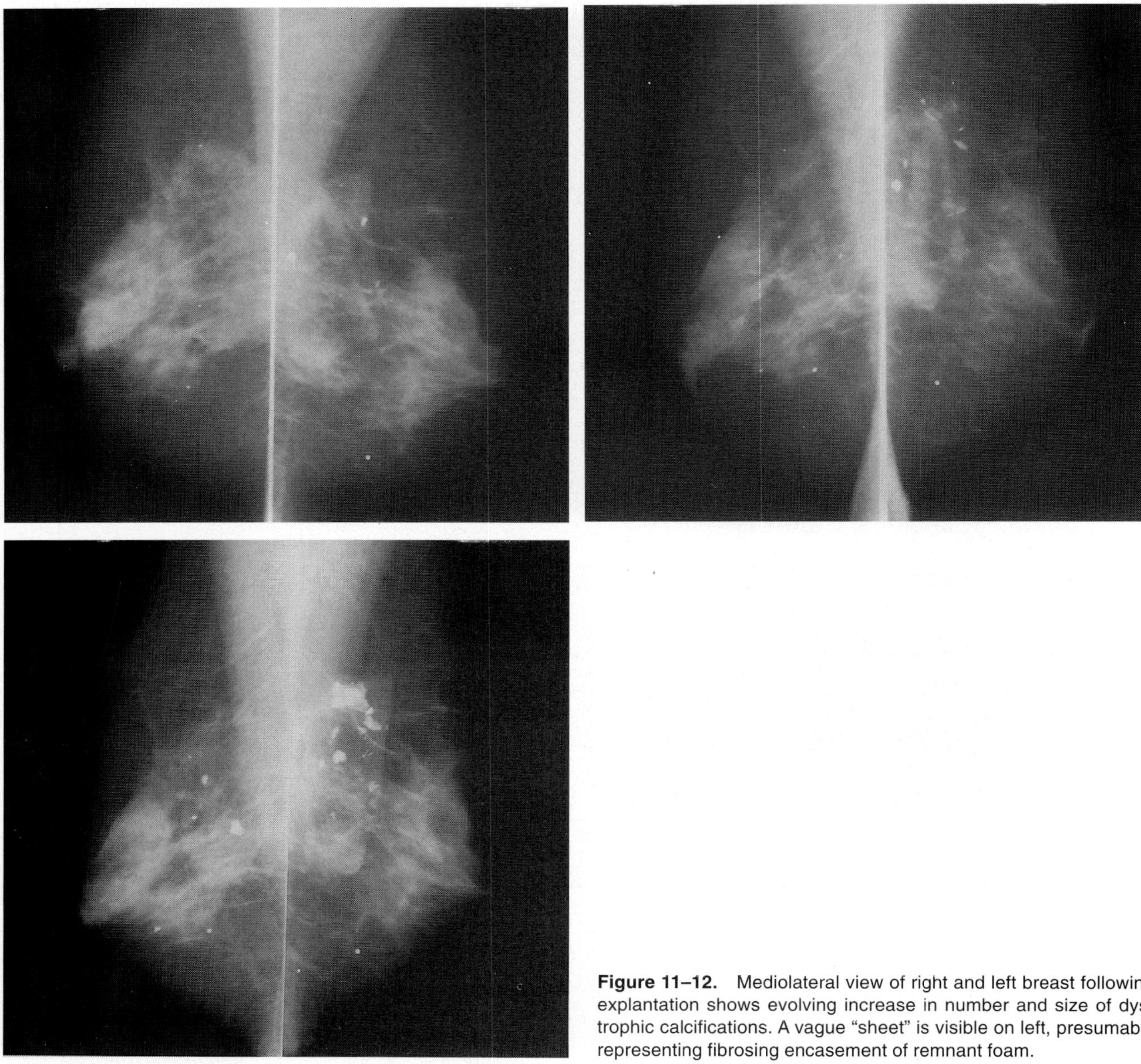

A B C

Figure 11–12. Mediolateral view of right and left breast following explantation shows evolving increase in number and size of dystrophic calcifications. A vague "sheet" is visible on left, presumably representing fibrosing encasement of remnant foam.

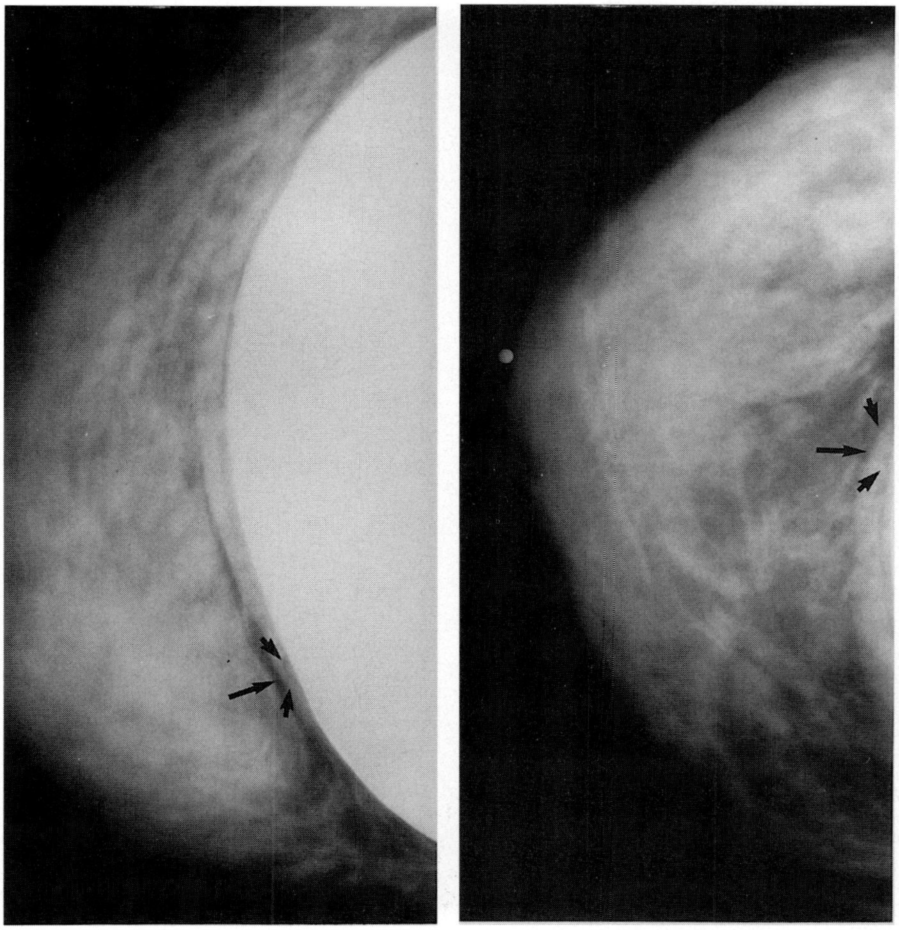

A B

Figure 11–13. Cranial-caudal mammographic view (**A**) shows only scattered microcalcifications, but implant displacement view (**B**) in same projection permits identification of the most superficial portion of a cluster of microcalcifications intimately associated with the fibrous capsule (arrows). *(continued)*

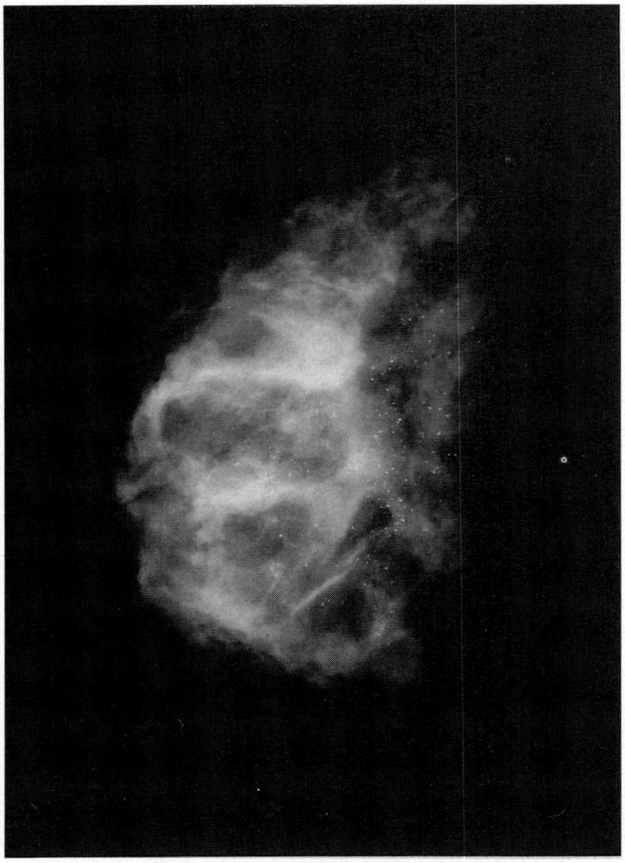

C

11–13. *(Continued)* (**C**) Following preoperative localization, extensive dystrophic calcifications are demonstrated in the specimen radiograph.

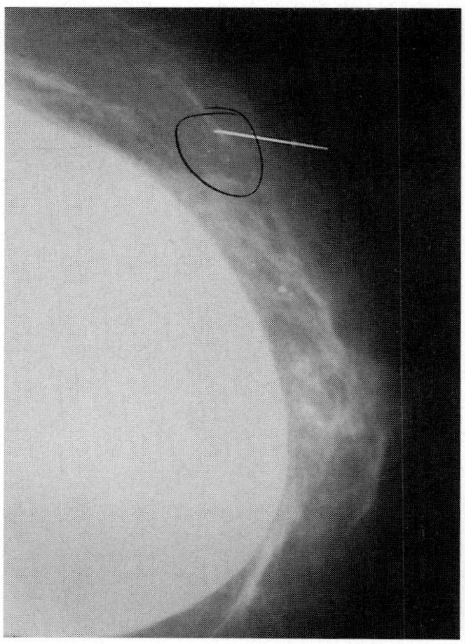

A

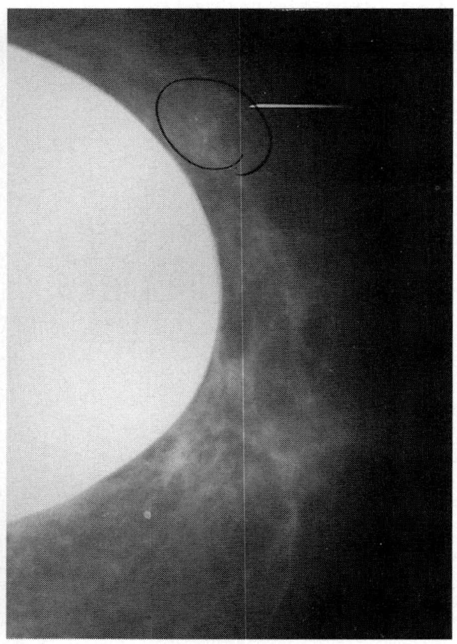

B

Figure 11–14. Preoperative localization using a hypodermic needle and methylene blue dye marker in the anteroposterior approach for this superficial cluster of microcalcifications. The needle tip is placed during implant displacement, but mediolateral (**A**) and cranial-caudal (**B**) nondisplacement views show the needle tip localizer in the proper location for excisional biopsy (circle).

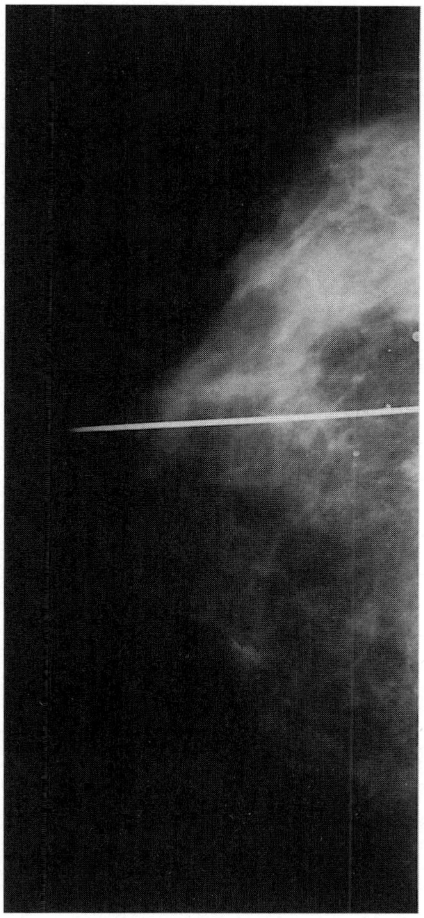

Figure 11–15. Calcifications deep within the breast, discussed in Figure 11–8, are localized in a manner similar to those in Figure 11–14. See specimen radiograph (Fig. 11–8B).

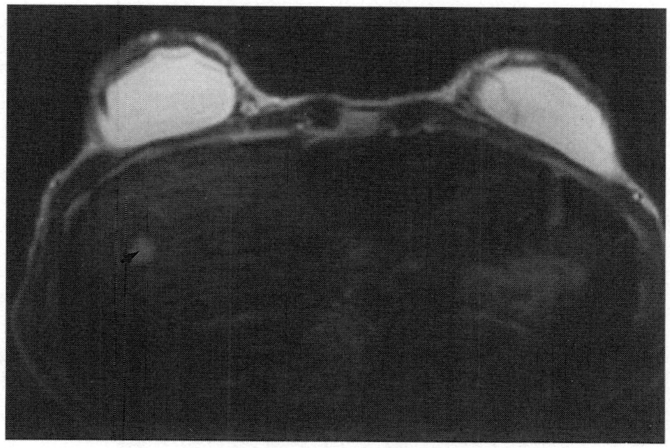

Figure 11–16. Localization MRI T2-weighted sequence depicts incidental lesion in the anterior segment of the right hepatic lobe (arrow). Presumptive diagnosis: hemangioma, or cyst.

ginning in 1987, the American Society of Plastic and Reconstructive Surgery encouraged physicians to refer patients with breast implants to skilled mammographers.[15] Such a recommendation remains particularly relevant at the present time.

REFERENCES

1. Thompson WD. Genetic epidemiology of breast cancer. *Cancer.* 1994;74(suppl):279–287.
2. Silverstein MJ, Handel N, Gamagami P. Breast cancer diagnosis and prognosis in women following augmentation with silicone gel-filled prostheses. *Eur J Cancer.* 1992;28:635–640.
3. Ouimet-Oliva D, Hebert G. Les protheses mammaires: a quelles conditions? *La Sein.* 1992;2:201–211.
4. Leibman AJ, Kruse B. Breast cancer: mammographic and sonographic findings after augmentation mammoplasty. *Radiology.* 1990;174:195–198.
5. Fajardo LL, Harvey JJ, McAleese KA, et al. Breast cancer diagnosis in women with subglandular silicone gel-filled augmentation implants. *Radiology.* 1995;194:859–862.
6. Destouet JM, Monsees BS, Oser RF, et al. Screening mammography in 350 women with breast implants: prevalence and findings of implant complications. *AJR.* 1992;159:973–978.
7. Morgenstern L, Gleishman SH, Michel SL. Relation of free silicone to human breast carcinoma. *Arch Surg.* 1985;120: 573–577.
8. Foster RS. Limitations of physical examination in the early diagnosis of breast cancer. *Surg Oncol Clin North Am.* 1994;3:55–67.
9. Brenner RJ, Pfaff JM. Mammographic findings after conservation therapy for malignant breast disease: serial standardized findings using regression analysis. *AJR.* (in press).
10. Dershaw DD, McCormick B, Cox L, et al. Differentiation of benign and malignant local tumor recurrence after lumpectomy. *AJR.* 1990;155:35–58.
11. Brenner RJ. Interventional procedures of the breast: medicolegal considerations. *Radiology.* 1995;195:611–615.
12. Mund DF, Wolfson P, Gorczyca DP, et al. Mammographically detected recurrent nonpalpable carcinoma developing in a transverse rectus abdominus myocutaneous flap. *Cancer.* 1994; 74:1804–2807.
13. Fajardo LL, Roberts CC, Hunt KR. Mammographic surveillance of breast cancer patients: should the mastectomy site be imaged? *AJR.* 1993;161:953–955.
14. Mitchell DG. Hepatic imaging: techniques and unique applications of magnetic resonance imaging. *Magn Reson Q.* 1993;9: 84–112.
15. Position statement: detection of breast pathology in women with breast implants. Arlington Heights, IL: American Society of Plastic and Reconstructive Surgery; 1987.

12

Breast Cancer Surgery in the Augmented Breast

J. MICHAEL GUENTHER AND ARMANDO E. GIULIANO

The surgical implantation of breast prostheses has become increasingly popular since the development of the silicone prosthesis in 1963. Nearly 150,000 women each year and more than 2,000,000 women to date have undergone cosmetic augmentation mammoplasty (AM).[1] Most achieve good or excellent cosmesis and a correspondingly improved self-image. The most common reasons for AM are cosmesis (75%) and reconstruction after mastectomy (25%).

■ IMPLANT MATERIAL AND LOCATION

Silicone is a polymer of silicon, an elemental metal chosen because of its nonreactive properties. The original silicone gel implants consisted of a thin silicone shell containing silicone gel, sealed with silicone adhesive. Modern prostheses are essentially unchanged; they may be filled with silicone gel or saline—or both, as in double-lumen concentric shells. Additionally, prostheses may be covered with polyurethane foam.

Extensive retrospective epidemiologic studies have failed to implicate silicone implants in the development of breast cancer,[2,3] nor have animal studies demonstrated an increased risk of breast cancer. Although rats have developed a wide variety of sarcomas in association with foreign materials, no carcinomas have been induced.

Breast prostheses may be placed in a subcutaneous pocket anterior to the pectoral muscles or in a retromuscular position beneath the muscles of the chest wall. When possible, placement of prostheses in a retromuscular position enhances mammographic visualization and improves cosmesis should breast-conserving surgery be necessary.

■ CAPSULAR CONTRACTURE

The incidence of capsular contracture is related to the soft tissue coverage of the implant. As noted by McGrath and Burkhardt,[3] "Any nondegradable, inert material will be encapsulated in a relatively acellular and avascular collagenous sheath." Thus, all types of breast prostheses have been associated with capsular contracture, including gel-filled, saline-filled, and combination prostheses of all shapes and sizes. Contracture has been linked to hematoma formation.[4,5] In addition, hematoma may precede a periprosthetic infection, which significantly contributes to fibrosis and firmness.

Several studies have reported that capsular contractures are more frequent in women with subcutaneous breast implants than in those with retromuscular implants. Ryu et al[6] found that none of their five patients with retromuscular implants experienced capsular contracture after radiation therapy. In our series, all six patients with retromuscular implants had excellent or good cosmesis, whereas 3 of the 14 patients with subcutaneous implants had fair or poor results.[7] The improved cosmesis associated with retromuscular implants has been ascribed to the muscular envelope's antibacterial properties and to simple mechanical action.

■ DIAGNOSIS OF BREAST CANCER IN WOMEN WITH AM

The incidence of breast cancer appears to be rising; an estimated one of every eight women will develop breast cancer in her lifetime. As the population of women with breast implants increases and ages, it is likely that the number of breast cancers in this group will also increase. Diagnosis and treatment of breast cancer in patients with AM is a significant clinical problem.

Mammographic imaging of the augmented breast is difficult and may delay the diagnosis of primary and recurrent breast malignancies. Hayes et al[8] reported that AM obscures 22 to 83% of glandular tissue examined with standard techniques. Silverstein et al[9] described a 49% decrease in measurable tissue area after AM; these authors concluded that mammography is not possible in most patients with silicone gel–filled implants. At the John Wayne Cancer Institute (JWCI) only 7 of 20 cancers in patients with AM were mammographically visualized.[7]

There are several mechanisms by which breast implants may impair mammography:

- Radiopaque implants, particularly silicone-filled implants, may obscure fine microcalcifications and soft tissue masses.[10]
- Implant compression of parenchyma, scarring, distortion, density, or calcification may interfere with the sensitivity of screening mammography.
- The augmented breast is less compliant and compressible, particularly when capsular contractures are present.[11] The more significant the contracture, the more marked the reduction in the area visualized.

Another consideration is the denser breast parenchyma of younger women, which limits the effectiveness of screening mammography. Because AM has only been performed with regularity for 25 to 30 years, many women with AM and breast cancer may be somewhat younger than the series of breast cancer patients without AM. The mean age at diagnosis for JWCI patients is 52 years. Handel et al[1] report a mean age of 47 years.

Although standard compression techniques are good for imaging posteriorly near the pectoralis muscles, they are not adequate for anterior breast tissue. Breast imaging in patients with AM has been significantly improved by posterior implant displacement (Eklund technique), which enables visualization of anterior tissues and thus more breast volume.[12] Displacement of the implant against the chest wall is facilitated by retromuscular implants and allows tissue to be pulled in front of the implant, improving compression. If capsular contracture limits the ability to flatten the implant and displace it posteriorly, addition of a 90°lateral projection may improve visualization of breast tissue above and below the implant. In general, a breast prosthesis in the retromuscular position will improve mammographic sensitivity, regardless of the size or type of implant used, and it should improve image quality by decreasing the incidence of capsular contracture.

The poor reliability of mammography in women with AM (particularly young women) and the proportion of patients with small but palpable lesions underscores the need for thorough breast examination in patients who have undergone AM. It has been proposed that AM may facilitate breast physical examination. Breast implants, particularly those in retromuscular positions, may provide a firm background against which a breast mass can be more easily appreciated. In our study, 15 of 20 breast cancers were palpable despite a mean tumor dimension of 1.43 cm.[7]

■ TREATMENT

The surgical treatment options for women with AM and early-stage breast cancer are mastectomy (with or without reconstruction) or breast-conserving therapy (BCT) consisting of local tumor excision plus axillary lymphadenectomy and whole-breast irradiation. Mastectomy allows patients with stage I or II breast cancer to avoid radiation therapy but leaves cosmetic and perhaps psychological deficits. In contrast, BCT is desirable for many breast cancer patients but requires postoperative radiotherapy. At least seven prospective randomized trials have demonstrated no significant difference in survival or local recurrence for patients undergoing BCT versus modified radical mastectomy (MRM).[13–19] MRM with implant removal is an acceptable and definitive treatment for women with prepectoral prostheses who desire mastectomy or who have contraindications to BCT. A patient with implants in a retromuscular position, however, need not undergo implant removal if the tumor is confined to the breast.

Despite equivalent rates of survival and local control, several authors have suggested that mastectomy should be considered for all breast cancer patients with AM, citing the high incidence of capsular contracture and overall poor cosmesis with BCT.[1,20] In their series of 15 women undergoing BCT for stage I or II breast cancer, Handel et al[1] reported that 10 (67%) patients experienced significant capsular contractures and 4 (27%) required surgical revision. The authors concluded that patients with breast prostheses should be considered for MRM with immediate reconstruction, thereby eliminating the need for radiation. A similar conclusion was reached by Halpern et al,[20] who reported that 8 of 11 patients with subcutaneous breast implants had only fair or poor cosmetic results after BCT. In contrast, 17 of 20 patients described in our study of women with AM undergoing BCT achieved excellent or good cosmetic results when evaluated using a scoring system recommended by the American College of Radiology, the American College of Surgeons,

Table 12–1 Four-Point Scoring System for Breast Cosmesis[21]

Excellent (9–10)	Treated breast almost identical to untreated breast
Good (7–8)	Minimal difference between treated and untreated breasts
Fair (5–6)	Obvious difference between treated and untreated breasts
Poor (1–4)	Major functional and aesthetic sequelae in treated breast

From Winchester and Cox.[21]

the College of American Pathologists, and the Society of Surgical Oncology (Table 12–1).[21] Of three patients with suboptimal cosmesis, one was discovered to have a ruptured implant with extensive fibrosis and she subsequently underwent surgical revision. There have been no local recurrences with a mean follow-up of nearly 4 years. We believe that our excellent cosmetic results reflect attention to four factors: (1) technical details of the surgical procedure, (2) total radiation dose to the whole breast, (3) use of a radiation boost to the tumor site, and (4) location of the implants.

■ SURGICAL TECHNIQUE

It has been our experience that postoperative, preradiation cosmesis is a strong predictor of postradiotherapy cosmesis. As a result, meticulous surgical technique is desirable. Breast incisions should be curvilinear and centered over the lesion; flap thickness is maintained. The tumor is excised with a rim of normal-appearing breast tissue; a 1-cm gross margin of normal breast tissue is recommended because unnecessarily wide margins often lead to poor cosmesis. The implant capsule should not be resected unless it abuts tumor margins. The specimen is carefully oriented for pathologic examination to allow identification and possible reexcision of a close or tumor-positive margin. Local hematoma, wound infection, or prosthetic leakage can increase the risk of capsular contracture and thereby impair cosmesis; careful attention to surgical technique should minimize the incidence of these problems.

The periphery of the wound is marked with titanium surgical clips to identify the precise target of a postoperative radiation boost (Fig. 12–1). To avoid unattractive dimpling or denting of the breast, deep reapproximation of breast tissue should not be performed. Tumor biopsy sites should not be drained or needlessly aspirated. Implants inadvertently ruptured or found to have malignant adhesions may be removed and exchanged concurrently with acceptable cosmesis.

An axillary lymph node dissection is performed through a separate, transverse incision beneath the hair-bearing portion of the axilla. Interestingly, the presence of a breast prosthesis does not affect intraoperative lymphatic mapping and sentinel lymphadenectomy to stage the axilla of patients with invasive breast cancer.[22]

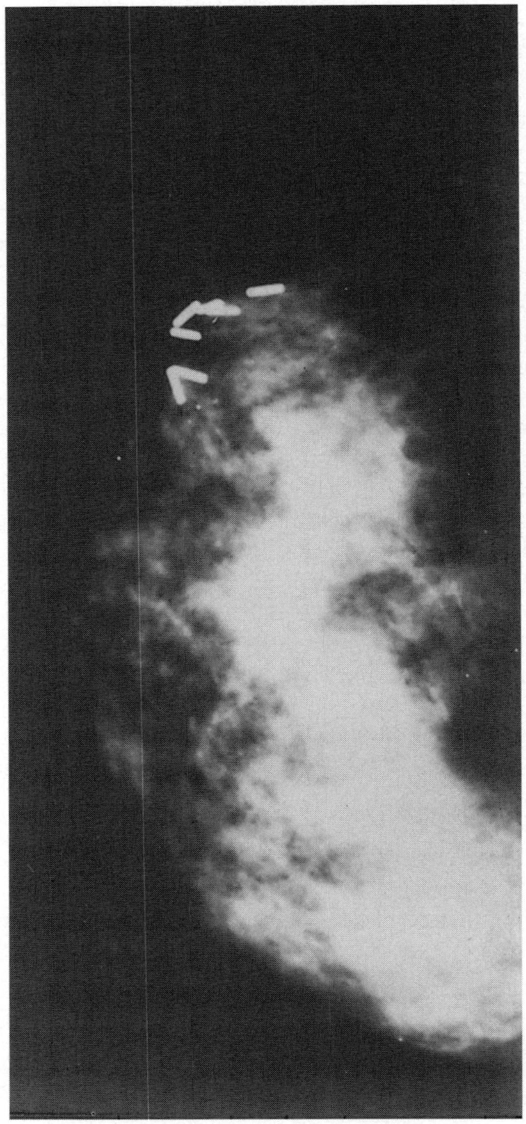

Figure 12–1. Titanium surgical clips mark the precise target for a radiation boost dose. (Reprinted with permission from Guenther et al.[7])

■ POSTOPERATIVE THERAPY

The presence of a breast implant requires minimal dose changes; Krishnan et al[23] and McGinley et al[24] found similar photon and electron dose distribution with radiation of a silicone prosthesis and a water phantom. As a result, postoperative radiation therapy is done in a standard fashion. A prescription volume is irradiated, using angles allowing incident, opposed tangential photon irradiation (4–6 MeV) of the whole breast. Wedges are used in each case. Half-beam

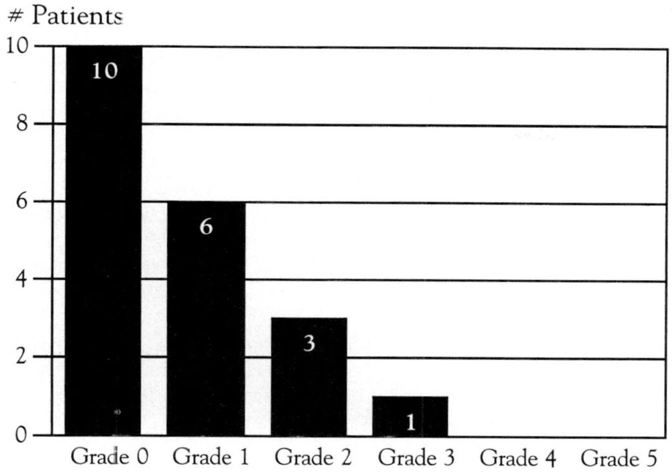

Figure 12–2. Distribution of Radiation Therapy Oncology Group/European Organization for Research on the Treatment of Cancer (RTOG/EORTC) scores for skin and subcutaneous tissue in 20 patients undergoing postoperative radiation therapy (6400 cGy including boost). (Reprinted with permission from Guenther et al.[7])

blocks are employed when possible to minimize radiation exposure to the heart and lungs. Unless the patient is to receive postoperative chemotherapy, radiation therapy is initiated 4 to 6 weeks after surgery. Nodal irradiation is not performed.

Patients with nodal metastases and those at high risk for metastases receive adjuvant systemic therapy for 2 to 4 months before undergoing radiation therapy. Our results offer no support for anecdotal reports linking postoperative chemotherapy to poor cosmesis. Five of six patients receiving chemotherapy in our study had excellent or good cosmetic outcomes.[7]

Boost Dose

It is not clear that a radiation boost dose to the tumor site is necessary; however, routine use of boost doses appears to improve local control. The 1991 National Institutes of Health consensus statement on treatment of early-stage breast cancer recommends limiting the boost to 15 cGy to minimize cosmetic impairment.[25] At the John Wayne Cancer Institute, most patients receive a boost of 12-MeV electrons. Because large boost areas have been associated with poor cosmesis, the area of the breast that is boosted should be no larger than that which encompasses the entire tumor bed. Marking the tumor site with surgical clips, as mentioned above, may be more accurate than estimating margins around the tumor bed, and is particularly important when the incision is not centered directly over the tumor.

Total Radiation Dose

The total dose of breast radiation (including boost) varies among different studies. Using 5000 cGy, the National Surgical Adjuvant Breast Project study reported local recurrence rates equivalent to those reported in other studies using up to 7500 cGy.[14–16,18] Other authors have noted that lower total doses tend to be associated with better cosmetic results. Total doses greater than 7000 cGy produce a higher rate of cutaneous and cosmetic complications. Since 1985 it has been our practice at the JWCI to limit the total dose (including boost) to 6400 cGy. Using these guidelines to assess the 20 patients in our study of BCT after AM revealed only one case of grade 3 radiation morbidity (Fig. 12–2) and no local recurrences after a 4-year median follow-up.[7]

■ SUMMARY

As the population of women with AM increases and ages, a significant number are likely to develop breast cancer. Careful physical examination in combination with conventional and displacement mammography is the standard means of surveillance and diagnosis.

Once diagnosed, patients with early-stage breast cancer (with or without AM) may be treated with mastectomy or BCT. For breast cancer patients with AM, the cosmetic results of BCT appear to depend primarily on the technical details of the surgical procedure, the radiation boost to the tumor site, the total radiation dose, and the location of the implants.

■ ACKNOWLEDGMENT

This work is supported by the Joyce and Ben Eisenberg Foundation.

REFERENCES

1. Handel N, Lewinsky B, Silverstein MJ, et al. Conservation therapy for breast cancer following augmentation mammaplasty. *Plast Reconstr Surg.* 1991;87:873–878.
2. Deapen DM, Pike MC, Casagrande JT, Brody GS. The relationship between breast cancer and augmentation mammo-

plasty: an epidemiologic study. *Plast Reconstr Surg.* 1986;77: 361–367.
3. McGrath MH, Burkhardt BR. The safety and efficacy of breast implants for augmentation mammaplasty. *Plast Reconstr Surg.* 1984;74:550–560.
4. Watson J. Some observations on breast augmentation procedures over the past two decades. *Aesthetic Plast Surg.* 1976;1:89.
5. Cronin TD, Persoff MM, Upton J. Augmentation mammaplasty: complications and etiology. In: Owsley JQ Jr, Peterson RA, eds. *Symposium on Aesthetic Surgery of the Breast.* St. Louis: CV Mosby; 1978:272–282.
6. Ryu J, Yahalom J, Shank B, et al. Radiation therapy after breast augmentation or reconstruction in early or recurrent breast cancer. *Cancer.* 1990;66:844–847.
7. Guenther JM, Tokita KM, Giuliano AE. Breast-conserving surgery and radiation after augmentation mammoplasty. *Cancer.* 1994;73:2613–2618.
8. Hayes H, Vandergrift J, Diner WC. Mammography and breast implants. *Plast Reconstr Surg.* 1988;82:1–8.
9. Silverstein MJ, Handel N, Gamagami P, et al. Mammographic measurements before and after augmentation mammaplasty. *Plast Reconstr Surg.* 1990;86:1126–1130.
10. Gumucio CA, Pin P, Young VL, et al. The effect of breast implants on the radiographic detection of microcalcification and soft tissue masses. *Plast Reconstr Surg.* 1989;84:772–780.
11. Monsees BS, Destouet JM. Mammography in aesthetic and reconstructive breast surgery. *Perspect Plast Surg.* 1991;5:103–119.
12. Eklund GW, Busby RC, Miller SH, Job JS. Improved imaging of the augmented breast. *AJR.* 1988;151:469–473.
13. Fisher B, Redmond C, Poisson R, et al. Eight-year results of a randomized clinical trial comparing total mastectomy and lumpectomy with or without irradiation in the treatment of breast cancer. *N Engl J Med.* 1989;320:822–828.
14. Veronesi U, Banfi A, Del Vecchio M, et al. Comparison of Halsted mastectomy with quadrantectomy, axillary dissection, and radiotherapy in early breast cancer: long term results. *Eur J Cancer Clin Oncol.* 1986;22:1085–1089.
15. Sarrazin D, Le MG, Arriagada R, et al. Ten-year results of a randomized trial comparing a conservative treatment to mastectomy in early breast cancer. *Radiother Oncol.* 1989;14: 177–184.
16. Blichert-Toft M, Rose C, Andersen JA. Danish randomized trial comparing breast conservation therapy with mastectomy: six years of life-table analysis. Danish Breast Cancer Cooperative Group. *Monogr Natl Cancer Inst.* 1992;11:19–25.
17. Straus K, Lichter A, Lippman M, et al. Results of the National Cancer Institute early breast cancer trial. *Monogr Natl Cancer Inst.* 1992;11:27–32.
18. van Dongen JA, Bartelink H, Fentiman IS, et al. Randomized clinical trial to assess the value of breast-conserving therapy in stage I and stage II breast cancer, EORTC 10801 trial. *Monogr Natl Cancer Inst.* 1992;11:8–15.
19. Habibollahi F, Fentiman IS, Chaudray MA, et al. Conservation treatment of operable breast cancer. *Proc Am Soc Clin Oncol.* 1987;6:A230.
20. Halpern J, McNeese MD, Kroll SS, Ellerbroek N. Irradiation of prosthetically augmented breast: a retrospective study on toxicity and cosmetic results. *Int J Radiat Oncol Biol Phys.* 1990;18:189–191.
21. Winchester DP, Cox JD, eds. Standards for breast-conservation treatment. *CA Cancer J Clin.* 1992;42:134–162.
22. Giuliano AE, Kirgan DM, Guenther JM, Morton DL. Lymphatic mapping and sentinel lymphadenectomy for breast cancer. *Ann Surg.* 1994;220:391–401.
23. Krishnan L, St George FJ, Mansfield WM, Krishnan EC. Effect of silicone gel breast prosthesis on electron and photon dose distribution. *Med Phys.* 1983;10:96–99.
24. McGinley PH, Powell WR, Bostwick J. Dosimetry of a silicone breast prosthesis. *Radiology.* 1980;135:223–224.
25. Treatment of early-stage breast cancer: NIH Consensus Conference. *JAMA.* 1991;265:391–395.

13

Pathology of the Failed Breast Implant

NIR KOSSOVSKY

In the common parlance of medicine, pathology (literally, the study of suffering) is a bridging discipline involving both basic science and clinical practice. Pathology studies structural and functional changes in cells, tissues, and organs that underlie "dis-eases."[1] This broad mandate acknowledges the pioneering role played by pathologic investigations:

1. Pathology uses basic science tools and incorporates basic science knowledge to advance the understanding of disease processes;
2. Pathology applies its knowledge and skill set to understand current clinical medical diseases; and
3. Pathology explores and defines features of new medical problems that manifest as states of "dis-ease," that is, the physical state in which a patient senses that "things are not normal."[2]

Over time, many of these states of "dis-ease" acquire formal names or eponyms, and the full range of clinical and pathologic features are subsequently assembled to produce clinicopathologic entities.

In the tradition of classical pathology, medical device pathology is a bridging discipline involving materials sciences, biophysics, and mechanics in addition to conventional biologic and chemical basic sciences. The breast implant is one of several hundred medical devices used to save, sustain, or enhance life. The pathology of a breast implant is similar to that of many other devices. There is pathology consequent to materials, design, and engineering factors; consequent to user factors; and consequent to biologic factors. There is also unique pathology. The breast implant is (generally) a permanently implanted device composed of a fluid or colloidal mixture of polymers of varying molecular weights and viscosities often encased in a rubber shell composed of a similar mix of materials. It is a cosmetic device, and it is most often implanted in young healthy women. These parameters introduce unique features to the general discourse of materials, user, and biologic factors.

■ MEDICAL DEVICE PATHOLOGY

Medical devices fail for one of three non–mutually exclusive reasons. First, failure may be a consequence of an intrinsic element of design or fabrication. Included in this category are failures due to insufficient mechanical strength, fatigue resistance, corrosion resistance, tear resistance, and fracture resistance. Also included in this category are the "freezing" of moving parts due to unanticipated expansion, swelling or wear debris accumulation. Second, failure may be due to an error in usage or application. Mismatched components of a multicomponent system, a reversal of polarity of electronic devices, a reversal of direction in the installation of a flow control device, size incompatibility, surgically induced tearing, and other induced forms of trauma all constitute extrinsic user-supplied causes of failure. Last, failure may be due to the consequences of one of four basic pathophysiologic phenomena: the promotion of infection, the induction of thrombosis, the stimulation of inflammation, or the induction and promotion of carcinogenesis.

To understand these basic principles, consider a cardiac valve prosthesis (Table 13–1). Heart valve replacement with a prosthesis is a common and generally lifesaving procedure used to treat surgically a functionally significant anatomical anomaly or acquired damage to a native heart valve. There are fairly specific indications for the procedure. Serious

Table 13–1. Medical Device Pathology

Sphere	*Exemplary Processes*	*Cardiac Valve Prosthesis*
Design or fabrication	Mechanical strength Fatigue resistance Corrosion resistance Tear resistance Fracture resistance Mechanical freezing Material swelling and degradation Debris spallation	Tissue leaflet degradation accelerated by tanning process Valve wear, swelling, and fracture
User error	Inappropriate placement Inappropriate indication Excessive contraindications Inappropriate auxiliary instrument utilization Component mismatch Surgically induced trauma	Implanted backward Excess suture impinges and freezes valve Residual valvular tissue impinges and freezes valve
Biologic and pathophysiologic processes	Promotion of infection Induction of thrombosis Stimulation of inflammation Induction and promotion of neoplasia	Thrombosis and thromboemboli Infective endocarditis Fibrosis of the AV node

medical device pathology arises in approximately 60% of heart valve replacement recipients within 10 years postoperatively.[3]

Design, Mechanical, and User Pathology

Bioprostheses, the valves fabricated from treated animal tissues, tend to degrade under the mechanical load of blood flow. Much of the natural elasticity and fatigue strength of natural tissues is lost by the chemical treatment process used to prepare the bioprosthetic valves. Consequently, over 30% of these valves become torn or calcified and require replacement within 10 years of implantation. Wear of the various moving parts of the mechanical valve; swelling, fracture, and escape of the poppet of ball-cage valves; and excessive noise are examples of the mechanical complications seen over the years with cardiac valve prostheses.

As to user complications, there are basically three. First, a valve may be implanted contrary to the direction of flow. Second, a valve may be sewn into the cardiac muscle and a residual strand of suture material may become lodged between one of the moving parts, causing the latter to stick. Third, a residual piece of cardiac valvular tissue, if not removed sufficiently, may also become lodged and impinge a moving component.

Biological Pathology

Of the four basic pathophysiologic process, induction of thrombosis and the potentiation of infection are the predominant complications affecting heart valves prostheses. Thromboembolic complications constitute the major problem with mechanical valves, which necessitate long-term anticoagulation in patients with these devices. Hemorrhagic complications, however, such as stroke or gastrointestinal bleeding, may arise secondarily in patients who receive long-term anticoagulation.[4]

Infective endocarditis, occurring at the interface between the prosthesis and the native heart muscle, is seen in about 6% of valve recipients within 5 years of implantation.[4] Extension of the infection from a paravalvular abscess to a frank perforation results in regurgitation of blood around the valve. If the valve becomes sufficiently loose, it may become completely dislodged. Common infecting organisms are staphylococci and streptococci.

Inflammation triggered by the materials of the valve sewing rings, usually polyethylene terephthalate (Dacron) can result in fibrosis that may affect the integrity of the atrioventricular node. Otherwise, inflammation is not currently felt to be a significant problem with heart valves. Neoplasms of the heart are exceedingly rare, and the specific induction of neoplasms in the heart by heart valves has not been shown.

■ BREAST IMPLANT PATHOLOGY

For many years breasts have been augmented by the injection or implantation of a number of materials. Waxes, oils, polyvinyl alcohol, and polyurethanes have all been used in the past 50 years.[5,6] Since the 1960s, formal devices fabricated primarily from silicones have been used almost exclusively.

In contrast to almost all other medical devices, the collection of data by the medical community on the performance and complication rate of breast implants has been complicated by an emotional and often rancorous public, political, legal, and medical debate.[7–12] Breast implants are cosmetic medical devices that are potentially life enhancing.[13–18] They are used almost exclusively by one gender, and the complication rate with these devices is largely unknown.

Structural Pathology

Breast implants are the most recognized of the many medical applications of silicone in modern medicine.[19] The chemistry of both silicon and silicones has been recently reviewed in detail in the medical literature,[20,21] and it is sufficient for this medical device pathology-oriented review to note that silicones are a family of polymers composed of an alternating silicon-oxygen atom backbone. Medical silicone, or more precisely poly(dimethylsiloxane) (PDMS), can be formulated in a number of different ways with the inclusion of a number of additives,[22] resulting in materials of varying structures and properties, such as in oils, gels, or rubbers. For the past 40 years, the medically relevant silicones have been synthesized mostly from starting blocks of octamethylcyclotetrasiloxane, more commonly written as D_4. The D_4 cyclic is linearized and the individual chains are polymerized by a catalyst to approximately 90% equilibrium favoring the polymer—an oil.[23] The PDMS oil is then cured or vulcanized in the manufacture of gels, elastomers, rubbers, and solids. In the production of elastomer, which is used to form the shell on both gel and saline filled breast implants, about 95% of the PDMS polymer chains are cross-linked. Fumed silica, which may compose up to 30% of the elastomer shell by mass, is added for strength. The remaining 5% silicone oil content in the shell provides suppleness and elasticity. The cured gel in the devices is composed of a loose network of chains that trap the oil molecules. The actual oil content in commercially sold medical devices ranges from about 9 to 80%.[23]

Silicone breast implants are a heterogeneous class of medical devices (Table 13–2). At least 10,000 different combinations of properties are possible. There is variability associated with the chemistry and with the implant construction. Variations include, but are not limited to, differences in gel viscosity, composition, and catalyst, and differences in outer envelope surface textures, thicknesses, and chemistry. At the most superficial level, silicone breast implants can be categorized in one of four broad structural groups:

- silicone rubber envelopes filled with saline
- silicone rubber envelopes filled with silicone gel
- silicone rubber envelopes covered with approximately 1.35-g of a 1-mm-thick polyester polyurethane foam coating and filled with silicone gel
- dual silicone rubber envelopes, the inner envelope containing silicone gel and the outer envelope filled with saline, surrounding the inner envelope.

MATERIAL DEGRADATION

While it first appeared that silicones might be resistant to degradation, evidence to the contrary was uncovered during metabolic studies of 2,6-*cis*diphylhexamethyltetrasiloxane. In 1980 it was observed that the cyclic silicone oligomer could be degraded into hydrophilic diols. Its two major metabolites, identified in both man and monkey, were dimethylsilanediol and phenylmethylsilanediol. Recent studies have reaffirmed the hydrolytic degradation potential of

Table 13–2. Breast Implant Variations

Components	*Minimum Number of Variables*	*Variables**
Fixation site	2	Present or not Usually fabricated from polyethylene terephthalate (Dacron)
Shell	1	350% minimum percent elongation Resistant to failure when stressed 200% for 10 seconds Backbone comprised of a siloxane polymer
	4	Bound to the siloxane backbone may be methyl, phenyl, vinyl, and fluoralkyl side groups appearing individually or in combination
	10	Shell fillers may include fumed silica, treated fumed silica, hydrated silica, diatomaceous earths, metal oxides, carbon, conductive metals, calcium carbonate, ground quartz, or none of these Variable thicknesses
Valves	3	None, or present in type I (single-lumen) and type II (double-lumen) variable volume prostheses Should not leak when subjected to retrograde pressure for 5 minutes
Silicone gel	1	Weight loss less than or equal to 1.0% at 150°C with a minimum 25 cm^2 surface area. Should meet minimum cohesion tests specifications Implant volume tolerance is 35%
Catalytic processing	7	2,4-dichlorobenzoyl peroxide, benzoyl peroxide, dicumyl peroxide, modified hexane, butylperbenzoate, platinum, or none of these
Sterilization processing	3	Ethylene oxide, autoclave or radiation

*Based on ASTM specifications F 604, F 703, and F 881. *Annual Book of Standards, vol 13.01, Medical Devices.* Philadelphia: American Society for Testing and Materials; 1989.

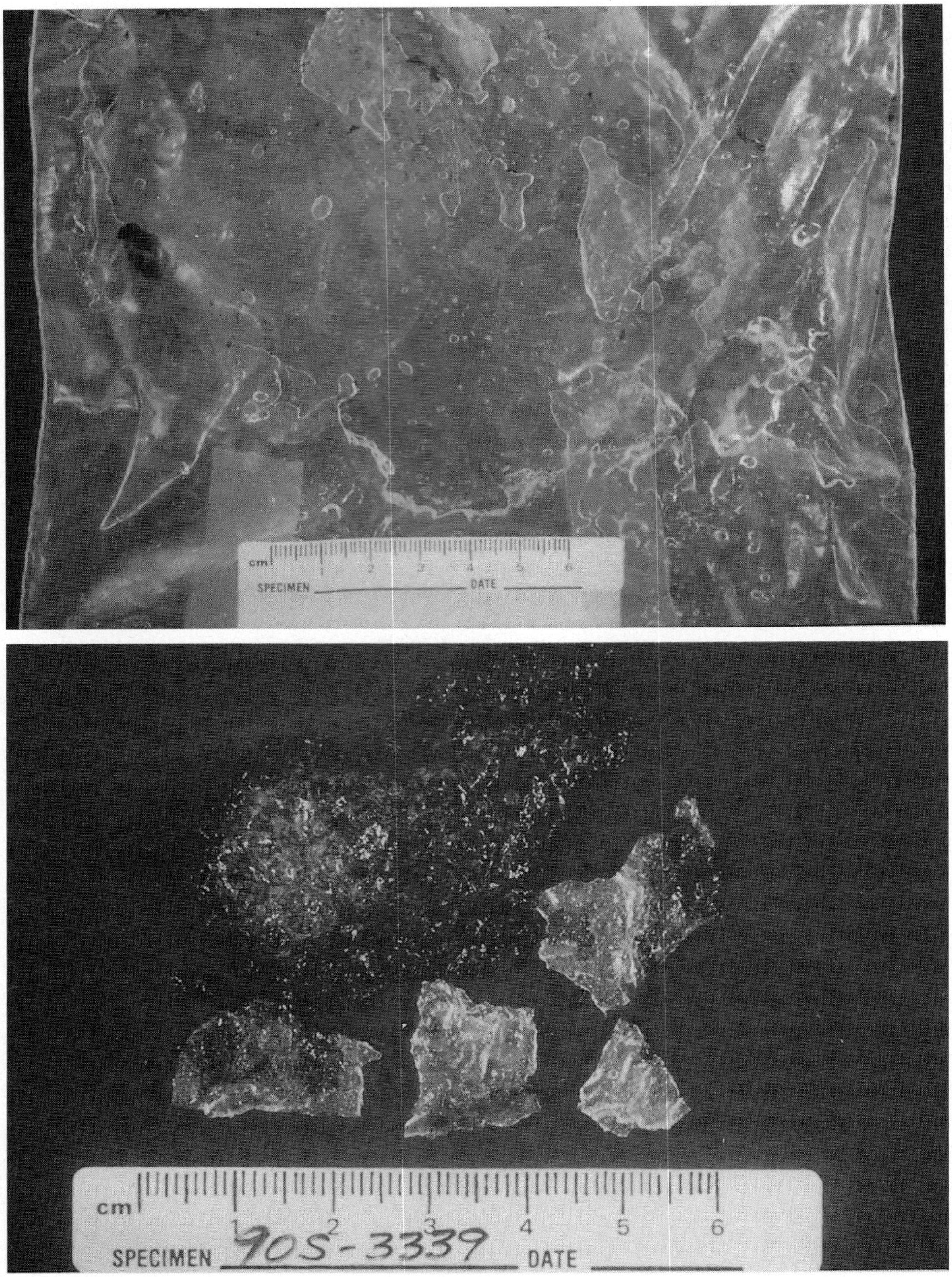

Figure 13–1. (**A**) Surgical pathology specimen of a gel-filled breast implant whose outer shell has undergone substantial material degradation. Seen is a specimen bag filled with gel and particulate rubber fragments. The scale at the bottom is in centimeters. (**B**) A specimen similar to the above, where the some glistening gel has been spread and four irregularly shaped silicone rubber fragments have been separated and arranged for display purposes. The scale at the bottom is in centimeters.

silicones and have established the activation energy for the Si-O bond at between 4.1 and 4.6 Kcal/mol.[24] Other degradative mechanisms, including oxidation, have been proposed. Recent in vivo data suggest that irrespective of the pathway, a family of reactive silicon intermediaries are established.[25–27] Si nuclear magnetic resonance (NMR) offers evidence that these reactive intermediaries in human tissue yield a full range of molecules, including native PDMS, hydrolyzed silicone, silica gel, and highly coordinated silicon.[28]

The exact elements that promote degradation are not well established. Hydrolysis simply by being in the presence of the aqueous biologic environment appears to be sufficient and can generate reactive hydroxyl moieties; however, even fungi have been shown to contribute to the erosion of implanted elastomeric materials.[27,29–33]

Other mechanisms of degradation may be related to the absorption of foreign macromolecules.[34,35] Studies in the mechanical properties of silicone rubber during static, nonloaded subcutaneous or intramuscular implantation showed an 8% reduction in tensile strength and embrittlement after only 24 months (Fig. 13–1).

DEVICE RUPTURE AND GEL BLEED

The mechanical strain on an implant is greatest at the periphery of the implant or points of folding of the shell where sudden changes of shape occurs.[36] The combination of weakened polymer from both degradation and embrittlement that is then challenged by mechanical strain makes failure of the implant shell almost inevitable. Time, presumably, is the principal variable separating low molecular weight silicone bleed through an intact elastomer shell from gross silicone gel spillage through a ruptured shell.[37–41] While the frequency of rupture and rate of bleed are still being characterized, implants appear to be much more likely to rupture beyond 10 years of implantation.

GROSS PATHOLOGIC EXAMINATION

Silicone bleed and device rupture with gross gel spillage are the extreme forms of device pathology evident in the gross or macroscopic state. In general, identifying gross structural abnormalities is best accomplished through a methodologic examination of the device upon its removal from the chest where it may have been residing in a subcutaneous, subglandular, or even submuscular position (Fig. 13–2).

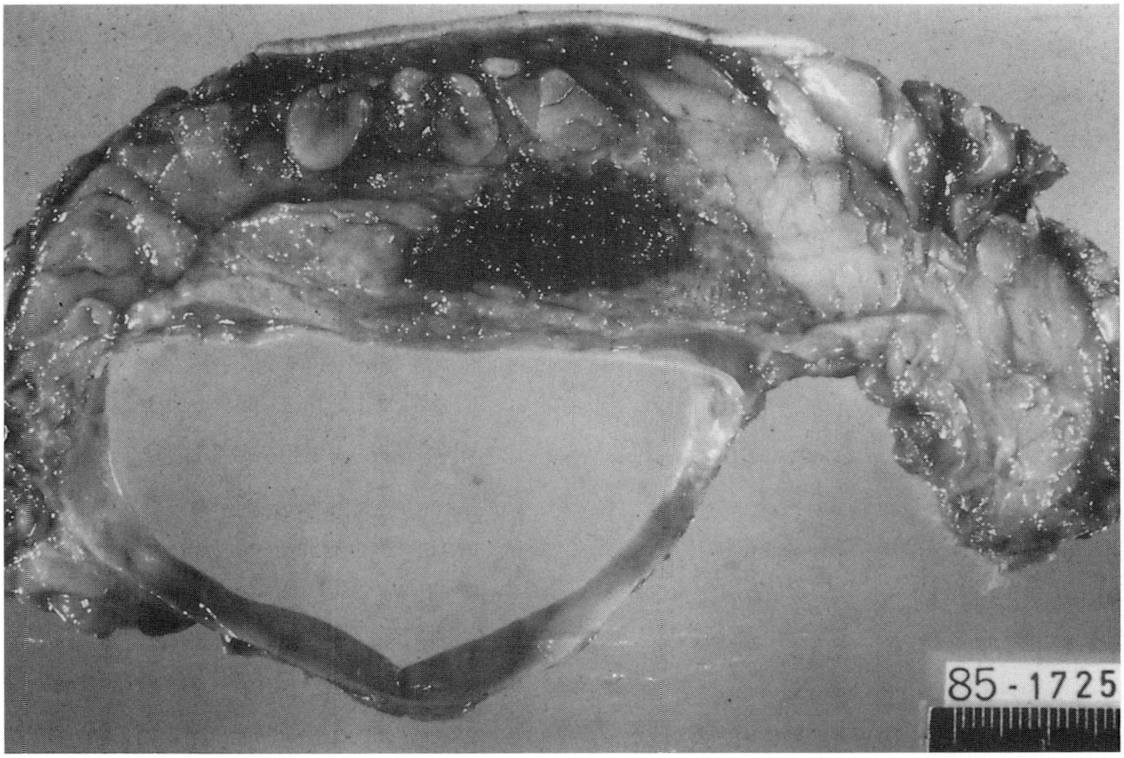

Figure 13–2. Sagittal section through a mastectomy specimen illustrating the relationship between capsule and (the now removed) submammary implant. The black oval in the center is residual hemorrhage from a biopsy cavity. An infiltrating ductal carcinoma abutting the implant capsule was the indication for mastectomy. The scale at bottom right is in centimeters.

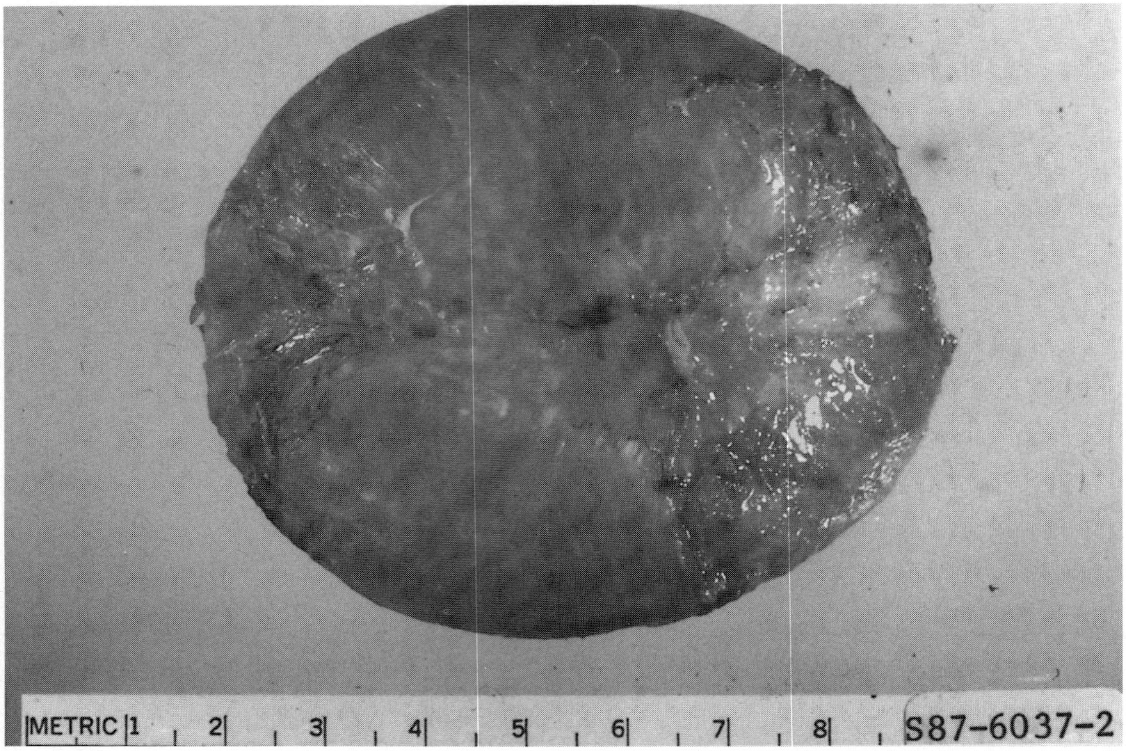

Figure 13–3. Gross appearance of an implant surrounded by a firmly adherent fibrous capsule. The scale at the bottom is in centimeters.

Note should be made of what is removed from the body and the status of the received materials, for example, a breast prosthesis and surrounding adherent capsular tissue (Fig. 13–3), a prosthesis and separate tissue capsule, a prosthesis only, or other materials. The prosthesis should be weighed and the integrity of the envelope (shell) noted. The contents may consist of gel, water, blood tinged gel, or other materials. The number of lumina and the presence of a valve should be noted. Inflatable devices received flat should be so described (Fig. 13–4).

The exterior surface may be smooth and white or translucent, transparent, or yellow tinted. It may be textured, and it may contain yellow brown flaking material or white gritty material. There may be inscriptions on the filling patch at the base.

The tissue mass should be weighed separately, and any abnormalities noted. A representative "jelly roll" should be prepared for histologic examination.

Biological Pathology

Despite differences among the various devices, there are common biologic phenomena associated with the implantation of silicone gel–filled beast prostheses. The macrophage-rich chronic inflammatory reaction to breast prostheses and other implants, often granulomatous in nature, has been described as a "nonspecific" foreign body reaction.[42,43] The clinical consequences of the inflammatory reaction have been at the center of considerable controversy for the past few years.[14,44–47] In addition to inflammation, there are three other major pathologic process that may be identified: thrombosis, infection, and neoplasia. With silicone breast implants, thrombosis is not a clinical concern and infection is relatively rare.[48] Neoplasia, while always of concern, currently seems to be exclusively an experimental phenomenon that has not been observed in humans.[49–52]

MICROSCOPIC EXAMINATION

Formal microscopic examination of the tissue consists of a sequential review of cut histologic sections with a view toward identifying inflammatory, infectious, or neoplastic features. The microscopic anatomical manifestations of direct exposure to silicone from breast implants are fairly characteristic. The tissue bed of an implanted silicone breast prosthesis is characterized by a fibrous scar capsule composed of dense collagen, fibroblasts, macrophages, giant cells, lymphocytes, and, in some cases, plasma cells (Fig. 13–5).[53] De-

(text continues on page 184)

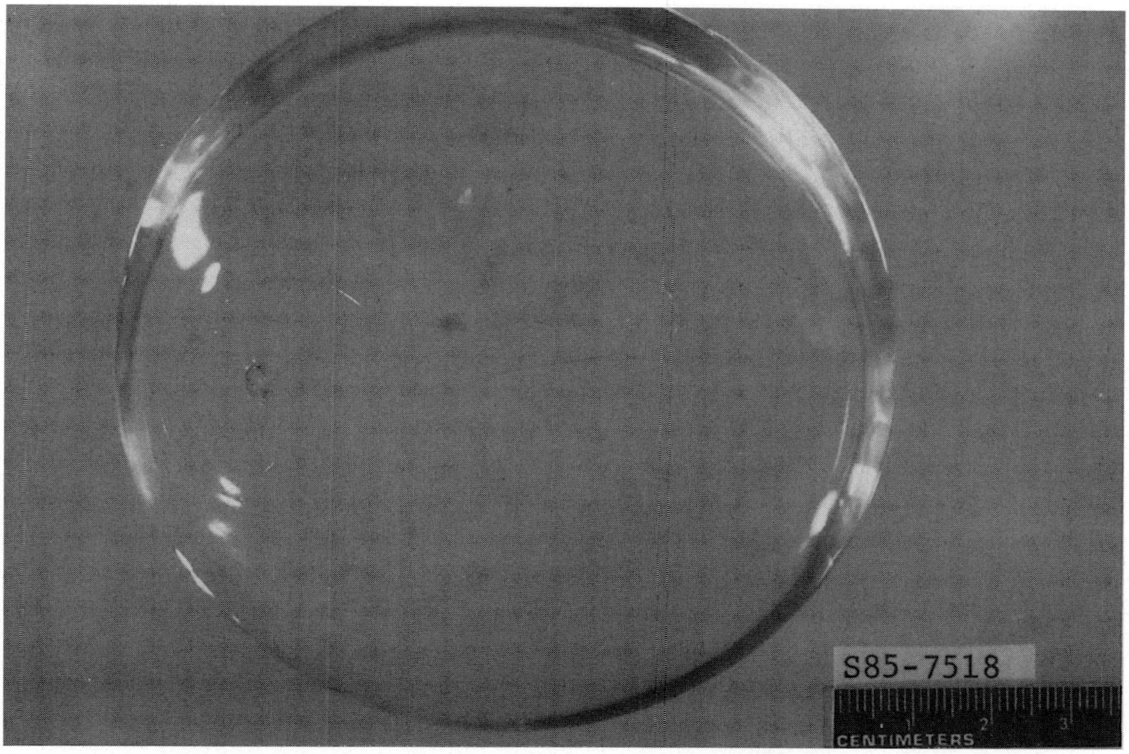

A

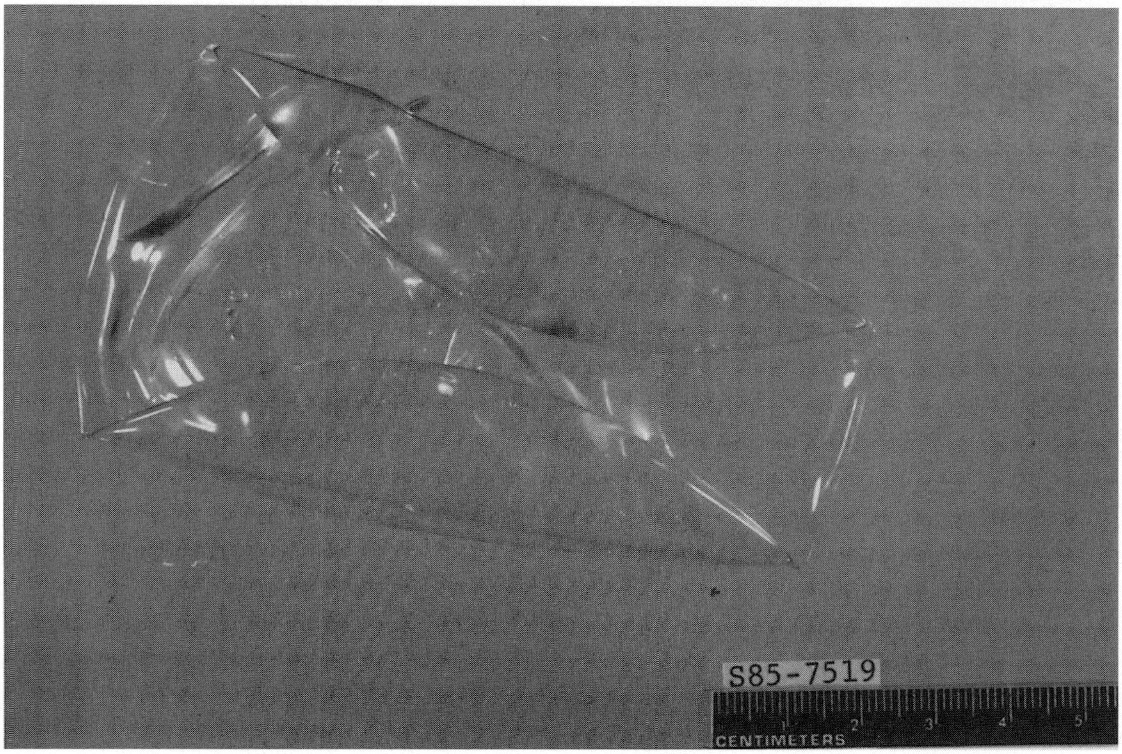

B

Figure 13–4. (**A**) First of a pair—inflatable saline-filled breast prosthesis, intact, recovered at surgery. (**B**) Second of a pair—inflatable saline-filled breast prosthesis, deflated and flat, recovered at surgery. *(continued)*

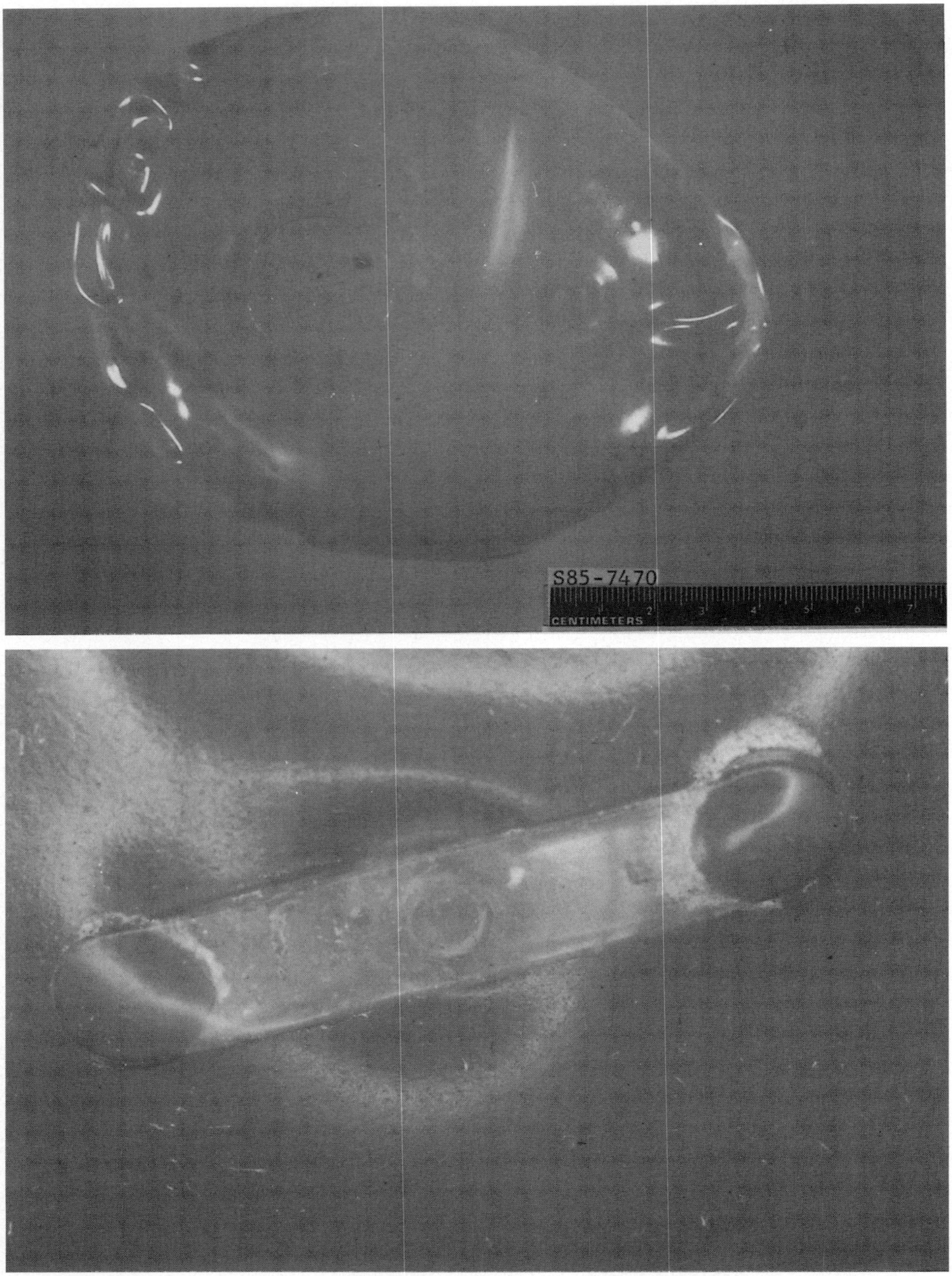

C

D

13–4. ***(Continued)*** (**C**) Another inflatable saline-filled breast prosthesis, partially deflated with a wrinkled shell, recovered at surgery. (**D**) Cover overlying the inflation port at the base of each of the above prostheses. There is no manufacturer inscription nor is their an identifying model number, lot number, or serial number. *(continued)*

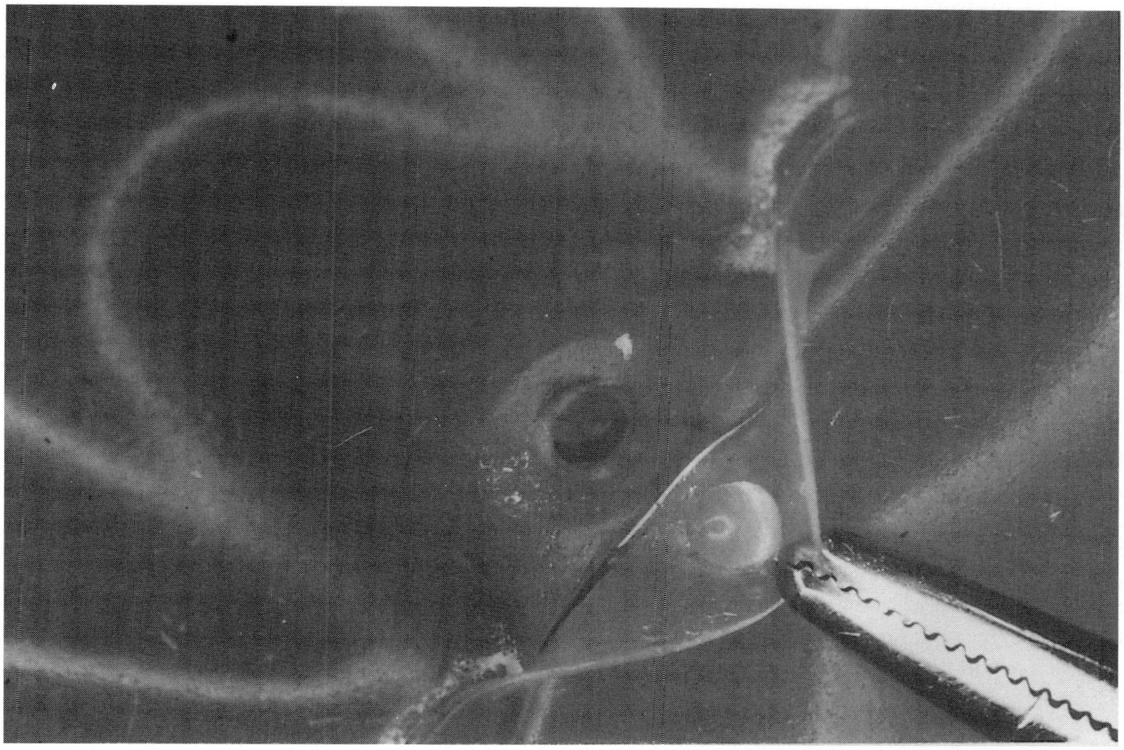

E

13–4. ***(Continued)*** (**E**) Under the cover is a simple valve constituting the inflation port of this model of prosthesis.

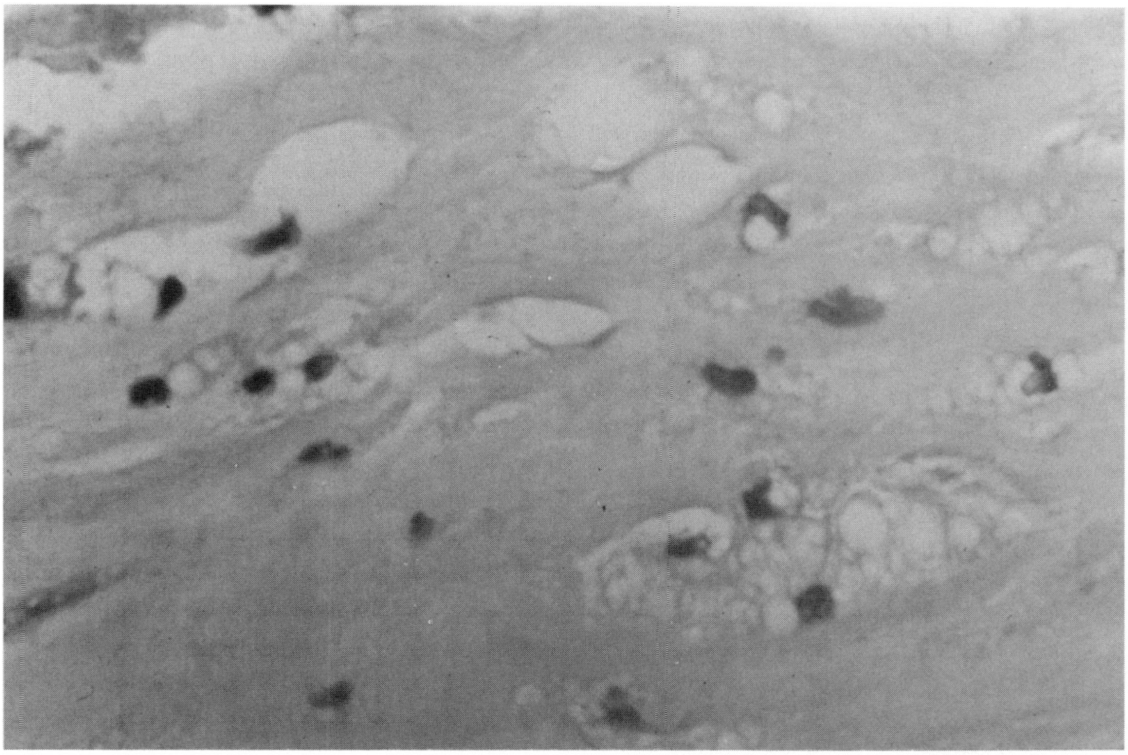

Figure 13–5. Characteristic histologic appearance of the fibrous periprosthetic capsule surrounding an "intact" gel-filled breast implant. Within the otherwise bland collagenous background are scattered macrophage nuclei and intracytoplasmic vacuoles characteristic of silicone. The silicone in these macrophages escapes from within the confines of the silicone rubber shell of the implant through a process described in the clinical literature as "bleeding." Original magnification ×100, hematoxylin and eosin.

vices coated with a layer of polyurethane foam tend to exhibit a similar pattern of inflammation, although giant cells tend to be more prevalent and both lymphocytes and plasma cells tend to be sparse (Fig. 13–6).[16,54,55] Scar capsular mineralization is common around devices that have been implanted for many years.[56] Saline-filled implants have not been studied extensively, although the tissue bed exhibits a predominantly fibroblastic reaction, with macrophages occupying primarily the interfacial zone between the fibrous scar and the silicone rubber surface. Detection of submicron-sized particulates of silicone in lymph nodes can be extremely challenging for the pathologist. While massive silicone deposition with sinus histiocytosis and abundant foamy macrophages may be obvious by light microscopy (Fig. 13–7) in the appropriate setting even by fine needle aspiration biopsy,[57] smaller quantities of silicone are more easily identified with ancillary techniques. The specialized analytic techniques discussed below are helpful in distinguishing silicone from other polymeric and alloyed materials that have been found in the lymph nodes of patients with prosthetic implants.[58]

SPECIAL ANALYTIC TECHNIQUES

There are many limitations to conventional light microscopic examination of hematoxylin and eosin stained paraffin embedded tissue. Positive identification of nonbiologic materials, especially those resistant to routine histologic staining, can be difficult. While x-ray spectroscopy (a.k.a. microprobe analysis) can identify silicon, it cannot distinguish between the carbon-rich organic molecular forms of silicon such as silicone and the inorganic mineral forms of silicon such as silica.[59] The conclusive technique for identifying organic silicon, or silicone, is infrared spectroscopy, where the molecule has an unambiguous absorption spectrum. Another technique that has been only recently shown to be useful when applied to human tissue is nuclear magnetic resonance.[60] At the research level, there are a variety of techniques. Spectroscopic methods include those using frequencies in the infrared, near infrared, and ultraviolet ranges, chromatography, nuclear magnetic resonance spectroscopy, mass spectrometry, atomic spectroscopy, and both Raman and x-ray spectroscopic techniques.[61]

■ PATHOPHYSIOLOGY OF BREAST IMPLANT INFLAMMATION

The most abundant materials available to elicit a biologic response following breast prosthesis implantation are silicone gel and, in some cases, polyurethane foam. Little is known

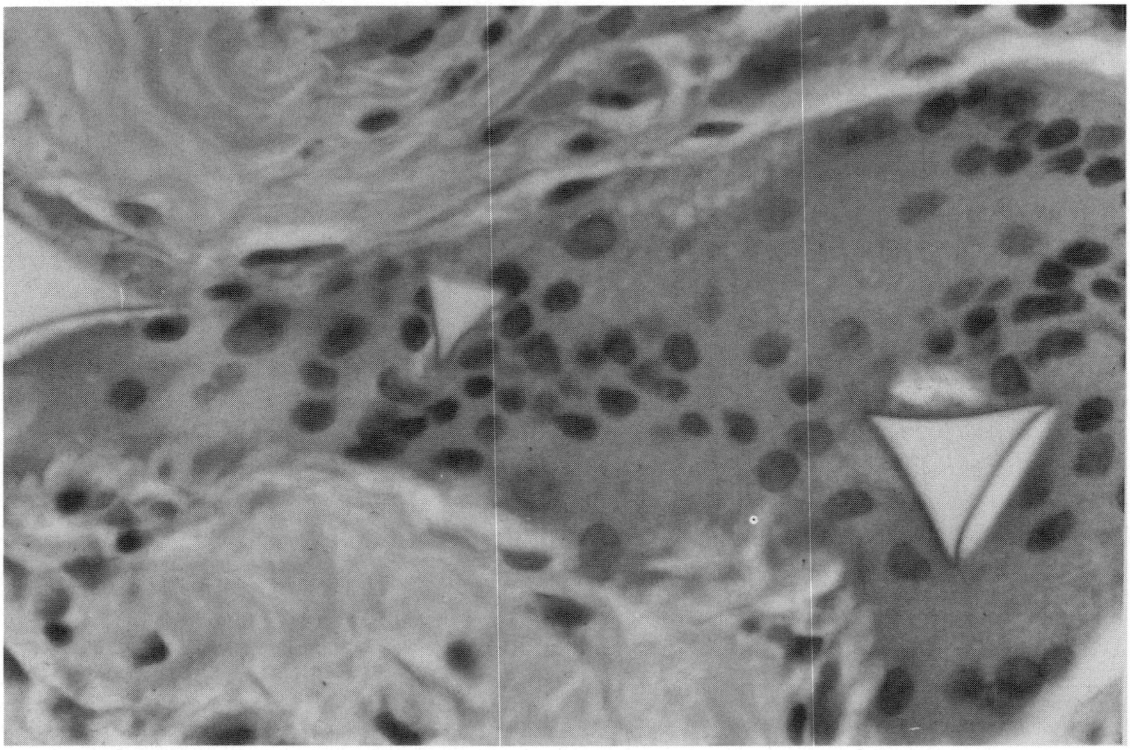

Figure 13–6. Periprosthetic capsule from a gel-filled foam-covered breast implant. Multinucleated giant cells surround curvilinear edged triangular polymeric fragments characteristic of the degradation products of polyurethane foam. Original magnification ×160, hematoxylin and eosin.

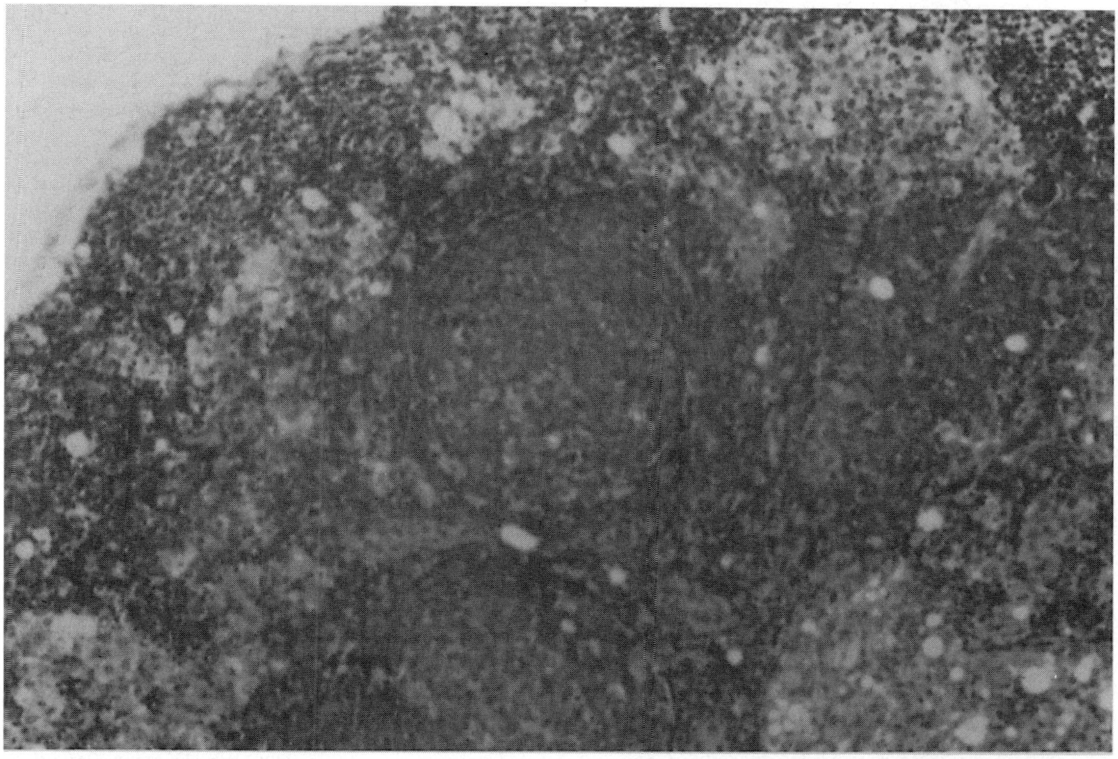

A

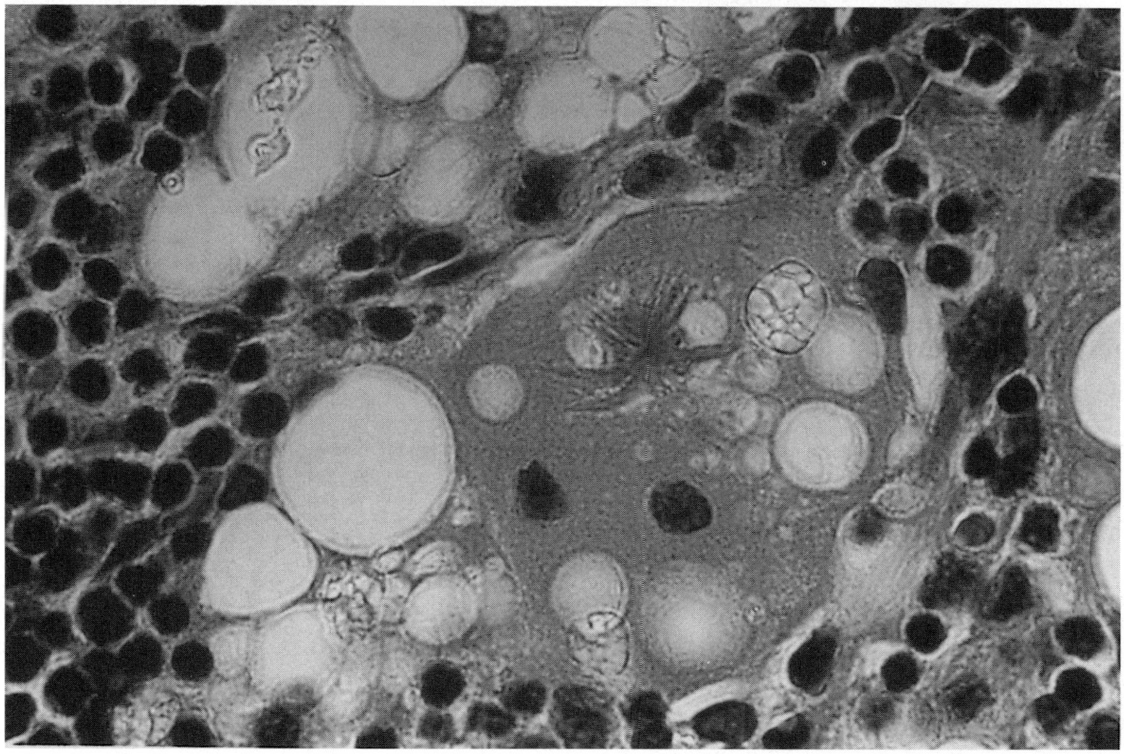

B

Figure 13–7. (**A**) Axillary lymph node exhibiting sinus histiocytosis, a pattern that often accompanies gross implant rupture and axillary silicone migration. The numerous vacuoles are consistent with silicone deposits. Original magnification ×16, hematoxylin and eosin. (**B**) Higher magnification featuring a giant cell filled with clear intracytoplasmic vacuoles consistent with silicone. Also within the macrophage is a stellate intracellular inclusion that is similar in appearance to the asteroid bodies of sarcoidosis. Original magnification ×250, hematoxylin and eosin.

about the silicone rubber component, and the saline component can be dismissed a priori. The biophysics of the interaction between silicones and biologic tissues have been reviewed extensively, and the experimental immunologic data may be found in several excellent summaries.[62]

Briefly, once freed from the envelope either by bleed or gross rupture, silicone gel tends to disperse[63] via soft tissue,[64] the lymph nodes,[65] or the vasculature,[66] possibly moving to more distal sites.[67,68] The local inflammatory processes have been well characterized. The systemic effects of local inflammation are well-known consequences of cytokine liberation, and there has been an extensive discussion of the pathophysiology of immunity and autoimmunity.[69–71] The range of diseases that have been attributed to silicone is broad. However, the magnitude of the range is not inconsistent with the range exhibited by another subtle chemical toxin, ethanol (Table 13–3).

■ CONCLUSION

The pathology of silicone breast implants has been reviewed. While the association of silicone with a distinct human disease state remains an epidemiologic challenge, there are ample doubts as to the medical safety of silicones. There are four primary driving forces for these persistent concerns:

1. There are *no* studies actually demonstrating the safety of silicone—only recent retrospective and controversial epidemiologic studies suggesting the absence of specific disease states over a relatively short time span.
2. There is a wealth of empirical small animal experimental research demonstrating broad range of adverse biologic effects and existing environmental chemistry models supporting a cause and effect relationship.
3. There is a wealth of basic physicochemical data providing evidence that silicones should cause immunologic reactions.
4. There is a growing body of evidence that humans exposed to silicone, primarily in the form of breast implants, do have both inflammatory and immunologic reactions.

REFERENCES

1. Cotran R. Cellular injury and death. In: Cotran R, Robbins SL, Kumar V, eds. *Robbin's Pathologic Basis of Disease,* 5th ed. Philadelphia: WB Saunders; 1994:1.
2. Spier RE. Therapeutic vaccines: a pandoric prospect. Presented at the 39th OHOLO conference, Eilat, Israel, May 1995.
3. Hammermeister KE, et al. A comparison of outcomes in men 11 years after heart-valve replacement with a mechanical valve or bioprosthesis. *N Engl J Med.* 1993;328:1289.
4. Schoen F. The heart. In: Cotran R, Robbins SL, Kumar V, ed. *Robbin's Pathologic Basis of Disease,* 5th ed. Philadelphia: WB Saunders; 1994:556–557.
5. Goldsmith M. Image of perfection one the goal—now some women just seek damages. *JAMA.* 1992;267:2439–2442.
6. Adler J. New bodies for sale. *Newsweek,* 27 May 1985; 64–69.
7. Human Resources and Intergovernmental Relations Subcommittee of the Committee on Government Operations, 102d Congress, 2d session, House of Representatives. *The FDA's Regulation of Silicone Breast Implants.* Washington, DC: GPO; 1993.
8. Fisher JC. The silicone controversy—when will science prevail? *N Engl J Med.* 1992;326:1696–1698.

Table 13–3. Range of Biologic Reactions Evoked by Subtle Chemical Toxins

	Ethanol[72]	*Silicone*
Range of biologic effects	Early: cognitive impairment and sedation Liver: insignificant histologic changes, alcoholic hepatitis and scarring/cirrhosis (only 10% of alcoholics actually progress to cirrhosis) Other: heart failure, muscle wasting, nerve conduction failure, structural changes in the brain, pancreatitis, and testicular atrophy	Brain: cognitive impairment and sedation (chronic lethargy) Breast: insignificant histologic changes to the tissues around a breast implant, silicone mastitis, and scarring/capsule formation and contracture (only 40% of breast implant patients have severe capsule formation) Other: muscle and joint pain, skin and hair changes, and other symptoms
Biophysical mechanisms	Direct: ethanol Indirect: one of the few metabolic products generated by liver enzyme processing of this simple 2-carbon compound; ethanol or one of its metabolites stimulates the liver's p450 microsomal oxidative system	Direct: silicone Indirect: one of the numerous metabolic products generated by liver enzyme processing of this complex polymer; silicones stimulate the liver's p450 microsomal oxidative system
Immunologic reactions	Both alcoholic hepatitis[73,74] and alcoholic heart muscle[75] diseases may be immunologic reactions[76] against native proteins denatured by alcohol	Some of the manifestations may be due to immunologic reactions against native proteins denatured by silicone

9. Lundberg GD. The breast implant controversy. A clash of ethics and law. *JAMA.* 1993;270:2608.
10. Angell M. Breast implants: protection or paternalism? *N Engl J Med.* 1992,326:1695–1696.
11. Kessler DA. The basis for the FDA's decision on breast implants. *N Engl J Med.* 1992;326:1713–1715.
12. Editorial. The American Disease. *Wall Street Journal,* January 20, 1992.
13. Shipley RH, O'Donnell JM, Bader KF. Personality characteristics of women seeking breast augmentation. *Plant Reconstr Surg.* 1977;60:369–376.
14. Zones JS. The political and social context of silicone breast implant use in the United States. *J Long-Term Effects Med Implants.* 1992;1:225–241.
15. Brody GS The breast-implant controversy (letter). *N Engl J Med.* 1993;328(10):732.
16. Lynch W. *Implants: Reconstructing the Human Body.* New York: Van Nostrand Reinhold; 1982.
17. Hatcher C, Brooks L, Love C. Breast cancer and silicone implants: psychological consequences for women. *J Natl Cancer Inst.* 1993:85:1361–1365.
18. Winer EP, Fee-Fulkerson K, Fulkerson CC, et al. Silicone controversy: a survey of women with breast cancer and silicone implants. *J Natl Cancer Inst.* 1993;85:1407–1411.
19. Kossovsky N, Heggers JP, Robson MC. The bioreactivity of silicone. In: Williams DF, ed. *CRC Critical Reviews in Biocompatibility.* Boca Raton: CRC Press; 1987;3:53–85.
20. Yoshida SH, Chang CC, Teuber SS, Gershwin ME. Silicon and silicone: theoretical and clinical implications of breast implants. *Regul Toxicol Pharmacol.* 1993;17:3–18.
21. Council on Scientific Affairs, American Medical Association. Silicone gel breast implants. *JAMA.* 1993;270:2602–2606.
22. Picha GJ, Goldstein JA. Analysis of the soft-tissue response to components used in the manufacture of breast implants: rat animal model. *Plast Reconstr Surg.* 1991;87(3):490–500.
23. Wilkerson P. Presented before the General and Plastic Surgery Devices Panel meeting, FDA, Feb. 18–20, 1992, Bethesda, MD.
24. Marotta J, DePalma, Batich C. *Trans Soc Biomat.* 1994;17: 148.
25. Kossovsky N, Heggers JP, Parsons RW, Robson MC. *Plast Reconstr Surg.* 1983;71:795.
26. Heggers JP, Kossovsky N, Parsons RW, Robson MC, Pelly RP, Raine TJ. *Ann Plast Surg.* 1983;11:38.
27. Garrido L, Pfleiderer B, Papisov M, Ackerman JL. *Magnetic Resonance Med.* 1993;29:839.
28. Garrido L, Pfleiderer B, et al. *Magnetic Resonance Med.* 1994;31:328.
29. Kallos G., Tou JC, Malczewski RM, Boley WF. *Am Ind Hygiene Assoc J.* 1991;52:259.
30. Roggendorf E. *J Biomed Mater Res.* 1976;10:123.
31. Neu TR, VanderMei HC, Busscher HJ, Dijk F, Verkerke GJ. *Biomaterials.* 1993;14:459.
32. Gent AN, Vondracek P. *J Appl Polymer Sci.* 1982;27:4537.
33. Vondracek P, Gent AN. *J Appl Polymer Sci.* 1982;27:4517.
34. *Dow Corning Med Materials Data Bull.* 1963;14:003.
35. Bischoff F. *Clin Chem.* 1972;18:869.
36. Schmidt GH. *Ann Plast Surg.* 1987;5:369.
37. Robinson OG. Annual Meeting of Southeastern Society of Plastic and Reconstructive Surgeons, Amelia Island, FL, June, 1992.
38. Robinson OG, Bradley EL, Wilson DS. *Ann Plast Surg.* 1995; 34:1.
39. Fisher JC. *Ann Plast Surg.* 1995;34:6.
40. Harris KM, Ganott MA. 77th Radiological Society of North America Annual Meeting, Chicago, IL, Dec., 1991.
41. de Camara DL, Sheridan JM, Kammer BA. *Plast Reconstr Surg.* 1993;91:828.
42. Coleman DL, King RN, Andrade JD. The foreign body reaction: a chronic inflammatory response. *J Biomed Mater Res.* 1974;8:199–211.
43. Kossovsky N. The demise of the non-specific foreign body giant cell reaction. *Trends Polymer Sci.* 1993;1:190–191.
44. Kossovsky N, Papasian N. Mammary implants: a clinical review. *J Appl Biomat.* 1992;3:239–242.
45. Sergott TJ, Limoli JP, Baldwin CM, Laub DR. Human adjuvant disease, possible autoimmune disease after silicone implantation. *Plast Reconstr Surg.* 1986;78:104–114.
46. Walsh FW, Solomon DA, Espinoza LR, Adams GD, Whitelocke JE. Human adjuvant disease: a new cause of chylous effusion. *Arch Intern Med.* 1989;149:1194–1196.
47. Varga J, Schumacher HR, Jiminez SA. Systemic sclerosis after augmentation mammoplasty with silicone implants. *Ann Intern Med.* 1989;111:377–383.
48. Freedman AM, Jackson IT. Infections in breast implants. *Infect Dis Clin North Am.* 1989;3:275–287.
49. Berkel H, Birdsell DC, Jenkins H. Breast augmentation: a risk factor for breast cancer? *N Engl J Med.* 1992;326:1649–1653.
50. Deapen DM, Brody GS. Augmentation mammaplasty and breast cancer: a 5-year update of the Los Angeles study. *Plast Reconstr Surg.* 1992;89:660–665.
51. Deapen DM, Brody GS. Breast augmentation and the risk of subsequent breast cancer. *N Engl J Med.* 1993;328:662–663.
52. Epstein SS. *Int J Occup Med Toxicol.* 1995;4:315.
53. Kossovsky N, Freiman CJ. Silicone breast implant pathology: clinical data and immunological consequences. *Arch Pathol Lab Med.* 1994;118:686–693.
54. Kossovsky N. Biomaterials and medical device pathology. I: Implantable breast prostheses. In: *ASCP Check Sample Special Topics. Am Soc Clin Pathol.* 1992;29:2.
55. Cocke WM, Leathers HK, Lynch JB. Foreign body reactions to polyurethane covers of some breast prostheses. *Plast Reconstr Surg.* 1975;56:527–530.
56. Rolland C, Lecoux R, Guidoin R, Marceau D. First observation of hopeite and parascholzite in fibrous capsules surrounding silicone breast implants. *In J Artif Organs.* 1989;12: 180–188.
57. Tabatowski K, Elson CE, Johnston WW. Silicone lymphadenopathy in a patient with a mammary prosthesis. Fine needle aspiration cytology, histology, and analytical electron microscopy. *Acta Cytol.* 1990;34:10–14.
58. Albores-Saavdera J, Vuitch F, Delgado R, Wiley E, Hagler H. Sinus histocytosis of pelvic lymph nodes after hip replacement. A histiocytic proliferation induced by cobalt-chromium and titanium. *Am J Surg Pathol.* 1994;18:83–90.
59. Rudolph R, Abraham J. Tissue effects of new silicone mammary-type implants in rabbits. *Ann Plast Surg.* 1980;4: 14–20.
60. Garrido L, Pfleiderer B, Papisov M, Ackerman JL. In vivo degradation of silicones. *MRM.* 1993;29:839–843.
61. Smith AL. *The Analytical Chemistry of Silicones.* New York: Wiley; 1991.
62. Kossovsky N. Non-covalent interactions between silicone and biological macromolecules yield bioreactive substances. *Appl Organometal Chem,* In press.
63. Rees TD, Ballantyne DL, Seidman I, Hawthorne GA. Visceral response to subcutaneous and intraperitoneal injections of silicone in mice. *Plast Reconstr Surg.* 1967;39:402–410.
64. Thomsen JL, Christensen L, Nielsen M, et al. Histologic changes and silicone concentrations in human breast tissue surrounding silicone breast prostheses. *Plast Reconstr Surg.* 1990;85:38–41.
65. Truong LD, Cartwright J, Goodman MD, Womichi D. Silicone lymphadenopathy associated with augmentation mamma-

plasty. Morphological features of nine cases. *Am J Surg Pathol.* 1988;12:484–491.

66. Travis WD, Balogh K, Abraham JL. Silicone granulomas: report of three cases and review of the literature. *Hum Pathol.* 1985;16:19–27.
67. Celli B, Textor S, Kovnat DM. Adult respiratory distress syndrome following mammary augmentation. *Am J Med Sci.* 1978;275:81–85.
68. Huang TT, Blackwell SJ, Lewis SR. Migration of silicone gel after the squeeze technique to rupture a contracted breast capsule. *Plast Reconstr Surg.* 1978;61:277–280.
69. Mena EA, Kossovsky N, Chu C, Hu C. Inflammatory intermediates produced by tissues encasing silicone breast prostheses. *J Invest Surg.* 1995;8:31–42.
70. Kossovsky N, Freiman CJ. Physicochemical and immunological basis of silicone pathology. *J Biomat Sci Polymer Ed.* 1995; 7:101–113.
71. Cotran R. Pathology of the liver. In: Cotran R, Robbins SL, Kumar V, eds. *Robbin's Pathologic Basis of Disease,* 5th ed. Philadelphia: WB Saunders; 1994:281.
72. Scholmerich J, Holstege A. Aetiology and pathophysiology of chronic liver disorders. *Drugs.* 1990;40(suppl 3):3–22.
73. Ruhland B, Walker L, Wollitzer AO, Peterson CM. Ethanol influences class I and class II MHC antigen expression on human fetal islet-like cell clusters. *Alcoholism, Clin Exp Res.* 1991;15:745–747.
74. Mishiro S, Hoshi Y, Takeda K, et al. Non-A, non-B hepatitis specific antibodies directed at host-derived epitope: Implication for an autoimmune process. *Lancet.* 1990;336(8728): 1400–1403.
75. Preedy VR, Richardson PJ. Ethanol-induced cardiovascular disease. *Br Med Bulletin.* 1994;50:152–163.
76. Paronetto F. Immunological reactions in alcoholic liver disease. *Semin Liver Dis.* 1993;13:183–195.

14

Immunologic and Clinical Aspects of Silicone in Women with Breast Implants

NACHMAN BRAUTBAR AND ARISTO VOJDANI

■ CHEMICALS AND THE IMMUNE SYSTEM

Silicone is a polymer of silica, oxygen, and methyl groups. The oxygen group contributes a significant electrical charge and the methyl group has binding capacity that could be responsible for absorption or binding to body macromolecules and thus, for potential immunologic effect, is mainly autoimmunity.[1] However, the exact cellular mechanism by which silicone exerts its immunologic effects until atypical autoimmune and neurologic diseases are developed is not clear yet.[2]

Elements of the Immune System

For understanding the mechanism of action of chemicals, such as silicone, on cell-mediated immunity, we need to become more familiar with the elements of the immune system. The human immune response is dependent on cells of the reticuloendothelial system and the lymphatic network. Products of the reticuloendothelial system include macrophages and monocytes. These cells identify, capture, and ingest invading pathogens. They are widely distributed in the body and include Kupffer's cells in the liver, microglial cells in the brain, osteoclasts in the bone, mesangial cells in the kidney, and alveolar macrophages in the lung.

These phagocytic cells play a key role in the stimulation of T lymphocytes and B lymphocytes, the primary immune cells of the lymphatic network. T cells originate in the bone marrow and become immunologically competent in the thymus. When mature, they enter the blood where they patrol, circulating from the blood to the lymph in tissues through the lymph nodes, and back to the blood via the thoracic duct. B cells originate and mature in bone marrow. Once released, they migrate to secondary lymphatic tissues, which include the lymph nodes, Waldeyer's ring, the spleen, and masses of tissue found in the small intestine, known as Peyer's patches.

Macrophages are the first line of defense that can trap, ingest, and digest invading pathogens and antigens, including silicone. The macrophage ingests these agents, processes them, and expresses their antigen on its surface membrane. This activates circulating T cells to recognize their specific antigen. For a cell-mediated immune response to occur, antigen-specific T cells must be stimulated. Interleukin-1, a product of activated macrophages, enhances this T-cell response. T-cell stimulation results in the clonal proliferation of helper T cells, cytotoxic (killer) T cells, suppressor T cells, and memory T cells. When activated, T cells produce and secrete a wide variety of immune products, including interleukin-2, gamma interferon, and B cell growth factors. These products, known as cytokines, recruit and activate nonspecific destructor cells such as natural killer (NK) cells, polymorphonuclear phagocytes (PMNs), and macrophages. Cytokines also stimulate the further growth and differentiation of T cells and B cells. In the presence of antigen and activated T cells, B cells proliferate, expand clonally, and differentiate into plasma cells and secrete antibody into the blood and lymph. The antibody binds to the antigen that stimulated its production. This response is also antigen-specific and is known as humoral immunity. There are five classes of immunoglobulins—IgG, IgA, IgM, IgD, and IgE—and many cytokines and lymphokines that play a very important role in cellular and humoral immunity. This complexity of the immune system and its connection with the endocrine and neurologic system, and the contact with many chemicals, makes the immune system and its cellular components target organs for general and/or selective chemical-induced immunotoxicity.

Immunologic Effects of Chemicals

Exposure to immunotoxicants at dose levels below those levels that induce severe organ toxicity can potentially effect the immune system as a primary target or can injure a secondary target system (lung, skin, nervous system, thyroid, etc.). Under the influence of modifying factors, such as hormonal imbalances, stress, and the presence of concurrent diseases, and nutritional status, altered immune function resulting from such exposure can potentially manifest itself in the form of hypersensitivity, autoimmunity, or immune deficiency with secondary increase in infections and/or neoplasia.[3] When the immune system is a primary target, the immunotoxicant may simultaneously act as an antigen sensitizing the host to future exposure, such as in the case of toluenediamine (a by-product of polyurethane), toluene diisocyanate, trimelytic anhydride, and formaldehyde.[4–11]

Examples of environmental/industrial agents and their interaction with the immune system include organic chemicals, such as diisocyanates and anhydrides that can induce asthma by acting as both irritants and allergens; certain drugs, such as phenytoin, which can induce selective toxicity for specific immunocompetent cells; and simple elements, such as beryllium salts that can induce delayed contact hypersensitivity.[5–11] Other elements and elemental salts, such as mercuric chloride, cadmium, and gold thiomalate, can induce non–organ-specific autoantibody formation, experimental autoimmune disease, and hypergammaglobulinemia.[3]

Mercuric chloride is known to induce autoimmune disease in rats and mice with production of autoantibody to the nuclear antigen fibrillen and hypergamaglobulinemia, particularly IgE. Cadmium has induced antinuclear antibody formation in approximately 90% of mice exposed orally to this agent in low concentrations. Many of these animals have developed amyloidosis and antiglomerular basement membrane antibody. Cadmium also has been known to have immunosuppressive effects in animal models. Gold thiomalate likewise has induced antinuclear antibody formation in experimental animals.[12–16]

It is well known that a group of systemic autoimmune diseases, including systemic lupus erythematosus (SLE,) Sjögren's syndrome, polymyositis/dermatomyositis, scleroderma, and mixed connective tissue diseases are associated with autoantibodies that react with nucleic acids and intracellular proteins. Initial studies of autoantibodies were concerned with those reactive with DNA and the histone components of deoxyribonucleoprotein. The immunologic specificity of autoantibodies to these antigens and their relationship to certain connective tissue diseases has also been thoroughly reviewed. It is believed that the latter antigens represent subcellular intranuclear protein-protein of protein-nucleic acid assemblies or particles collectively referred to as small nuclear ribonucleoproteins (RNPs). Evidence suggests that small nuclear RNPs regulate such important intracellular events as pre–messenger RNA (mRNA) splicing. Other nuclear protein autoantigens and their respective autoantibodies have been important in studying mechanisms of DNA synthesis and replication. Functioning sites of these particles appear to be stimulating immune responses, and there is speculation that perturbation of these subcellular particles by environmental agents, such as toxins or infectious agents, might render them immunogenic. Thus, it is reasonable to hypothesize that the immune response to these autoantigens may be primarily driven or directed by external environmental agents. Some clinical evidence may be provided from mercuric chloride–, cadmium-, and gold thiomalate–induced autoantibody formation and from the antihistone antibodies of drug-induced SLE.[17–24]

Chemicals and Autoimmune Disease

The mechanisms of immunologic unresponsiveness afford the body tissues a large measure of protection against an immune system developed for the destruction or elimination of antigenically foreign substances. Nevertheless, a number of well-established clinical syndromes exist in which the self-recognition process apparently fails, and the immune response is directed against autologous antigens.[20,25,26] The autoantibodies that appear in these disease states demonstrate different degrees of specificity with respect to both tissues and species. Tissue-specific autoantibodies include those that react against erythrocyte stromal antigens, platelets, antihemophilic globulin, thyroid tissue and other tissues, and Y-globulin (rheumatoid factor). Autoantibodies without tissue specificity include antinuclear, antinucleoprotein, anti-DNA, and anticytoplasmic antibodies. Autoantibodies directed against the formed elements of the blood can undoubtedly induce disease by causing the destruction and removal of these cells from the circulation.[27–31] Most studies of autoantibodies in both humans and animals have concentrated on the reactivity of humoral constituents. However, it should be remembered that the cell-mediated immune response is far more efficient in terms of tissue destruction. Because humoral antibodies have been shown, under appropriate circumstances, to prevent cell-mediated tissue damage, it is conceivable that they may have a protective, rather than a destructive function. Therefore, measurement of cell-mediated immunity is much more diagnostic than detection of humoral antibodies due to chemical exposure.[32–34] There is presently no indication whether the autoantibodies detected in human disease represent a primary manifestation of the disease itself or a secondary event stimulated by an underlying, but unrelated, abnormality. In either event, the mechanisms that may be responsible for the abrogation of natural immunologic tolerance are worthy of consideration. Five general mechanisms have been proposed in the pathogenesis of autoantibody production:

1. alterations in the structure or distribution of antigens;
2. formation of cross-reactive antibodies following exposure to extrinsic antigens;
3. release of sequestered antigens;
4. abnormalities of immunologic responsiveness;
5. adjuvant effect.

One or all of the above mechanisms may be involved in the pathogenesis of implant-induced autoimmune reactivity.[35–41]

■ SILICONE BREAST IMPLANTS AND IMMUNE-MEDIATED DISEASE

In recent years, concern has been raised about the safety of silicone breast implants. Several experimental animal studies dating back to 1967, patient case reports, and patient controlled studies, as well as in vivo and in vitro studies indicate that silicone is associated with immunologic abnormalities and systemic symptomatology, and, in some cases, disease processes. These above studies coupled with a public concern led the Food and Drug Administration (FDA) to ban the use of silicone breast implants for cosmetic purposes effective 1992. Recent epidemiologic studies concluded that there is no association between silicone breast implants and typical autoimmune disease.

This section summarizes the available experimental animal data, in vitro studies, in vivo studies, case reports, clinical studies, and recent epidemiologic studies, and reviews the criteria necessary to establish medical causation.

Experimental Animal Data

Subcutaneous and intraperitoneal injections of silicone in experimental animals demonstrated that silicone fluid (injected) is deposited in the spleen, liver, adrenals, pancreas, ovaries, abdominal lymph nodes, and kidneys.[42] A likely mechanism is phagocytosis by histiocytes and generalized deposition in the reticuloendothelial system similar to the distribution of carbon particles. The effects of silicone droplets have been studied by Ben-Hur et al,[43] who have shown lymphocytic infiltration in response to deposits of the silicone. The injected silicone was engulfed by histiocytes, transported to the region of the lymph node, and eventually distributed throughout the reticuloendothelial system.

Brody and Fray[44] demonstrated that intraperitoneal silicone caused a significant inflammatory reaction, and concluded that liquid silicone "not be used" intraperitoneally in humans until "further long-term studies" were completed. Interestingly enough, documents from Dow Corning[45] show a study conducted in mice, utilizing linear 3,4- and cyclic 4,5-silicone. The investigators concluded that parenterally administered silicone caused a transient response in the lymphoreticular system with a maximum at 48 hours. This response was found to involve macrophages, and depressed the carbon clearance of the reticuloendothelial system. The researchers concluded that silicone caused a direct effect on the immune system in experimental animals.

The experimental studies in these animals show (1) an immunologic reaction with production of an inflammatory reaction including phagocytosis; (2) transported by the lymphatic system into the reticuloendothelial system, liver, spleen, kidney, and pancreatic lymph glands; (3) direct influence on the function of the reticuloendothelial system.

Laboratory and Clinical Data Demonstrating that Implants "Bleed" (Leak)

Barker et al[46] have shown that the implants leak without rupture. Thomsen et al[47] have studied histologic changes and silicone concentrations present in human breast tissue surrounding silicone breast prostheses, and utilized scanning electron microscopy and energy dispersive analysis of x-rays to quantitatively measure silicone in the tissue that developed around the implants. They concluded that the silicone prostheses provoked an inflammatory response not only because they act as a foreign body, but also because of silicone leakage through the membranes. That this is indeed the chain of events, and that silicone leaks from the implants, has been shown in 1978 by Housner et al,[48] who studied a 24-year-old woman in good general health who had bilateral augmentation mammoplasty without any complication. In July 1977 she noted a lump in the upper inner quadrant of her right breast. During surgery, the prosthesis was found to be encapsulated by dense fibrous tissue and no ruptures of the prosthetic envelope could be found. (In other words, intact envelope of the implants.) Random section of the fibrous capsule adjacent to the implant prepared from formalin-fixed and paraffin-embedded tissue showed focal accumulation of large histiocytes with foamy vacuolated cytoplasm. Vacuoles within the histiocytes contained a refractile material microscopically identical to the gel that was adherent to the inside of the envelope in the sections. Two of the lymph nodes studied contained many multinucleated giant cells. Many of the vacuoles were filled with refractile material, optically identical to both the gel and the intrahistiocytic material adjacent to the prosthesis.

The investigators concluded that their data show (1) the envelope of the implant was intact; (2) there was leakage of silicone through the intact envelope; (3) silicone was transferred via the lymphatic system and was found in lymph nodes in the axilla; (4) this was associated with phagocytosis by the histiocytes at the site of introduction.

Recent studies[49] utilizing nuclear magnetic resonance technology with in vivo spectroscopy of the livers of animals with long-term (10–12 months) silicone implants, reveal the presence of silicone in the liver. Ex vivo, spectroscopy of the liver, spleen, and capsule from 9 to 12 months after implantation, also demonstrate that free silicone migrates from silicone gel–filled implants. These investigators also showed that silicones are not metabolically inert, and biodegradation in tissue may occur within the implant and can be monitored after 9 to 12 months of implantation. The animal findings were supported by those obtained by atomic absorption spectroscopy. The three-dimensional structure of the gel disintegrates, increasing the molecular mobility of the polymer, and consequently its proton values. Measurements of the soluble fraction extracted with chloroform from silicone gel implants at various implantation sites 12 months after the implantation with no rupture and with intact implant membrane were associated with significant reduction of silicone gel contents, clearly demonstrating leakage of the silicone, without a rupture.[50]

Thus, data suggest that (1) silicone leaks through the intact gel membrane, (2) the leaked silicone particles are phagocytosed and then transferred via the lymphatic system to lymph nodes and distant organs, and (3) silicone is biodegradable after being released from the gel through the intact membrane and forms various silicones and silicates.

Clinical Autoimmune Disease and Immune Dysfunction, and Data from Human Case Reports and Controlled Studies

Chronic arthropathy after silicone augmentation mammoplasty was described in three women who developed fibrous capsular contractures.[51] Kaiser et al[52] describe a patient who presented with immunologic features of systemic lupus erythematosus 11 years after silicone augmentation. After explantation, antinuclear antibody titers decreased and the patient improved. The dramatic improvement upon removal of the silicone indicated that silicone is reactive probably via an immunologic reaction. Following clinical findings in a small series, 18 patients and a review of 28 published Japanese patients, Kumagai et al[53] describe patients with defined connective tissue disease; 12 had scleroderma including eight with progressive systemic sclerosis; six with rheumatoid arthritis; five with systemic lupus erythematosus, and one with polymyositis; 22 patients had human adjuvant disease, with some symptoms, signs, and laboratory abnormalities suggestive but not diagnostic of connective tissue disease. The authors conclude that (1) progressive systemic sclerosis is approximately three times more frequent in women with silicone injection and implants; (2) progressive systemic sclerosis developed primarily in individuals injected with paraffin; and (3) injected substances may induce immunologic disorders by acting as adjuvants. Other investigators have described autoimmune disease in patients after mammoplasty. Van Nunen et al[54] describe three patients in whom autoimmune connective tissue disease developed within 2 1/2 years after cosmetic mammary augmentation with silicone gel–filled elastomer envelope-type prosthesis. They suggest that silicone gel–filled mammary implants could precipitate connective tissue disease in a susceptible host.

Additional case reports showing effects of silicone breast implants on other organ systems have been described. Celli et al[55] describe adult respiratory distress syndrome immediately following mammary augmentation. This was associated with sudden hypoxemia and pulmonary infiltrates following intramammary injection of silicone. The findings of birefringent particles in the alveolar macrophages indicate entrance of silicone into the vascular compartment and migration across the damaged alveolar capillary membrane. The authors conclude that silicone droplets gained access into the circulation through the lymphatic system, and through that into the pulmonary system, causing respiratory distress syndrome.

The original description of the association between silicone and connective tissue disease was found in the Japanese literature by Myoshi et al.[56] This phenomenon was described as human adjuvant disease (HAD). Such a clinical condition in humans with silicone gel–filled implants has been determined to be an autoimmune reaction to silicone.

Epidemiologic Data Claiming "No Association" Between Silicone Implants and Immune Disease.

Several larger scale studies have been performed claiming the absence of a significant association between silicone breast implants and a variety of connective tissue disorders. A review by Sanchez-Guererro et al[57] concluded that the clinical, immunologic, and epidemiologic evidence indicates little or no association between silicone breast implants and connective tissue disease or unique arthralgia, myalgia, or fibromyalgia syndrome. Silicone may elicit a local inflammatory response but this appears to be mild or transient. Most of the serologic abnormalities identified are similar to those in patients with an idiopathic form of different connective tissue syndrome, with the exception of an apparent lower frequency of anti-SC1-70, and higher frequency of anti-centromere antibodies in patients with silicone breast implants anad scleroderma.

Sanchez-Guerrero[58] conducts a large-scale questionnaire study of matched cohorts of female nurses between the ages of 30 and 55 and found no significant association between those with silicone breast implants and reported symptoms of connective tissue disease. Based on the responses of 1000 women, they found no demonstrable increased risk of women with silicone implants developing connective tissue disease, noting, however, that they did not include so-called atypical disease in their study.

While silicone-related reaction has been described as an atypical disease in patients with silicone breast implants and autoimmune reaction, the investigators of this study did not include atypical disease, indicating that "since the specification criteria for connective tissue disease excluded patients with milder or atypical cases and those who did not fulfill the criteria earlier in the disease, the true incidence of the disease could have been underestimated."

Claman and Robertson[59] performed a cross-sectional survey of 150 women, of whom 131 had implants. They studied four groups: group 1 consisted of 19 volunteer women without breast implants who felt healthy; group 2 consisted of 82 women with implants who had various symptoms; and group 3 consisted of 11 women with implants and autoimmune disease. Scleroderma was overrepresented in group 3, found in 6 out of 11. Antinuclear antibodies were determined on hep-2 cells using serum dilutions of 116, 164, and 1/256. A positive test was indicated by +1 or more fluorescence at 1 : 1/256 dilution. Antinuclear antibody tests were positive in none of group 0, 18 % of group 1 ($p < .05$ compared with group 0); 26 % of group 2; and 64% of group 3. These findings suggest that patients with silicone breast implants have higher levels of antinuclear antibodies, especially when they are symptomatic.

Gabriel et al[60] attempted to evaluate the anticipated risk of women with implants in developing connective tissue disease using retrospective review of medical records in a large number of patients. They found no appreciable association between silicone implants and the development of disease.

Strom et al[62] conducted telephone interviews and some personal interviews with 219 patients diagnosed with one specific form of connective tissue disease, namely systemic lupus erythematosus (SLE). Using case-control methodologies, they concluded that there was no association between silicone breast implants and the development of SLE.

Evidence that Silicone is Immunogenic

Naim and Lanzafame[63] compared the immune potentiation effects of silicone gel with that of Freund's adjuvant, using bovine serum albumin as the test antigen in rats. They found that silicone gel is a potent immunologic adjuvant and concluded that silicone gel may mediate an autoimmune reaction.

Press et al[64] studied antinuclear antibodies in women with silicone breast implants. Of 11 patients who had symptoms and signs of autoimmune disease, seven had scleroderma or a subset of this disorder, and others had systemic lupus erythematosus, rheumatoid arthritis, or overlapping autoimmune disease. High antinuclear antibody (ANA) titers were present in 10 of these 11 patients, and the ANA specificities were similar to those found in idiopathic forms of the corresponding autoimmune disease. Traumatic rupture of implants accelerated the onset of symptoms in 13 other patients who had autoimmune disorder of a less clearly defined nature, and a low titer of antinuclear antibodies. These findings indicate a dose-response relationship. They concluded that antinuclear antibodies are associated with the development of autoimmune complications in women with silicone breast implants.

Silicone polymer precursors and prosthesis components were recently studied by Picha and Goldstein,[65] who subcutaneously implanted silicone shells, shells extracted from their low molecular weight components, silica-free silicone, silicone oil, fumed silica, and silicone extracts. They measured the intensity of the cellular and capsular response. They have shown that the intensity of the cellular and capsular response was lowest for the silicone oil and increased as the material molecular weight increased and material compliance decreased. Fumed silica elicited the most highly reactive cellular response.

They concluded that the polymer's molecular weight influences its migrations, encapsulation, and intensity of cellular response. Furthermore, the silicone extract distillate elicited a highly intense cellular response with pronounced lymphocyte invasion. This study indicates that silica is immunogenic, and that the silicone oil, the low molecular weight species, is prone to site migration as well as to introducing a foreign body response with the presence of macrophages, fibroblasts, and lymphocytes. The degree of fibrosis, however, is lower for the oil than the gel, and subsequently lower for the solid polymer sheath. By comparing the silica-free silicone and the extracted implant ready shells, a correlation was made regarding the effects of silica filler. The histologic response to the fumed silica represents the most intense cellular response compared with those of the other materials. Thus silicone is biodegradable with immunogenic silica released from the gel.[49,50]

Crystalline silica is known to stimulate production of antibodies of various isotopes to the T-dependent antigen. Mansino et al[66] have shown silicone is an adjuvant that was found for TPN-KLH, an antigen with a high degree of macrophage-dependency. Silica induces selected toxic effects on macrophages and its adjuvant activity is prevented by treatment of animals with the macrophage stabilizing material and oxide.[67,68] These observations suggest that silica may play a role in the immunogenicity of the shell of the implants.

Bridges et al[69] studied 156 women with silicone breast implants and rheumatic disease complaints. They measured various immunoglobulins, complement C-reactive protein, rheumatoid factor, and autoantibodies by indirect immunofluorescence, immune diffusion, and Western blot. Three subgroups of patients based on clinical and laboratory findings were defined. Joint and muscle pain was seen in 95 patients, joint swelling in 32 patients, and connective tissue disease in 29 patients. Most women had normal immunologic studies. The patients with joint swelling had mild asymmetric rheumatoid factor and negative synovitis that did not meet American College of Rheumatology criteria for rheumatoid arthritis. Fourteen patients had a scleroderma-like illness, and anticentromere and anti-PMSCI antibodies by Western blot.

Ten patients had a positive Western blot for BB polypeptide, a small nuclear ribonucleoprotein, but did not meet criteria for systemic lupus erythematosus. No antibodies to known disease-related polypeptides were detected on Western blot in the control group. The authors concluded that most women with silicone implants and rheumatic complaints had normal serologic tests, and nonspecific symptoms suggesting no serious connective tissue disease. However, a subset of women had clinical signs and serologic tests that were unusual, even for referral patients.

Vojdani et al[70] studied 40 women with silicone breast implants and various symptomatology in comparison with a control group of 40 normal women. They measured autoantibodies including antinuclear antibodies, as well as lymphocyte subset analysis and natural killer cell cytotoxic activity, which are markers for immune compatibility. Significant elevations of myelin-basic protein, a marker of antibodies against the myelin sheath of the nervous system were found, together with significant T-helper/suppressor ratio abnormalities, with distributions toward the lower end and upper ends that were statistically and significantly different from control patients. Lymphocytic mitogenic response was also abnormal in silicone-exposed patients. These studies suggest that silicone triggers autoimmunity as well as lymphocyte subcellular response, resulting in the production of an antibody to silicone, native macromolecule, or their combination.

Goldblum et al[71] describe two patients demonstrating immunologic reaction to silicone tubing used for ventricular peritoneal shunts. They concluded that elastomers of silicone elicit specific silicone antibodies. Wolf et al,[72] in a large study, found specific antisilicone IgG antibodies in those patients who had implants, the highest levels in patients with rupture or leakage of the implants. They conclude that sufficiently high antisilicone antibody levels indicate systemic exposure to silicone.

Immunologic Effects of Silicone

A variety of immunologic tests are employed for the testing of humoral and cell-mediated immunity. The picture is not complete until the important interacting cells in various immune functions (ie, macrophages) are also considered. The macrophages play an important role in both humoral and cellular immune responses by cooperating with selective immunocytes. The awareness of the role of macrophages in immunotoxicity is becoming more important and interesting. Undoubtedly, more tests of different kinds have been performed including natural killer cytotoxic factor, lymphokine production, and lymphocyte blastogenic responses to the T-cell and B-cell mitogens. In many cases, the reactivity of specific cells to surface-acting agents can be evaluated in vitro by using the mitogens. Direct effects of chemicals can be evaluated by their addition to cultures but should be viewed with caution. A number of chemicals decrease the response of lymphocytes to blastogenic agents by virtue of being cytotoxic. On the other hand, some chemicals may have nonspecific mitogenic properties themselves. Interaction of chemicals with mitogens in the medium may modify their function. Similar effects can be produced if the interfering molecules in the medium, such as specific fractions of serum proteins, are neutralized or altered by the presence of these chemicals. Selection of these tests is based on the following seven steps and immune pathways that are likely to be affected by the chemical:

1. Antigen contact and processing
2. Antigen recognition
3. Cell proliferation
4. Clonal proliferation
5. Antibody production
6. Release of factors
7. Effects or action.

The end results of this effect could be degradation, sedimentation, and tissue damage.[73–75]

Immunologic Markers for Silicone

In recent years, there have been many reports that breast augmentation procedures led to clinical syndromes, some of which resemble systemic lupus erythematosus, rheumatoid arthritis, Sjögren's syndrome, scleroderma, polymyositis, polymyositis-scleroderma overlap syndrome, and other rheumatic diseases. Other patients have clinical syndromes that are less clearly defined for which the term *atypical disease* or *disease-like syndrome* has been used. The nature of the humoral and cellular immune responses in immunologic disorders associated with breast augmentation has recently been assessed and abnormalities at the level of T-cell, B-cell, helper cell, suppressor cell, and NK cell activity was reported.[2,76,77] Based on the above findings and experience with analysis of thousands of blood samples from patients with silicone breast implants and the degree of variability of this immunologic picture, there is no single blood test to assist in the diagnosis of SIIDS. Rather, assessment of both humoral and cellular compartments of the immune system are needed for the diagnosis of this complex disease. Only those markers that were found to be significantly different in silicone implant patients are discussed.

Evaluation of Cellular Immunity in Relation to Silicone

FLOW CYTOMETRY ANALYSIS OF T-HELPER AND T-SUPPRESSOR LYMPHOCYTES

The number and functional capacity of circulating peripheral blood leukocytes reflect the overall state of immune competence of an individual. In a variety of clinical situations, tests for granulocyte, lymphocyte, and monocyte number and function have become routine in the diagnosis of disease and in monitoring immunosuppressive and immunorestorative treatments. In recent years, flow cytometric tests for lymphocyte subsets have begun to be recognized as useful diagnostic and prognostic indicators in several clinical situations, including bone marrow and organ transplantation, diagnosis of leukemias and lymphomas, and evaluation of immune deficiency disorders. Flow cytometric measurements allow the enumeration of different types of lymphocytes, which are known to have distinctive functional activities.

HELPER/SUPPRESSOR RATIO

Disease-related changes in T4+(helper) and T8+(suppressor) lymphocyte levels may alter T4/T8 inducer : suppressor/cytotoxic cell ratios. As a result, T4/T8 ratios may also be useful as diagnostic and/or prognostic indicators of immune competence.

T4/T8 ratios in conjunction with T4+lymphocyte cell numbers have been the most widely used laboratory parameters for the evaluation of AIDS-related complex and AIDS. T4/T8 ratios fall toward zero in advanced-AIDS patients with no detectable levels of T4+lymphocytes. In such cases, T8+lymphocyte levels may be normal, increased, or decreased.

Modulations in T4/T8 ratios and T4+and T9+lymphocyte levels may occur in autoimmune diseases, such as multiple sclerosis (MS) and systemic lupus erythematosus (SLE). Increased T4/T8 ratios and decreased numbers of T4+and T8+lymphocytes have been observed in patients with progressive (active) MS. The lymphocyte response pattern in SLE, however, appears to reflect clinical disease activity and the level of the organ involvement in the SLE disease process. To illustrate, high T4/T8 ratios and elevated T4+lymphocyte percentages have been found in active/inactive SLE patients with multisystem disease, including lymphadenopathy, although little or no renal disease has been detected. High T4/T8 ratios, but decreased percentages of T8+lymphocytes, have also been documented in similarly active SLE patients. Additionally, high T4+and low T8+lymphocyte percentages have been measured in active SLE patients with central nervous system disease but with no renal disease. In contrast, low T4/T8 ratios and decreased T4+lymphocyte percentages have been noted in active/inactive patients with SLE manifested by severe renal disease and/or thrombocytopenia. In other active/inactive SLE patients, both low T4+and high T8+lymphocyte percentages have been recorded.

This pattern of immunologic abnormalities, including immune dysfunctions and dysregulations, has been detected following exposure to pentachlorophenol, chlordane, benzene, formaldehyde, polycyclic aromatic hydrocarbons, and solvents, and could extend to other chemicals. In fact, the nature of the humoral and cellular immune responses in immunologic disorders associated with breast augmentation has recently been assessed, and abnormalities at the level of T-cell, B-cell, helper cell, suppressor cell, and NK cell activity was reported. Elevated T helper suppressor ratios in about 50% of silicone implant patients and decreased T helper suppressor ratios in about 10% of these patients may have been the impetus for the induction of autoantibodies and autoimmune condition in some individuals.[76]

NATURAL KILLER (NK) CELL ACTIVITY

Natural killer (NK) cells appear to play a role in a variety of human diseases. Compromised or absent natural immunity, as measured in vitro by decreased NK cell activity and/or depressed absolute numbers of circulating NK cells, has been linked to the development and progression of cancer, to chronic and acute viral infections, including AIDS, to chronic fatigue syndrome, psychologic dysfunction, various immunodeficiencies, and certain autoimmune diseases. Recent evidence indicates that NK cells may be involved in multiple effector, regulatory, and developmental activities of the immune system and that deficiencies or abnormalities in NK cell function may contribute to, or be a biologic marker for, disease. For the above reasons, it is important to reliably detect abnormalities in NK cell function. Furthermore, recent evidence indicates that there is a relationship between an individual's reaction to emotional stress and NK cell activity. The role of NK cells in viral disease has been known for a long time. The correlation between low NK cell activity and serious viral infections in immunocompromised hosts, for example, in AIDS, after transplantation, and in certain congenital immunodeficiencies, has been well documented. Abnormalities in NK cell function have been described in a variety of autoimmune diseases and, because these diseases are frequently associated with serious viral infections and malignancy, low levels of NK cell activity may be biologically important in individuals with autoimmune disorders. Finally, chronic fatigue immune dysfunction syndrome (CFIDS) is characterized by a number of immunologic abnormalities, the most consistent being a significant depression of NK cell activity.[7] A similar phenomenon (low NK cell cytotoxic activity) was very recently reported by our laboratory and others in patients who have a history of toxic chemical exposure and silicone breast implants.[76,78] In the latter group, 65% showed low NK cell activity of below 20 lytic units, while similar abnormalities of low NK cell activity were found in only 17% of controls.[76] In individuals who had chosen to remove their implants when this assay was repeated a year postexplanation, reversal to a normal NK cell activity was observed in 60% of explanted patients.[79] This improvement in the NK cell activity after explantation is sufficient evidence for causation and effect.

Similar results were reported in previous studies and indicated that NK cell activity was suppressed in female B6C3F1 mice exposed to silicone gel. Silicone gel was also found to suppress NK cell activity in female Fischer 344 rats. Very recently, this study was further extended to NK cell function of spleen and peripheral blood. It was found that NK cell was suppressed 38 to 61% as early as 17 days after implant. There was a biphasic dose response with a nadir at doses between 50 and 100 mL/kg of silicone gel. NK suppression was reversed after silicone gel removal.[80] These studies indicate the following: (1) spontaneous NKI cell activity is suppressed following exposure to silicone gel, (2) suppression is reversed following removal of the implants, and (3) NK cells from silicone gel–implanted rats are capable of exhibiting augmented lytic activity in response to Poly-I : C, which is a stimulator of interferon.

T-CELL AND B-CELL FUNCTION

Lymphocyte proliferation or transformation is the process whereby new DNA synthesis and cell division take place in lymphocytes after a stimulus of some type, resulting in a series of changes. The lymphocytes increase in size, the cytoplasm becomes more extensive, the nucleoli are visible in the nucleus, and the lymphocytes resemble blast cells. The term *blast transformation* is also sometimes applied to this process.

MEMORY LYMPHOCYTE IMMUNE FUNCTION ASSAY (MELIFA)

Antibodies produced in vitro by activated lymphocytes following autogenic stimulus and cultured for 5 to 7 days are evaluated by a method called MELISA and MELIFA. This new generation of laboratory tests should result in a more effective method for the diagnosis of SIIDS. During the past 5 years, these tests have been successfully applied to many haptens and antigens, including dietary antigens and metals. The application of this knowledge from scientific journals to silicon dioxide and silicone further demonstrates the importance of memory lymphocytes and their measurements for the diagnosis of immunologic disorders induced by chemicals.

MEASUREMENTS OF HUMORAL IMMUNITY

As immunoserologic markers for silicone, humoral immunity is dealing with different materials that are present in plasma or serum. These factors play an important role in natural body defense and their concentrations may be increased or decreased during an inflammatory response. Examples of such humoral factors, whose concentration varies in patients with implants, are C3, C4 complement, rheumatoid factor, and immune complexes.

Other humoral factors that are produced by lymphocytes and secreted into circulation are antibodies. These antibodies (IgG and IgM) may be directed specifically or nonspecifically against nuclear material (ANA) or tissue antigens such as striated muscle, smooth muscle, thyroid, immunoglobulins, or brain, or directly against silicone after its binding to these tissue antigens. During additional immunostimulation, produced antibodies at high concentration form immune complexes and bind to complement. Immune complexes by binding complement become activated complexes that directly or indirectly cause membrane damage to the cells of target organ. The end result of this autoimmune reaction is partial or complete loss of functioning capacity of that target organ. Therefore, measurements of humoral factors are important for evaluation of immunologic abnormalities and treatment of patients with silicone implants.

ANTINUCLEAR ANTIBODY (ANA)

ANA is another non specific factor that was found to be elevated in 25 to 64% of patients with silicone breast implants.[79] Using this test, it is possible to examine the relationship between breast implants and autoimmunity. For example a cross-sectional survey was recently conducted that included 150 women, 131 of whom had implants. Group 1 was composed of healthy women without implants and group 2 was composed of women with breast implants who felt healthy. Women with implants who had various symptoms, including fatigue, were placed in group 3, and group 4 included women with implants who had autoimmune disease. In these groups, 0%, 18%, 26%, and 64%, respectively, demonstrated positive ANA antibodies. The authors concluded that women with breast implants may be at risk for development of antinuclear antibodies and autoimmunities.[58] Therefore, the detection of circulating antibodies to nuclear antigens is an important tool in the investigation of systemic rheumatic disease in patients with implants. Antinuclear antibodies may be classified biochemically according to whether they bind nucleic acid per se, a chromatic component such as a histone, a ribonucleoprotein (RNP), or some other nuclear constituent. Antibodies within each class can be detected readily in assays based on immunofluorescence using the hep-2 cell line, enzyme immunoassay, and Western blot assays using biochemically purified antigens.[58,69]

Detection of an antibody to extractable nuclear antigens (ENA) or non histone nuclear antigens are helpful in the evaluation of patients with SLE, mixed connective tissue disease (MCTD), scleroderma, Sjögren's syndrome (SS), dermatopolymyositis, and rheumatoid arthritis (RA). These antibodies include SM and n-RNP; SS-A/Ro and SS-B/La; Scl-70; Pm-1 and Jo-1; PCNA; RANA; and MA. Detection of these antibodies is possible by taking the ANA test one step further by using biochemically purified antigens and enzyme-linked immunosorbent assay (ELISA) or Western blot assays. If the ELISA-ANA (EANA) is positive for ANA, it is important to determine the immunologic specificity of the ANA. In many cases when the implants were removed, the ANA titered was reduced significantly and the symptomatology either improved or disappeared.[81–84] The improvement in the laboratory markers and symptomatologies strongly suggests the adverse causes of silicone. Another phenomenon that was described recently relates to the nonspecific clinical feature or atypical autoimmune illness in patients with silicone breast implants. For example, a large group of patients with asymmetric arthritis were seronegative, and only 12 out of 97 had a positive rheumatoid factor.[89]

A high proportion of patients with a scleroderma-like illness showed symptoms consistent with connective tissue disease, which has been associated with silicone implants. These observations support a hypothesis that silicone may, like other occupational and environmental exposures, "trigger" scleroderma-like illness.[69] These atypical clinical and serologic features of the patients with a scleroderma-like illness also support an association between silicone implants and scleroderma. The clinical and serologic features of patients with this scleroderma-like illness and silicone implants differed from classical scleroderma reported in the scientific literature. Such features may indicate a unique difference in autoantibodies of patients with silicone breast implants. An additional atypical marker that was found to be abnormal is BB polypeptide.[69] BB polypeptide is a member of the small nuclear ribonucleoproteins (SmRNP); autoantibodies to this polypeptide are found characteristically in SLE associated with Sm antigen, but may be found in MCTD or scleroderma associated with RNP antigen reactivity. About 25 to 30% of patients with silicone breast implants with nonspecific clinical features have a negative or low-titer ANA test, and do not have defined criteria for lupus MCTD or scleroderma. However, they do demonstrate an antibody to BB polypeptide with reaction with Sm, which is unusual. Whether these patients have an early SLE or they represent a new subgroup of patients with connective tissue disease is unclear. The finding of this marker is important because these women did not have laboratory evidence of connective tissue disease until autoantibodies were assessed by Western blot assay. The authors concluded that sensitive testing by Western blot assay is necessary to detect atypical tissue autoantibodies suggestive of atypical connective tissue disease in patients with silicone implants.[69]

THYROID ANTIBODIES

Autoimmune thyroid gland disorders are characterized by detection of antithyroid antibodies, primarily against thyroglobulin and microsomal thyroid antigens. Recently it has been shown that thyroid peroxidase (TPO) is the protein responsible for microsomal antigenicity. Thyroid microsomal autoantibodies occur in sera of most autoimmune thyroid disease patients, and levels correlate with the degree of lymphoid infiltration of the thyroid gland. Thyroid antibodies (TA) are a characteristic finding in patients with Hashimoto's and Graves' diseases. The presence of TA in the sera of 80% of patients with these two diseases led to the recommendation that some type of TA testing should be a feature of the workup of any patient with a goiter. Although TA are predominately associated with Hashimoto's or Graves' diseases, they may be found in the sera of patients with other diseases such as myxedema, granulomatous thyroiditis, nontoxic modular goiter thyroid carcinoma and silicone implants.[85–87] TAs are also found in most cases of lymphocytic thyroiditis in children and rarely in patients with pernicious anemia. Most TAs are of the IgG class. However, IgA and IgM type TA have been observed. As described below, there are three recognized thyroid organ–specific and antigen antibody systems: thyroglobulin antibodies directed against the thyroglobulin present in the lumen of thyroid tissue follicles; microsomal antibodies found in the cytoplasm of the columnar epithelium lining the follicles; and second colloid antigen antibodies localized in some, but not all, follicles.

The presence of thyroglobulin and/or microsomal antibodies in patient's sera at titers greater than 1 : 10 is significant in patients with thyroid disease. Titers greater than 1 : 1000 are frequently found in patients with Hashimoto's and Graves' diseases, but are rarely detected in those with other diseases. The clinical significance of antibodies for the second colloid antigen is unknown. Although the incidence of Hashimoto's disease is not precisely known, the disease is four times as common in white as in black persons and is four times as common in women.[85,86].

RHEUMATOID FACTOR

Rheumatoid arthritis (RA) is a disease that affects approximately 3% of the population and results in considerable morbidity and debility. Rheumatoid factors represent a group of immunoglobulins (IgG, IgM, IgA) that are characterized by their ability to react with antigenic determinants or the FC portion of immunoglobulin G (IgG). This factor is most frequently utilized to aid in the differentiation of RA from other chronic inflammatory arthritides. It may also aid in substantiating the existence of an immunologically mediated disease in a patient with SLE or subacute bacterial endocarditis. The standard methods used to detect rheumatoid factor (RF) are based on the ability of RF to bind to IgG-coated erythrocytes or latex, and agglutinate them. Because these assays do not detect the nonagglutinating RFs, by utilizing radioimmunoassay or enzyme immunoassay, new tests have been developed. These new tests are very sensitive and reproducible, and correlate more than 80% with clinical features of RA. Additionally, these tests can measure the IgG RF, which may be associated with pathogenesis of glomerulonephritis. Also, immune deposits containing this factor were demonstrated in rejected human renal allografts.[87–90]

MYELIN BASIC PROTEIN, ASIALOGANGLIOSIDE GM_1, AND SULFATIDE ANTIBODIES

There is currently strong interest in the relation between immunologic disorders and neuropsychiatric manifestation. There is also much interest in how psychosocial factors affect autoimmune processes. Several studies have suggested, for example, that autoimmune phenomena may lead to events precipitating Alzheimer's disease,[91] Parkinson disease,[92] and AIDS dementia.[93] A recent study[94] clearly demonstrated the association between autoimmune processes, central nervous system functioning, and psychological processes in SLE and RA. Sera drawn from 14 RA patients, at biweekly intervals over three months, showed the presence of antibodies against transmembrane proteins. These antibodies correlated positively with rheumatoid factor and joint swelling. There was a trend toward a correlation between depression and daily mood scores and the number of antibodies reactive with brain. In addition, a correlation between cognitive coping styles in RA patients and autoantibodies was found. There was also evidence for a subpopulation of pathogenic antibodies. Therefore, the antibrain antibodies correlated with disease activity. These antibodies are mainly produced against myelin basic protein including myelin-associated glycoprotein (MAG), asialoganglioside GM_1, and sulfatide, which are present in multiple sclerosis.[91–94] Myelin is a multimellar membrane surrounding nerve fibers in both the central and the peripheral nervous system. It is derived from the plasma membrane of the oligodendrocyte in the central nervous system and the Schwann cell in the peripheral nervous system. Myelin consists of approximately 70% lipid and 30% protein by weight. The proteins, the proteolipids, and the basic proteins constitute 85% of the total protein of the membrane of which the myelin basic proteins (MBPs) are the most completely characterized.

Antibodies (IgG, IgM, IgA) against MBP and gangliosides, including GM_1, GD_{1a}, GD_{1b}, GT_{1b}, and LM_1, and other acidic glycolipids, including LK_1 and sulfatide, of human brain and peripheral nerve, have been observed in a high percentage of patients with the following neurologic conditions: multiple sclerosis, Guillain-Bar¥re syndrome, chronic inflammatory demyelinating polyradiculoneuropathy, motor neuron disease or peripheral neuropathies, peripheral neuropathy associated with monoclonal IgM antibody (IgM gammopathy), vascular multiinfarct dementia, Alzheimer's, RA, toxic chemical exposure, and silicone adjuvant disease.[76,78,94,95] Chronic inflammatory demyelinating polyradiculoneuropathy, motor neuron disease or peripheral neuropathies, and peripheral neuropathy are associated with monoclonal IgM antibody.[86,97–100] After receiving silicone gel implants, a certain percentage of women develop serious rheumatologic and neurologic symptoms.[2,76,101] When sural nerve biopsies are performed, neurogenic atrophy, myositis, vasculitis, and demyelination are detected.[121] Therefore, the demonstration of high levels of anti-MBP antibodies in greater than 50% of patients with silicone breast implants, which was reported 2 years ago by our laboratory, further corroborates the autoimmune phenomenon with possible involvement of the central and peripheral nervous system.[2,76]

By extending these measurements to MAG, asialoganglioside GM_1, sulfatide and chondroitin sulfate, we have shown first that only patients with IgM or IgA anti-MBP demonstrated antibodies against all or some of the above antigens, and second, levels of these antibodies are correlated with neurologic abnormalities including abnormal single photon emission computed tomography (SPECT) scans and other neurophysiologic testing. The mechanism by which these antibodies are produced is not yet clear. One proposed possibility is that the silicone breast implant oozes or bleeds small silicone particles, which are then absorbed or bind to macromolecules surrounding the silicone bag. The combined tissue antigen with silicon spheres are presented to the macrophages. After cooperation between T-helper cells and B cells, specific antibodies are produced that may react specifically to silicone and tissues from which antigens originate. As another possibility, because silicone is a synthetic polymer containing a silicon-oxide backbone and is an essential constituent of glycosaminoglycans such as chondroitin sulfate and sulfatides (a component of connective tissues), antibodies produced against silicone dioxide may cross-react with the connective tissue antigens.[52] Antibodies against MBP, MAG, ganglioside, and sulfatides as is done in our laboratory, should be measured quantitatively by ELISA and not by histologic staining and microscopical examination, because histologic staining for antibodies includes a high degree of false-positivity. Moreover, a yes or no answer may not enable the clinicians to follow improvements in their patients' conditions due to certain treatments that are still considered experimental in nature. In conclusion, neurologic antibodies should be measured by quantitative ELISA, in some cases combined with qualitative assay by thin layer chromatography and Western blot assay.

Silicone Antibody

Evidence for antigenicity and adjuvant effect of silicone was presented in several recent studies.[2,41,71,72,76,101] Silicone-specific antibodies are very important serologic factors that confirm immunologic reaction and, if accompanied by symptomatology and pathology, may suggest an association between symptomatologies and the exposure. Since 1992 we have been testing silicone-specific IgG, IgM, IgA, and IgE antibodies. We found that up to 60% of symptomatic patients produce antisilicone antibodies, some may produce IgG antibodies, while still others may produce IgM, IgA, or IgE antibodies to silicone. The pathologic meaning of these antibodies is not yet clear but certainly it means a specific immunologic response to silicone and possibly different tissue antigens.[2] Recently, detection of silicone-antibody (only IgG) was confirmed by two different investigators. As already mentioned, Goldblum et al[71] described two patients who exhibited immunologic reaction to silicone ventricular peritoneal shunts. Wolf et al[72] showed a relationship between systemic exposure to silicone and antisilicone antibodies. The highest antisilicone antibody levels were measured in implanted women with either frank implant ruptures or leakage of their implants.

In a different study, Kossovsky et al[102] describe a surface-dependent antigen identified by high binding avidity of serum antibodies in a subpopulation of patients with breast prostheses. Significant IgG acidities were found against silicone surfaces treated with fibronectin-laminin, phospholipids, and fibrinogen when compared with sera obtained from healthy, age-matched, nonimplanted women and a population of nonimplanted women with previously diagnosed autoimmune diseases. Moreover, the sera from approximately 15% of the positive responders were found to react to matrix proteins independent of the siloxane polymer. From these data, the authors suggest that human antibody production to native macromolecules with antibody avidity was related to molecular conformation. Silicone may function as an adjuvant by inducing changes in the conformation of native molecules. Our data indicate that antibodies are produced against silicone and body macromolecules, and a combination of silicone plus the macromolecules.[2] However, in contrast to the Wolf et al[72] study, in our investigation no correlation between the levels of antibodies and ruptured implants were detected. In fact, we had many cases with ruptured implants but nondetected levels of antibodies and in contrast high levels of antibodies were detected in individuals who had perfect implants. Therefore, as mentioned in this chapter, the results of silicone antibodies should be interpreted with many other laboratory examinations that are classified under cellular and humoral immunity.

Mechanism of Silicone-Induced Immune Disease

The exact mechanism of silicone-induced atypical connective tissue disease is not clear yet. However, there is little doubt that both cellular and humoral immunity are involved in the pathogenesis of this disease. On the basis of current knowledge, the following sequence of immunologic events can be hypothesized: silicone droplets are released from a silicone bag where they will be processed by histiocytes and macrophages. Breakdown of silicone to small spheres is followed by release of lymphokines, which may activate cell-mediated immunity. Silicone droplets come in contact with many tissue antigens including collagen, IgG, proteoglycans, and nucleic acids. Some of these antigens may bind, adhere, or even penetrate the silicone droplets and form liposome-like–containing antigens. This new antigen is presented by the antigen presenting cells (APCs) to specific helper T lymphocytes, resulting in their activation. For this activation to occur, T cells must recognize both the antigen and the DR determinants present on the APC membrane, and interleukin-1 (IL-1) must be released by monocytes/macrophages. Formation of the trimolecular (antigen/DR/T-cell receptor) complex results in the expression of IL-2 receptors on the T-cell surface. Synthesis and secretion of IL-2, which binds to these receptors, then lead to cell mitosis. The proliferation of this clone of T cells will continue as long as the specific antigen or silicone remains in the microenvironment. Activated T cells will secrete numerous other lymphokines in addition to IL-2. These include interferon, tumor necrosis factor B, IL-3, IL-4 (B-cell differentiating factor), and a host of mediators acting on macrophages to increase their enzymatic contents and phagocytic activity and to degrade more silicone droplets.

Signals transmitted from helper lymphocytes to B lymphocytes lead to the proliferation and activation of the B lymphocytes into antibody-producing cells. Evidence indicates that IL-1 (released by macrophages), IL-2, and IL-4 (released from activated T cells) are also needed for B-cell activation to occur. The antibodies produced will, after binding to their respective antigens, form immune complexes that can diffuse freely into the joint space, where they will fix complement and be phagocytosed by polymorphonuclear (PMN) leukocytes. Phagocytosis by the PMN will be accompanied by the generation and liberation of oxygen-derived free radicals, leukotrienes, prostaglandins, and neutral proteases. The end result of these immmunologic reactions is damage to the connective tissue.

MECHANISMS OF SILICONE-INDUCED AUTOIMMUNE NEUROLOGIC DISORDER

Similar to connective tissue disease both cellular and humoral immunity are involved in the pathogenesis of an atypical neurologic disorder induced by silicone. During this process silicone droplets are released from the bag where they are phagocytosed by histiocytes and macrophages. Histiocytes and macrophages break down silicone to many smaller spheres, after which further phagocytosis may occur and significant amounts of lymphokines such as IL-1 and tumor necrosis factor are released. High levels of lymphokines and cytokine through specific receptors may damage neurons, which results in the appearance of neuronal antigens such as myelin basic protein in circulation. Silicone droplets come in contact with these neuronal antigens and form a liposome-like–containing antigen. This highly antigenic material is presented to helper T lymphocytes, resulting in their activation and proliferation. Similarly to autoimmunity in which T cells, through a homing mechanism, travel from the thymus to the blood and hence to the target organ, these activated lymphocytes with neuronal antigens must travel to the nervous system and penetrate the blood-brain barrier. Once they arrive at the target, leukocytes—mainly T cells—acquire a foothold with the help of intracellular adhesion molecules called integrins. These molecules, which sit on the T cells, bear receptors that can be likened to Velcro fasteners. Counterreceptors belonging to the immunoglobulin supergene family constitute the other half of the Velcro bond. The counterreceptors grow from the endothelial lining of blood vessels at points that have been exposed to such cytokines as γ-2-interferon and tumor necrosis factor. These cytokines are produced on the spot by activated T cells and macrophages. Therefore, when a T cell rolls down a blood vessel and meets a counterreceptor, it sticks. The process of sticking causes the T cell to secrete proteases, enzymes that help to create a hole in the blood vessel and enable the T cell to tighten its cytoskeleton so that it can squeeze through the tiny hole. In this manner, leukocytes break through the blood-brain barrier to cause multiple sclerosis, penetrate the synovial lining to cause rheumatoid arthritis, and so on for all the other autoimmune diseases.

Destruction begins when a T cell encounters its antigen in the cleft of a human leukocyte antigen (HLA) molecule and releases proteins and peptides, including tumor necrosis factor, a chemical relative called lymphotoxin, and α-interferon. These chemicals have been identified as the proximate cause of demyelination. Macrophages then speed the process, partly by secreting tumor necrosis factor and partly by mounting a direct attack. Investigators have shown that macrophages actually strip fragments of myelin from the sheath encasing the nerve axons. One might suppose that autoimmune disease, once started, would proceed without interruption. Yet in multiple sclerosis, rheumatoid arthritis, systemic lupus erythematosus, and myasthenia gravis, periods of deterioration usually alternate with remission. In all these diseases the pattern of decline has been shown to correlate strongly with three factors in the environment: female hormones, infection, and stress. Obviously, these factors may contribute to the worsening of clinical conditions of patients with implants. However, one may ask why patients with silicone implants simultaneously produce antibodies against components of connective tissue and neurologic system. A partial answer may be given from an examination of the chemical structure of silicone and silicone-oxide backbone, which is an essential component of connective neurologic tissues. These include glycosaminoglycans such as chondroitin sulfate and sulfatides. Also, silicone, after its release from the bag, may be disintegrated by enzymatic contents of histiocyte vacuoles to silicone-oxide and the methyl group, which has binding capacity that could be responsible for binding to the body macromolecules, such as myelin or chondroitin sulfate. Based on this, both immunopathologic reactions shown in Figures 14–1 and 14–2 are possible.

What is Medical Causation?

REQUIREMENTS FOR MEDICAL CAUSATION

In 1964 the US Surgeon General's Advisory Group on Smoking and Health published a set of five criteria for assessing causation and epidemiology in their influential report on Smoking and Lung Cancer. Sir Austin Bradford Hill[103] published similar criteria for occupational cancer in 1965. Together these criteria have been widely influential in epidemiology, and provided the starting point for scientists seeking to determine whether a purported association reflects scientific knowledge or is merely speculative. Commonly known as the Bradford Hill Criteria these standards have been used by scientists to determine exactly what causation means. In his very eloquent and logical analysis of causation, and addressing occupational exposures and disease, Sir Bradford Hill stated that the fact that one cannot experiment with humans makes one rely on observations of the relationships that occur in nature before the clinician's eye. Faced with a clear and significant association between some form of sickness and some features of the environment, one should consider, in drawing conclusions about the nature of relationship causation or merely association, the following criteria:

1. Strength of the association.
2. Consistency of the observed association: Has it been repeatedly observed by different persons in different places, under different circumstances and times?
3. Specificity of the association: If the association is limited to specific workers in this case, or specific exposures, particular sites, and types of diseases, and there is no association between work and other modes of dying, then clearly that is a strong argument in favor of causation.
4. The relationship in time of the observed association: Which is the cart and which is the horse? This is a question that might be particularly relevant with diseases of slow development. Does a particular occupation or environment promote infection by tubercle bacillus or are the men and women who selected that kind of work more liable to contract tuberculosis?
5. The dose-response curve can reveal the biologic gradient.
6. Biologic plausibility: It would be helpful if the causation that is suspected is biologically plausible, although this is a feature that we cannot always demand. What is biologically plausible depends upon the biologic knowledge of the day.
7. Coherence of the evidence: The cause and effect interpretation of an association should not seriously conflict with the general known facts of the natural history and biology of a disease. It should have coherence.

With respect to published data on silicone and autoimmunity, we conclude that causation has been clearly established. Based on these data, one does not need "large" epidemiologic studies to conclude causation.

EVALUATION OF THE HILL CRITERIA IN LIGHT OF THE ABOVE LITERATURE

1. Multiple case reports and population studies show the strength of association.
2. The association is consistent. Silicone exposure has been associated with a spectrum of rheumatic diseases as a result of immune response, and reported by several independent investigators.
3. The association is specific for silicone, is reversible upon removal of the silicone, and the antibodies to silicone are specific.
4. Recovery of patients upon removal of the impacts clearly show a temporal relationship.

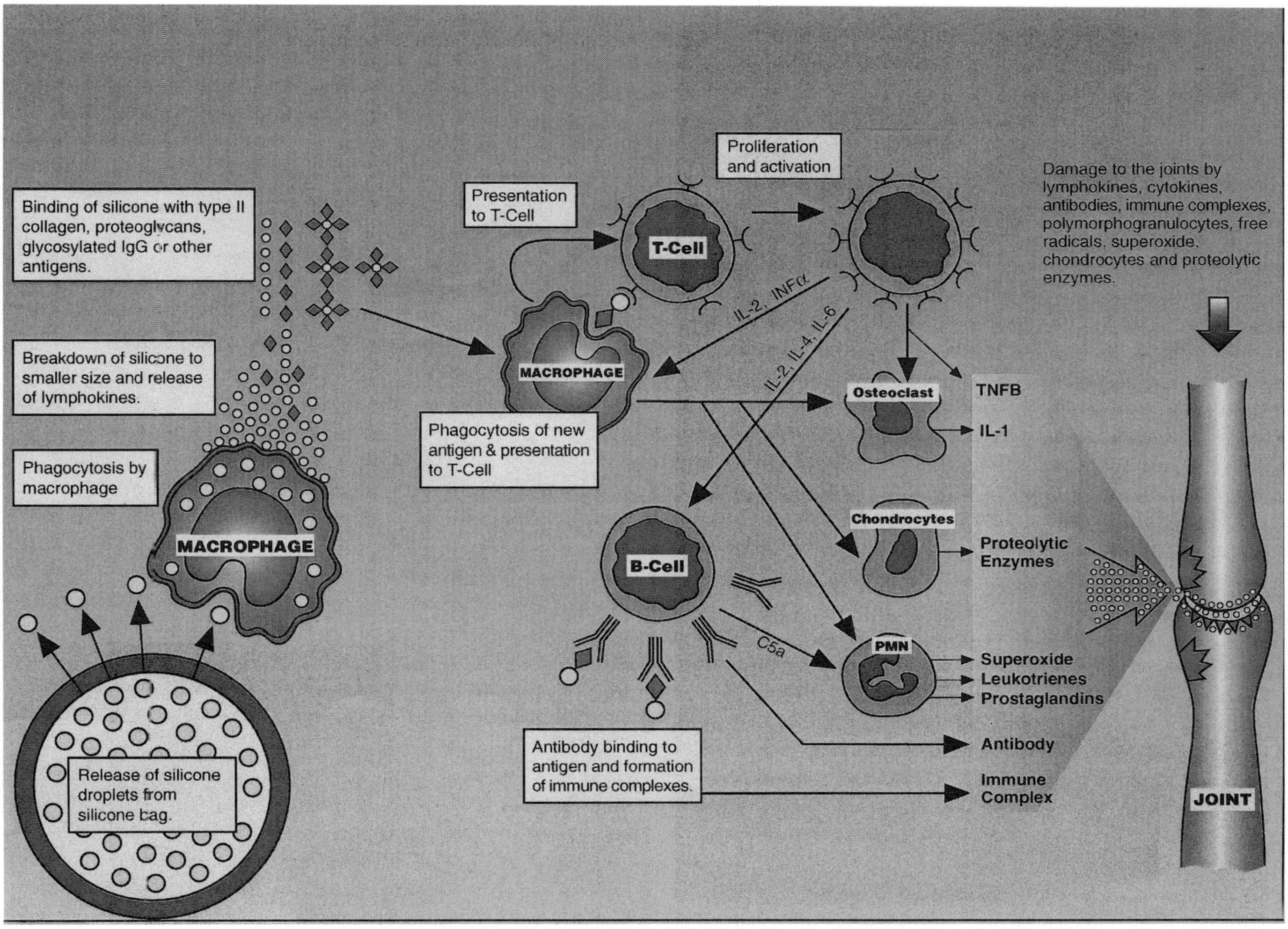

Figure 14–1. Proposed molecular cellular immunological reaction to silicone: Rheumatological disease.

5. The plausibility is shown in the in vivo and in vitro studies that silicone is immunogenic.

From a medical point of view, to establish causation for the practicing clinician and physician, one should be guided by the criteria presented by Sir Austin Bradford Hill, to the Royal Academy of Medicine in 1965, as described above. We need not forget that in medicine causation is concluded from three or four of the Bradford Hill criteria, mainly based on clinical observations supported by experimental studies in animals.

Genetic Predisposition Theory

A recent study by Young et al[104] concludes that "a small percentage of our patients with silicone breast implants do suffer from real physical complaints." They further examined human leukocyte antigen (HLA) and typing in different groups of patients with silicone breast implants. Brautbar et al[92] in 1992 suggested a genetic predisposition, due to the fact that some patients with silicone breast implants do develop a real physical disease, and others do not. Young et al conclude that symptomatic patients with implants share important genetic characteristics that differentiate them from their asymptomatic counterparts. Their findings and our investigation in 1992 clearly indicate that some patients who have a genetic predisposition are somehow more prone to develop a symptomatic disease. Is this something new in medicine or medical toxicology? Clearly not, because we know that in many disease entities the generic predisposition makes the patient more prone "or sensitive" to develop a reaction or a disease in response to environmental factors.

Finally Hennekens et al[105] studied a large retrospective cohort and concluded that "the self-reported data from this large cohort . . . suggests a small but statistically significant increased risk of the combined end point of any connective tissue disease . . . being either significant (other connective tissue disease) . . . or of borderline significance (rheumatoid

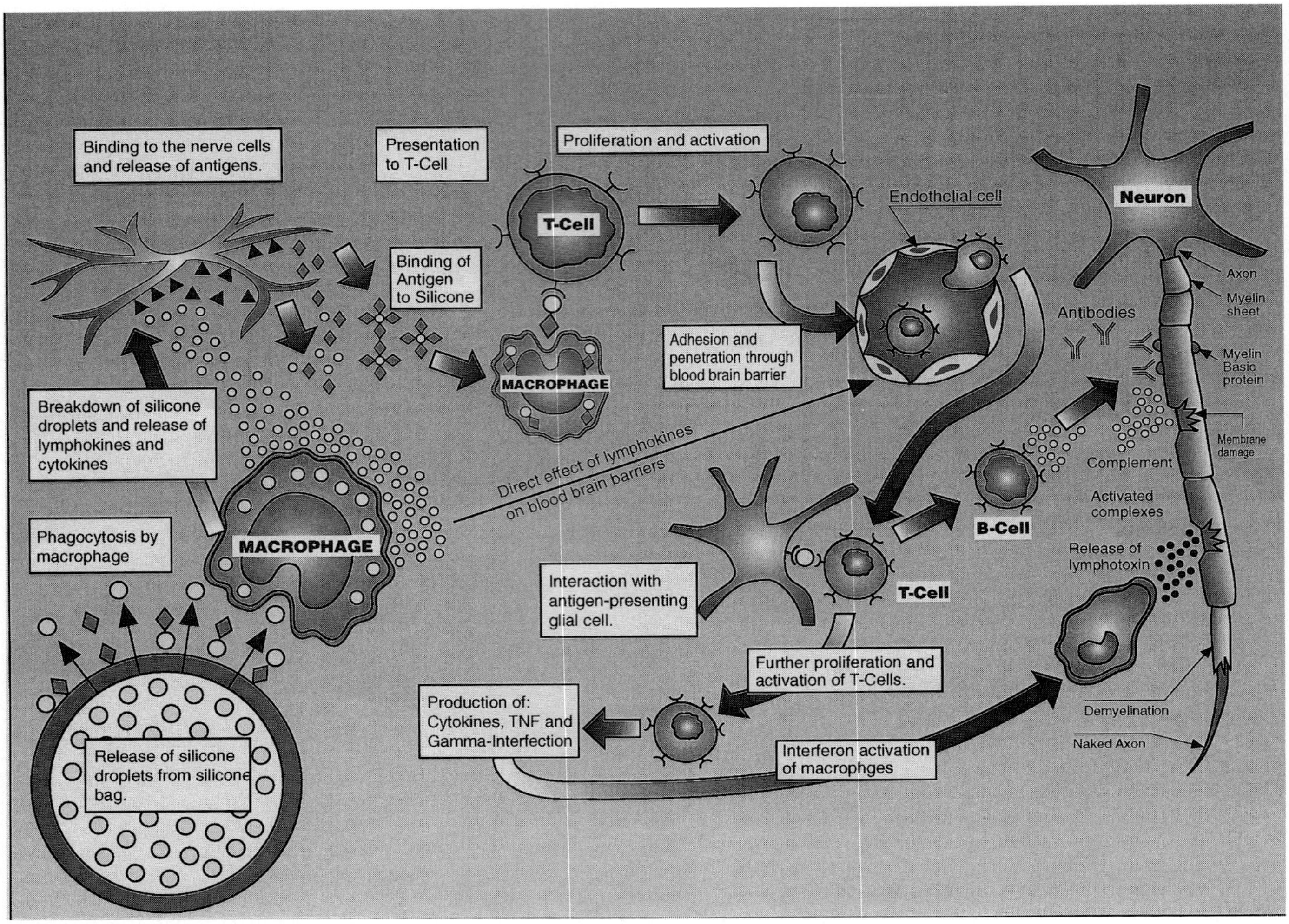

Figure 14–2. Proposed molecular cellular immunological reaction to silicone: Neurological disease.

arthritis, Sjögren's syndrome, dermatomyositis or polymyositis, and scleroderma)." It seems clear that all studies agree that (1) there is a *risk* assessed as small but significant, (2) there seems to be a genetic predisposition of these patients, and (3) medical causation has been shown in those cases.

■ ACKNOWLEDGMENT

The authors wish to thank Ms. Sally I. Loomis for her help in all aspects of transcription, editing, and structure.

REFERENCES

1. RÏotchild BM. Silicone breast implants: souvenir of youth or harbinger for the future? *Hosp Phys.* 1994;50:42–45.
2. Vojdani A, Brautbar N, Campbell AW. Antibody to silicone and native macromolecules in women with silicone breast implants. *J Immunopharmocol Immunotoxicol.* 1994;16:497–523.
3. Salvaggio JE. The impact of allergy and immunology on our expanding industrial environment. *J Allergy Clin Immunol.* 1990;85:689–699.
4. Chan SC, Bridsell, Gradeen CY. Detection of toluene-diamines in the urine of a patient with polyurethane-covered breast implants. *Clin Chem.* 1991;37:756–758.
5. Patterson R, Harris KE, Grammer LC. Canine antibodies against formaldehyde–dog serum albumin conjugates: induction, measurement, and specificity. *J Lab Clin Med.* 1985; 106:93–100.
6. Pien LC, Zeiss CR, Leach CL, et al. Antibody response to trimellitic hemoglobin in trimellitic anhydride induced lung injury. *J Allergy Clin Immunol.* 1988;82:1093–1103.
7. Thrasher JD, Vojdani A, Heuser G, Cheung G. Evidence for formaldehyde antibodies and altered cellular immunity in subjects exposed to formaldehyde in mobile homes–a brief communication. *Arch Environ Health.* 1987;42:347–350.
8. Bokina AI, Eksler ND, Semenenko AD, Merkuryeva RV. Investigation of the mechanism of action of atmospheric pollutants on the central nervous system and comparative evalua-

tion of methods of study. *Environ Health Perspect.* 1976;13: 37–42.

9. Zeiss CR, Patterson R, Pruzansky JJ, Miller MM, Rosenberg M, Levitz D. Trimellitic anhydride-induced airway syndromes. Clinical and immunological studies. *J Allergy Clin Immunol.* 1977;60:96–103.
10. Zeiss CR, Kanellakes TM, Bellone JD, Levitz D, Pruzansky JJ, Patterson R. Immunoglobulin E-mediated asthma and hypersensitivity pneumonitis with precipitating antihapten antibodies due to diphenylmethane diisocyanante exposure. *J Allergy Clin Immunol.* 1980;65:346–352.
11. Dewar MA, Baur X. Studies on antigens useful for detection of IgE antibodies in isocyanante-sensitized workers. *J Clin Chem Clin Biochem.* 1982;20:337–340.
12. Jones J, Amas H. Contact sensitivity in vitro: activation of actively allergized lymphocytes by a beryllium complex. *Int Arch Allergy Appl Immunol.* 1974;46:161.
13. Pelletier L, Pasquier R, Rossert J, Vial M-C, Chantal M, Druet P. Autoreactive T cells in mercury-induced autoimmunity: ability to induce the autoimmune disease. *J Immunol.* 1988;140:750–754.
14. Ohsawa M, Takahashi K, Otsuka F. Induction of antinuclear antibodies in mice orally exposed to cadmium at low concentrations. *Clin Exp Immunol.* 1988;73:98–102.
15. Robinson C, Egorov I, Balazo T. Strain differences in the induction of antinuclear antibodies by mercuric chloride, gold sodium thiomalata, and D-penicillamine in inbred mice. *Fed Proc.* 1983;42:1213.
16. Tan EM. Autoantibodies to nuclear antigens (ANA): their immunobiology and medicine. *Adv Immunol.* 1982;33:165–240.
17. Harmon CE. Antinuclear antibodies in autoimmune disease. *Med Clin North Am.* 1985;69:547–563.
18. Tan EM. Interactions between autoimmunity and molecular and cell biology: bridges between clinical and basic sciences. *J Clin Invest.* 1989;84:1–6.
19. Hirsch F, Couderc J, Sapin C, Fournie G, Druet P. Polyclonal effect of $HgCl_2$ in the rat, its possible role in an experimental autoimmune disease. *Eur J Immunol.* 1982;12:620.
20. Bigazzi PE. Mechanisms of chemical-induced autoimmunity In: Dean JH, Luster MI, Munson AE, Amos H, eds. *Immunotoxicity and Immunopharmacology.* New York: Raven Press; 1985:277.
21. Allison AC, Harrington JS, Birbeck M. An examination of the cytotoxic effects of silica on macrophages. *J Exp Med.* 1966;124:141–152.
22. Stankus RP, Salvaggio JE. Bronchopulmonary humoral and cellular enhancement in experimental silicosis. *J Reticuloendothel Soc.* 1981;29:153–161.
23. Jones RN, Turner-Warwick M, Ziskind M, Weill H. High prevalence of antinuclear antibodies in sandblasters' silicosis. *Am Rev Respir Dis.* 1976;113:393.
24. Rodnan GP, Benedek TB, Medsger TA, Cammarata RJ. The association of progressive systemic sclerosis (scleroderma) with coal miners' pneumoconiosis and other forms of silicosis. *Ann Intern Med.* 1967;66:323.
25. Dean JH, Luster M, Boorman C. Methods and approaches for assessing immunotoxicity: an overview. *Env Health Perspect.* 1982;43:27–33.
26. Turk JL, Parker D. *Drugs and Immunoresponsiveness.* London and Basingstoke: Macmillan; 1979.
27. Lange A, Smolik R, Zatonski W, et al. Autoantibodies and serum immunoglobulin levels in asbestos workers. *Int Arch Arbeitsmed.* 1974;32:313–325.
28. Lange A, Nineham LJ, Garncarek D, et al. Circulating immune complexes and antiglobulins (IgG and IgM) in asbestos-induced lung fibrosis. *Environ Res.* 1983;31:287–295.
29. Neilsen J, Welinder H, Schutz A, Skerfving S. Specific serum antibodies against phthalic anhydride in occupationally exposed subjects. *J Allergy Clin Immunol.* 1988;82:126–133.
30. Lee SL, Chase PH. Drug-induced systemic lupus erythematous: a critical review. *Semin Arthritis Rheum.* 1975;5: 83–103.
31. Russell AS, Lindstrom JM. Penicillamine-induced myasthenia gravis associated with antibodies to acetylcholine receptor. *Neurology.* 1978;28:347–849.
32. Levin A, Byers VS. Environmental illness: a disorder of immune regulation. In: Cullen MR, ed. Philadelphia: Hanley and Belfus; 1987:681–699.
33. Sharma RP, Zeeman MG. Immunologic alterations by environmental chemicals: relevance of studying mechanisms versus effects. *J Immunopharmacol.* 1980;2:285.
34. Vojdani A, Ghoneum M, Brautbar N. Immune alteration associated with exposure toxic chemicals. *Toxicol Ind health.* 1992;5:239–254.
35. McGrath KG, Zeiss CR, Patterson R. Allergic reactions to industrial chemicals. *Clin Immunol Rev.* 1983;2:1–58.
36. Lewis RE, Cruse JM, Johnson WW, Mohammad A. Histopathology and cell-mediated immune reactivity in halothane-associated lymphomagenesis and autoimmunity in BXSB/Mp and MRL/Mp mice. *Exp Mol Pathol.* 1982;36: 378–395.
37. Robbins A. Chemically induced illnesses: an overview. *Osteopath Med News.* 1989;6:19–20.
38. Zetterstrom O, Nordvall SL, Bjorksten B, Ahlstedt S, Stelander M. Increased IgE antibody responses in rats exposed to tobacco smoke. *J Allergy Clin Immunol.* 1985;75:594–598.
39. Muranaka M, Suzoki S, Koizumi K, et al. Adjuvant activity of diesel exhaust particulates for the production of IgE antibody in mice. *J Allergy Clin Immunol.* 1986;77:616.
40. Okano Y, Nichikai M, Sato A. Scleroderma, primary biliary cirrhosis and Sjogren's syndrome after cosmetic breast augmentation with silicone injection: a case report of possible human adjuvant disease. *Ann Rheum Dis.* 1984;43:520–522.
41. Naim JO, Lanzafame RJ. The adjuvant effect of silicone gel on antibody formation in rats. *Immunol Invest.* 1993;22(2): 151–161.
42. Rees TD, Ballantyne DL, Seidman I, Hawthorne GA. Visceral response to subcutaneous and intraperitoneal injections of silicone in mice. *Plast Reconstr Surg.* 1967;39:402–410.
43. Ben-Hur N, Ballantyne DL, Rees TD, Seidman I. Local and systemic effects of dimethylpolysiloxane in fluid in mice. *Plast Reconstr Surg.* 1967;29:423–425.
44. Brody GL, Fray CF. Peritoneal response to silicone fluid, histologic study. *Arch Surg.* 1968;96:241–277.
45. Lake RS, Radonovich MF. Action of polydimethylsiloxane on the reticuloendothelial system of mice: basic cellular interaction and structure activity relationship. Dow Corning, Bioscience Lab, Midland, Michigan, Internal Document, 1975.
46. Barker DE, Gretsky MI, Schultz SS. Bleeding of silicone from bag gel breast implants and its clinical relation to fibrous capsule reaction. *Plast Reconstr Surg.* 1978;61:836–841.
47. Thomsen JL, Christensen L, Nielsen M, et al. Histologic changes and silicone concentrations in human breast tissue surrounding silicone breast prostheses. *Plast Reconstr Surg.* 1990;85:38–41.
48. Housner RJ, Schoen FJ, Pierson K. Foreign body reaction to silicone gel in axillary lymph nodes after an augmentation mammoplasty. *Plast Reconstr Surg.* 1978;62:381–384.
49. Pfleiderer B, Ackerman JL, Garrido L. Migration and biodegradation of free silicone from silicone gel-filled implants

after long term implantation. *Magn Reson Med.* 1993;30: 534–543.
50. Garrido L, Pfleiderer B, Papisov M, Ackerman JL. In vivo degradation of silicones. *Magn Reson Med.* 1993;29:639–643.
51. Weiner SR, Clements PJ, Paulus HH. Connective tissue disease after augmentation mammoplasty. *Arthritis Rheum.* 1989;23:23–24.
52. Kaiser W, Biesenbach G, Stubby U, Graffinger P, Zazgornik J. Human adjuvant disease: remission of silicone induced disease after explantation of breast augmentation. *Eur J Surg Oncol.* 1990;16:468–469.
53. Kumagai Y, Shiokawa Y, Medsger TA Jr, Rodnan GP. Clinical spectrum of connective tissue disease after cosmetic surgery. *Arthritis Rheum.* 1984;2791:9–12.
54. Van Nunen SA, Gateby PA, Basten A. Post mammoplasty connective tissue disease. *Arthritis Rheum.* 1982;25(6): 694–697.
55. Celli B, Textor S, Covnat DM. Adult respiratory distress syndrome following mammary augmentation. *Am J Med Sci.* 1978;275:81–85.
56. Myoshi K, Shiragami H, Yoshida K. Adjuvant disease of men. *Clin Immunol.* 1973;5:785–794.
57. Sanchez-Guerrero J, Schur PH, Sergent JS, Liang MH. Silicone breast implants and rheumatic disease. *Arthritis Rheum.* 1994;37:158–168.
58. Sanchez-Guerrero J. Silicone breast implants and risk of connective tissue diseases and symptoms. *N Engl J Med.* 1995; 332:1666–1670.
59. Claman HN, Robertson AD. Antinuclear antibodies and breast implants. *West J Med.* 1994;160:225–228.
60. Gabriel SE, O'Fallon WM, Kurland LT, Beard CM, Woods JE, Melton LJ. Risk of connective-tissue diseases and other disorders after breast implantation. *N Engl J Med.* 1994; 330:1697–1702.
61. Angell M. Do breast implants cause systemic disease? (Editorial). *N Engl J Med.* 1994;330:1748–1749.
62. Strom BL, Reidengerg M, Freundrich B, Schinnar R. Breast silicone implants and risk of systemic lupus erythematous. *J Clin Epidemiol.* 1994;47(10):1211–1214.
63. Naim JO, Lanzafame RJ. The adjuvant effect of silicone gel on antibody formation in rats. *Immunol Invest.* 1993;22:151–161.
64. Press RI, Peebles CL, Kumagai Y, Ochs RL, Tan NM. Antinuclear autoantibodies in women with silicone breast implants. *Lancet.* 340:1304–1307.
65. Picha GJ, Goldstein JA. Analysis of the soft tissue response to components used in the manufacture of breast implants, rat animal model. *Plast Reconstr Surg.* 1991;87:490–500.
66. Mansino D, Vuotto ML, Minucci M. Effects of crystalline silica on antibody production to T-dependent and T-independent antigens in bulb/C mice. *Int Arch Allergy Appl Immunol.* 1984;73:10–13.
67. Kettle RWI, Monacco L, Marchisio MA. The specificity of the cytotoxic action of silica, a study in vitro. *Br J Exp Pathol.* 1963;44:351–364.
68. Allison AC, Harrington JS, Birbeck M. An examination of the cytotoxic effects of silica on macrophages. *J Exp Med.* 1966;124:141–153.
69. Bridges AJ, Connelly C, Wong G, Burns DE, Vassey FB. A clinical and immunological evaluation of women with silicone breast implants and symptoms of rheumatic disease. *Ann Intern Med.* 1993;118:929–936.
70. Vojdani A, Campbell A, Brautbar N. Immune functional impairment in patients with clinical abnormalities and silicone breast implants. *Toxicol Ind Health.* 1992;8:415–429.
71. Goldblum RM, Pelley RP, O'Donnell AA, Pyron D, Heggers JP. Antibodies to silicone elastomers and reactions to ventricular peritoneal shunts. *Lancet.* 1992;340:510–513.
72. Wolf LE, Leppe M, Patterson RD, Ezralison EG. Human immune response to polydimethylisolloxane silicone screening. *FASEB J.* In press.
73. Sharma RP, Reddy RV. Toxic effects of chemicals on the immune system. In: *Handbook of Toxicology.* Haley TJ, Brendt WO, eds. Washington, DC: Hemisphere; 1987:294–331.
74. Vojdani A, Alfred L. In vitro effects of certain polycyclic aromatic hydrocarbons on mitogen activation of mouse lymphocytes: action of histamine. *Cell Immunol.* 1983;77:132–142.
75. Sergott TJ, Limoli JP, Baldwin CM Jr, Laub DR. Human adjuvant disease, possible autoimmune disease after silicone implantation: a review of the literature, case studies, and speculation for the future. *Plast Reconstr Surg.* 1986;78: 104–114.
76. Vojdani A, Brautbar N, Campbell A. Immune functional abnormalities and autoimmunity in patients with silicone breast implants. *J Immunol.* 1993;150:157A.
77. Raso DS. Breast prostheses, the immune response, and B and T-lymphocytes. *Plast Reconstr Surg.* 1994;93:649–650.
78. Vojdani A, Ghoneum M, Brautbar N. Immune alteration associated with exposure to toxic chemical. *Toxicol Ind Health.* 1992;8:231–246.
79. Campbell A, Brautbar N, Vojdani A. Suppressed natural killer cell activity in patients with silicone breast implants: reversal upon explantation. *Toxicol Ind Health.* 1994; (in press).
80. Smith SD, Gerber PC, Meade BJ, et al. Natural killer cell activity is suppressed following exposure to silicone gel. *Soc Toxicol.* 1994.
81. Baldwin CM JR, Kaplan EN. Silicone-induced human adjuvant disease? *Ann Plast Surg.* 1983;10:270–273.
82. Spiera H. Scleroderma after silicone augmentation mammoplasty. *JAMA.* 1988;260:236–238.
83. Weisman MH, Vecchione RR, Albert D, Moore LT, Mueller MR. Connective tissue disease following breast augmentation: a preliminary test of the human adjuvant disease hypothesis. *Plast Reconstr Surg.* 1988;82:626–630.
84. Gutierrez FJ, Espinoza LR. Progressive systemic sclerosis complicated by severe hypertension: reversal after silicone implant removal. *Am J Med.* 1990;89:390–392.
85. Cowchock S, Dehoratius RD, Wapner RJ, Jackson LG. Subclinical autoimmune disease and unexplained abortion. *Am J Obstet Gynecol.* 1984;150:367–371.
86. Saliv M, Fukazawa H, Bernard N, Hiromatsu Y, How J, Wall JR. Role of autoantibodies in the pathogenesis and association of endocrine autoimmune disorders. *Endocr Rev.* 1988; 9:450–465.
87. Faith RE, Luster MI, Vos JG. Effects of immunocompetence by chemicals of an environmental cancer. In: *Reviews of Biochemical Toxicology*, vol 2. Hodgson JR, Bend R, Philpot RM, eds. New York: Elsevier North Holland; 1980:173–211.
88. Holoborow EJ. Autoantibodies in the rheumatic diseases. In: *Copeman's Test Book of the Rheumatic Disease,* 6th ed. Scott JT, ed. New York: Churchill-Livingstone; 1986:355–375.
89. Linker JB III, Williams RC. Tests for detection of rheumatoid factors. In: *Manual of Clinical Laboratory Immunology,* 34th ed. Rose NR, Friedman H, Fahey JL, eds. Washington, DC: American Society of Microbiology; 1986:759–761.
90. Miyata M, Milgrom F. Enzyme immunoassay for IgG rheumatoid factor combining with homologous IgG. *Immunol Invest.* 1988;17:561–565.
91. Forster MJ, Retz KL, Lal H. Learning and memory deficits associated with autoimmunity: significance in aging and Alzheimer's disease. *Drug Dev Res* 1988;15:253–273.

92. Pouplard A, Emle J, Pouplard F, Hurez D. Parkinsonism and autoimmunity: antibody against human symphathetic ganglion cells in Parkinson's disease. *Adv Neurol.* 1979;24: 321–326.
93. Kumar M, Resnick L, Lowenstein DA, Berger J, Eisdorfer C. Brain-reactive antibodies and the AIDS dementia complex. *J Acquired Immune Defic Syndr.* 1989;2:469–471.
94. Maag TJ, Hoffman A. Anti-brain antibodies in the sera of rheumatoid arthritis patients: relation to disease activity and psychological status. *J Neuro Immunol.* 1993;45:37–46.
95. Koski CL, Humphrey R, Shin ML. Anti-peripheral myelin antibody in patients with demyelinating neuropathy: quantitative and kinetic determination of serum antibody of complement component 1 fixation. *Proc Natl Acad Sci USA.* 1985; 32:905–909.
96. Baba H, Duane GC, Illyasi AA, et al. Anti GM_1, ganglioside antibodies with differing fine specificities in patients with multifocal motor neuropathy. *J Neuroimmunol.* 1989;25:143–150.
97. Voumvourakis C, Rombos A, Konstantoulakis MM, Segditsa I, Papageorgio C. Serum and anti-GM, and anti-GD1a antibodies in patients with motor neuron disease. *Acta Neurol Scand.* 1992;86:599–602.
98. Fredman P, Lycke J, Andersen O, Vrethem M, Ernerud H, Svennerholm L. Peripheral neuropathy associated with monoclonal IgM antibody to glycolipids with a terminal glucuronyl-3-sulfate epitope. *J Neurol.* 1993;240:381–387.
99. Zhou SR, Whitaker JN, Wood DD, Moscarello A. Immunological analysis of the amino terminal and the C8 isomer of human myelin basis protein. *J Neurol Immunol.* 1993;46: 91–96.
100. Horvath E, Edwards AM, Bell JC, Braun PE. Chemical deglycosylation on a micro-scale of membrane glycoproteins with retention of phosphoryl-protein linkage. *J Neuro Sci.* 1989;24:398–401.
101. Ostermeyer, Shoaib B, Patten BM, Calkins DS. Adjuvant breast disease: an evaluation of 100 symptomatic women with breast implants or silicone fluid injections. *Keio J Med.* 1994;43:79–87.
102. Kossovsky N, Zeidler Z, Chun G, et al. Surface dependent antigens identified by high binding avidity of serum antibodies in a subpopulation of patients with breast prostheses. *J Appl Biomaterials.* 1993;4:281–288.
103. Hill AB. The environment and disease: Association or causation? President's Address. *Proc R Soc Med.* 1965;9: 295–300.
104. Young L, Nemececk JR, Schultz BD, Phelan DL, Schoer MW. HLA typing in women with breast implants. *Plast Reconstr Surg.* 1995;96;1497–1519.
105. Hennekens CH, Lee IM, Cook NR. Self-reported breast implants and connective-tissue diseases in female health professionals. *JAMA.* 1996;275(8):516–621.

15

Medical-Legal Aspects of Breast Implants: A Primer

R. JAMES BRENNER

In 1995 a consortium of medical liability carriers pooled their claims data and reported in June of that year that delay in diagnosis of breast cancer was the leading reason that physicians were sued for "malpractice."[1] The reasons are manifold but an important component of the analysis is that women are probably better informed about breast disease and well-being than about many other maladies that threaten their health. The emphasis on breast disease in lay press publications has provided a forum for education and discussion.

There is another public discussion concerning breast disease that has prompted thousands of individual and scores of class action lawsuits, primarily involving nearly 2 million women who have undergone breast augmentation with the use of silicone implants, and has invited scrutiny from many aspects of society. The medical-legal aspects of lawsuits against physicians and manufacturers in many ways illustrate basic notions of civil law, and in other ways are virtually unique.

Chapter 16 summarizes the kinds of litigation that have evolved, especially during the past 10 years, regarding silicone implants. Much of the discussion is substantive, focusing on aspects of legal cases that need to be shown to prevail in court. Other aspects of the discussion illustrate procedural problems involved in such cases.

The preceding chapters in this text have been devoted to providing analysis of many of the factual considerations involved in the controversies surrounding silicone breast implants. This chapter therefore serves as a transition. Basic notions of law are discussed to provide the interested reader with an overview of the legal system so that the directed focus of discussion in the next chapter will be more meaningful. Readers versed in the material of the prior chapters may then judge for themselves the relative merits and deficiencies of the legal arguments that are highlighted subsequently, regarding the contentions and positions advanced by plaintiffs and defendants in court. This discussion is not an attempt to provide a full comprehension of civil law, but rather it is to enable the reader to deal with concepts that are discussed in the next chapter.

■ ORIGINS OF THE LAW

The law is a compilation of many different disciplines representing various aspects of society for which a "social contract" has been consensually developed. Thus areas of contract law, criminal law, maritime law, and communications law, for example, have emerged, each with different substantive theories, types of penalties, and standards of proof required to support a given contention. Criminal law, for example, represents rules of conduct designed to protect the interests of society as a whole and thus cases such as "the State versus. . . ." or "the County versus . . ." emerge where the complaining party represents an institutional interest. Because loss of basic freedoms (eg, incarceration) may be imposed, the highest standards of proof are required in criminal cases.

In contrast, civil law is that code of conduct that governs relationships between parties. The standards or "burden" of proof are not as high as in criminal law, and the remedies sought are usually focused on restitution, usually in the form of money damages, although other remedies in "equity" may be sought, such as restraining orders. Proof of a case is sought through introduction of evidence, the governing rules of which vary with each state. When cases are brought in federal court, the Federal Rules of Evidence apply uniformly, although there is latitude even in federal court for incorporating state law in that jurisdiction where the federal court may be situated.

Sometimes actions may be brought in different courts for the same action. For example, the loss of life may be pursued in criminal court as a manslaughter charge for which incarceration is the usual remedy and which case is pursued by the state. Concomitantly, a "wrongful death" action may be pursued by an aggrieved party in civil court against the defendant for money damages.

Although many lawsuits are resolved by mutual consent "settlements," others proceed to a trial court. A trial is an attempt to establish the truth from various facts that are disputed by the respective parties; it is not an attempt to establish the law. Thus the "trier of fact" may be a judge or jury that considers the evidence and the standards of proof required, and renders a decision as to whether or not sufficient facts establish or fail to establish the complaining party's contention. Experts may be called upon by the court (by each party) to help establish appropriate facts. A recent United States Supreme Court decision redefined the parameters involving the qualifications and introduction of experts, although the implications of the decision are still controversial.[2] Where issues of law are disputed following the establishment of a decision by the trier of fact, the case may be appealed to a higher court. Higher courts are generally not concerned with the facts of the case, although such facts are frequently reviewed in deciding issues of law. States and the federal government have at least two levels of higher courts, generally referred to as appellate courts. The highest federal court is the United States Supreme Court. Appellate courts publish their decisions, which are compiled and available in most law libraries. Appellate court decisions direct themselves to the given case, but the legal decisions rendered by such courts are binding on future cases in the area of jurisdiction assigned to that court.

Civil actions, often called "torts," are governed by two sources of law: statutory law and common law. Statutory law is passed by governmental legislative bodies, including local, state, and federal (ie, Congress) entities. These laws are published and available in most law libraries and are presumably "known" by the citizenry. Statutory law is usually implemented by agencies that develop regulations and are often charged with enforcement of the law. The Food and Drug Administration (FDA) is an example of a federal regulatory agency, and one of the areas of its jurisdiction is the monitoring and public protection of medical devices. By contrast, medical licensure is governed by state medical boards. Disputes arising between affected parties and regulatory agencies may be appealed to courts of law.

Civil law that is not expressly addressed by statutory provisions is called "common law." American common law is derived from eighteenth century common law whereby decision of judges established rules of conduct to be followed where similar circumstances would arise again. In a doctrine known as stare decisis, subsequent decisions would attempt as much as reasonably possible to defer to the prior decision so that proper forms of conduct would become anticipated. Trial court decisions, which are directed toward the resolution of a factual dispute, are not binding on any other trial court. Appellate court decisions, however, establish rules of law that are binding in that jurisdiction, as already mentioned, and are the ones that lend themselves to the doctrine of stare decisis. Oftentimes, principles derived from common law decisions will be formally enacted into statutory law.

■ TORT LAW AND MEDICAL PRACTICE

The relationship between law and medicine is neither new nor uniquely American. Although not the first to address the subject, Professor Andrew Duncan Sr.[3] of the institutes of medicine at the University of Edinburgh popularized the term *medical jurisprudence* in 1971. The term was incorporated into lectures in the United States first by James S. Stringham at Columbia College of Physicians and Surgeons in 1804 and later by Benjamin Rush in Philadelphia in 1810.[4] The term *medical jurisprudence* means medical law and may in fact be a misnomer for two reasons. First, discussions in jurisprudence are generally concerned with philosophies of law; second, most law dealing with the medical community is not specifically medical law, but law applying to medicine, although some laws (eg, Federal Food, Drug and Cosmetic Act, 21 U.S.C. Sec 321(h)(2), commonly referred to as the Medical Device Act) do address specific aspects of the medical profession.

There are several areas of civil law that are applicable to cases involving silicone breast implants, and a brief description is worth considering. Readers interested in exploring any of these areas in depth are referred to legal treatises and texts on the subject.

Intentional torts are those actions that a party intends to perpetrate on another and in fact does so. Battery is an example of an intentional tort, the intentional inexcusable contact with another person, to be distinguished from "incidental touchings" in a crowded room for which no intent can be shown. Virtually all invasive medical procedures—eg, surgery—raise the issue of battery. Consent by the party being touched, however, is a complete defense to the charge of battery, a notion derived from the Latin *volenti non fit injuria,* "to he/she who consents, there is no injury." Intentional misrepresentation ("fraud") is another such tort and in fact, like battery, may be pursued in both criminal and civil courts. In civil cases, withholding or misrepresentation of important (material) information may also extend or "toll" the statute of limitations, the time limit following discovery of injury (or when a person should have discovered an injury) after which a lawsuit may not be filed. (The rationale for such provisions are beyond the scope of this discussion.) Punitive damages are not infrequently awarded in cases of intentional torts, as such conduct is seen as preventively reprehensible such that the presumed punishing and deterrent effect of such awards are meant to prevent future actions.

The most common tort involved in medical practice is that of negligence.[5] Again derived from eighteenth century English common law notions whereby certain public callings would be held to a level of acceptable conduct (eg, innkeepers, physicians), a lawsuit in negligence is established by four elements: duty, breach of duty, causation, and damages. Where a duty between parties is established, and the breach of that duty is causative of injury, negligence will be found. Where actual damages can be shown, a cause of action or formal charge or complaint may be filed, and often several related "causes of action" are filed as part of the overall complaint. Two of these elements have been the subject of extensive commentary. The first is duty, which is defined by reasonable conduct of a person in similar circumstances.[6] Identified by the law as an "objective standard," experts are often called upon during trial to help establish what constitutes reasonable conduct. The second is causation. Often referred to as "cause in fact and proximate cause" or substantial causative relationship, causation is the element that links (provides a "nexus" between) the defendant's behavior or conduct to the harm or damage claimed. In lawsuits for negligence it is the conduct of the defendant that is at issue, not the consequences of that conduct. Nonetheless, it is in fact the consequences of that conduct that triggers most lawsuits because the element of damages is frequently the measure by which both patients are restituted and attorneys representing plaintiffs are compensated under the contingency fee system. As discussed in previous chapters and in Chapter 16, causation is the most controversial and perplexing issue in the field of alleged medical complications from silicone breast implants.

When dealing with corporate entities, the issue of duty and breach of duty become difficult to establish when a product is marketed to the public at large. The law addresses this problem, in part, in the form of strict liability and products liability as well as warranty. Reduced to simplest terms, a manufacturer represents a product as being reasonably safe when applied for its intended use. If the plaintiff shows evidence of a manufacturing defect, design defect, failure to warn (or breach of warranty), the defendant manufacturer may be held liable for damages. All three of these aspects regarding silicone breast implants are discussed in Chapter 16.

As has been discussed in previous chapters, many implants cannot be identified with respect to their manufacturer, either by imaging while the implant is within the breast or even after it has been explanted. Complicating these circumstances is the fact that many plastic surgeons have implanted several different types of silicone gel prostheses and may have not direct record of which one was used in a particular patient. Thus identification of the origin of the implant is difficult, compromising the plaintiff's position under the theory of strict liability in tort. Consequently, other theories have developed, successfully employed at times in other types of product liability cases. One is called market share liability. Where diethylstilbesterone (DES) was sold by Abbott Laboratories as a preventative for miscarriages with no warning to pregnant women following an order by the FDA to so warn, and with an overwhelming market share, the plaintiff was able to meet her standard of proof to indicate that the DES she took was manufactured by Abbott Laboratories.[7] Given the absence of convincing market share by any one manufacturer of silicone implants, this theory has not prevailed.

A second theory has been enterprise liability and a related theory of "concert in action," whereby a group of manufacturers or an entire industry is held accountable for harm. The procedural aspects of such an approach where there are several manufacturers, many of which have changed because of mergers, acquisitions, and changes of ownership, are such that this theory has not found wide acceptance in implant litigation.[8]

The law of negligence is also relevant to the subject of informed consent. Recall that simple consent by a plaintiff obviates a lawsuit for the intentional tort of battery. However, for more sophisticated acts, such as surgery and in this case augmentation surgery, physicians are held to a standard of care in obtaining the consent whereby the patient is reasonably informed of the risks and benefits (as well as alternatives) of the procedure. Different jurisdictions modify the measure of reasonableness, namely, what a reasonable physician would disclose or what a reasonable patient would need to know. Materiality of risks, or those risks that are either severe or likely to occur (or both) is essential in informed consent, which is often evidenced by a signed form. The process of obtaining such consent, therefore, is usually evaluated under the law of negligence. This aspect of litigation becomes even more important because manufacturers are often relieved of liability to warn if they have sufficiently warned the treating physician of potential risks. The physician is then considered a "learned intermediary" and charged with informing the patient of known risks. To the extent that manufacturers have insufficiently warned physicians, the strict liability claims of failure to warn may be sustained. Inherent within this discussion is the nature of research conducted by manufacturers and the element of disclosure. These aspects of litigation are discussed in Chapter 16.

The subject of silicone breast implants and litigation challenges multiple aspects of jurisprudence. When judges and juries look to legal precedent and standard regulatory procedures, and there are no analogous precedents and standard regulatory procedures have not taken place, then questions of law are difficult to resolve. When the court looks to science and medicine to evaluate the merits of a particular claim for appropriate disposition, and the studies and experts reach antithetical conclusions, then questions of fact remain unanswered. When a public places its trust in a court system to resolve disputes, and cases are resolved in no predictable manner, confusion and even cynicism emerge. The volatile issues inherent in litigation involving silicone breast implants offer solace to few. Perhaps time and ongoing studies will unravel the controversies regarding silicone implants because issues are unlikely to be solved until the facts are clarified. Science may help to establish those facts. Until such time, the courts will be asked to settle disputes by means of an adversarial system with the hope that truth—to the extent that it can be reckoned presently—will emerge.

REFERENCES

1. The Physicians Association of America. *Breast Cancer Study of 1995.* Washington, DC: Physicians Association of America; 1995.
2. *Daubert v Merrill Dow Pharmaceutical, Inc.,* 509 U.S., 113 S.Ct. 2786 (1993).
3. Duncan A. *Heads of Lectures on Medical Jurisprudence, or Institutiones Medicines Legalis.* Edinburgh: Neill and Co.; 1792.
4. Curran WJ, Shapiro ED. *Law, Medicine, and Forensic Science,* 3rd ed. Boston: Little, Brown; 1982.
5. Brenner RJ. Medicolegal implications of breast imaging in screening and diagnosis of breast cancer. *Surg Clin North Am.* 1994;3:67–83.
6. *Sheffington v Bradley,* 366 Mich 522, 115 N.W.2d 303 (Mich 1962).
7. *Sindell v Abbott Laboratories,* 26 Cal.3d 588, 163 Cal.Rptr 132, 607 P.2d 924 (1980), cert denied 449 U.S. 912, 101 S.Ct.285 (1980).
8. *Lee v Baxter Healthcare Corp.,* 721 F.Supp 89 (D.Md., 1989).

16

Medical-Legal Aspects of Breast Implants: A Review

DANIEL J. HERLING

During the early 1980s, breast implants, like any other medical product, were the subject of occasional product liability lawsuits. By 1987 only 50 such lawsuits had been filed. However, beginning in 1992 the scope of the litigation dramatically changed. Looking only at the lawsuits filed against one manufacturer, the Dow Corning Corporation, just over 100 were filed in 1990 and 1991, more than 3000 were filed in 1992, more than 8000 in 1993, and more than 7000 in 1994. By early 1995 Dow Corning alone was a defendant (either as a manufacturer or as a supplier of raw materials) in 45 putative class action lawsuits and more than 19,000 individual lawsuits involving more than 36,000 claimants. Almost uniformly, these claims alleged that breast implants had caused autoimmune diseases of one type or another. The damages sought in these individual cases were substantial, ranging from hundreds of thousands to tens of millions of dollars in compensatory and punitive damages.

The controversy surrounding breast implants is unlike the controversy that has surrounded any other product that has been embroiled in mass tort claims. For example, the emergence of asbestos claims as a mass tort can be traced to epidemiologic studies by Irving Selikoff and others that purported to show a strong link between asbestos exposure and disease. By contrast, breast implants appeared on the mass tort scene without the benefit of a single controlled scientific study showing that breast implants caused the diseases being claimed. Beneath the reams of paper and the thousands of words, in both the print and visual media, discussing the "breast implant controversy," are three issues that must be addressed each time a case goes to trial before a judge: causation, liability, and damages.

■ CAUSATION

The plaintiff must prove that her exposure to silicone breast implants (generally through the phenomena of gel bleed and/or rupture) caused her claimed autoimmune disease. If she cannot prove her implants caused her disease, the case is over—or should be. Without such proof, it should not be necessary for the trier of fact (the judge or jury) to determine whether the manufacturer of the implant, the supplier of the raw materials, and/or the plastic surgeon were liable, and the plaintiff should be precluded from asking the judge or jury to determine the damages that she is entitled to as a result of her exposure. Consequently, the issue of causation is paramount.

The medical community has long known of certain risks of breast implants, including complications from the surgery itself (as with any surgery), infections, and hemorrhage.[1] It has also been known that very small amounts of silicone fluid from the gel could leak or "bleed" through the outer envelope of the implant, and that a capsule of scar tissue could form and then contract excessively, distorting and hardening the breasts and causing discomfort. Additionally, surveys have shown that the plastic surgery community also knew that about 5% of women receiving breast implants experienced ruptures, which release the silicone gel into the surrounding tissues and flatten the breasts.[1] Early breast implant cases, preceding the emergence of the autoimmune issue, often centered on these issues; even today, plastic surgeons named as defendants are frequently asked to address these issues, particularly in the area of informed consent allegations.

The issue of whether a plaintiff's exposure to silicone breast implants can cause an immune disease, however, is the issue that has resulted in the verdicts adverse to the manufacturers. The plaintiffs' argument is that silicone gel–filled implants are responsible for a constellation of disorders described by various physicians and/or plaintiff's counsel as connective tissue disease, mixed connective tissue disease, silicone-associated disease (SAD), human adjuvant disease (HAD), and/or silicone arthroprothy.

Initially, the conventional wisdom among the manufacturers' lawyers was that cases in which the plaintiff was complaining of a disease recognized by the American College of Rheumatology (ACR), for example, systemic lupus erythematosus (SLE), rheumatoid arthritis, and scleroderma; would be the most difficult to defend, as it would be up to the defendants to establish that the particular plaintiff's exposure to silicone gel–filled breast implants did not cause the disease. This, in fact, has not been the case. Instead, the epidemiologic studies that have been completed to date have resulted in the ACR issuing a statement that the studies provide "compelling evidence that silicone implants expose patients to no demonstrable additional risk for connective tissue or rheumatic disease. Anecdotal evidence should no longer be used to support this relationship in the courts or by the FDA [Food and Drug Administration]."[2]

Plaintiffs respond to the defense argument of the lack of epidemiologic studies by usually choosing one of two avenues in attempting to establish their causation burden. First, a plaintiff may allege having contracted a disease so extremely rare that the epidemiologic studies did not cover it. Despite the conventional wisdom of the defense attorneys discussed above, cases that have resulted in the largest verdicts against manufacturers have generally involved claims of diffuse, nonspecific "flu-like" symptoms without a differential diagnosis of an ACR-recognized disease. Such claims are attractive on several levels. Most jurors can relate to the description of "flu-like" symptoms and would find empathy for a woman who has had to incur such symptoms over a lengthy period of time. Perhaps more importantly, a nonspecific diagnosis allows the plaintiffs' treating physicians and experts to argue that the epidemiologic studies are not relevant, as the studies did not evaluate and/or analyze the particular rare disease alleged by the plaintiff. It appears to be important for plaintiffs' counsel to avoid or deflect the significance of these studies, as the studies are now continuing to call into question the plaintiffs' arguments that exposure to implants can pose major health hazards. These studies also reduce the impact of anecdotal evidence that has been used on a continuing basis by the plaintiffs' experts to support their various theories of how silicone caused the particular plaintiff's problems.

A second approach, which can be used concurrently, is to challenge the studies on the merits, attacking them for not studying the proper disease, taking issue with the protocol followed in the study, and/or arguing that the authors of the study are biased because of the source of funding for the studies. This latter issue has taken on heightened significance and has resulted in modifications to the reporting of such studies. For example, the report relating to the Harvard Nurses Study included a detailed disclosure statement and prompted an editor's note in the *New England Journal of Medicine* stating that "this disclosure statement is in accord with our usual policy with somewhat more detail because of the intense public controversy over the health effects of breast implants."[3] Additionally, in its statement that recent studies provide compelling evidence that silicone implants expose patients to no demonstrable additional risk, the ACR included the following note: "Clinicians, scientists, academicians, and editors who have been harassed by plaintiffs' attorneys through their involvement in scientific research efforts related to silicone implants deserve the continued support of their institutions and professional societies."[4] Such statements are unprecedented and, although not directly related to the validity of the studies, appear to reflect that the second approach of attacking the studies' authors for bias has attracted the attention of the scientific and research communities. Whether such an attack will ultimately result in persuading a jury to disregard a study remains to be seen.

In addition to relying on the epidemiologic studies to support the defendants' position that silicone breast implants do not cause claimed autoimmune disease, the defendants in these cases do have alternative and/or additional defenses available.

For example, in responding to vague complaints of aches and pains in a plaintiff between the ages of 45 and 60, defendants can establish through expert opinion that it is difficult, if not impossible, to differentiate between the symptoms of the alleged silicone-induced disease and the constellation of aches and pains that relate to the female aging process, menopause, and/or chemical imbalance issues.

Additionally, no reasonable evaluation of causation can be made without an analysis of a plaintiff's psychiatric records, if any, as preexisting psychological symptoms are highly relevant to the issue of medical causation. Generally, plaintiffs argue that they never had a psychological problem until implantation, but have suffered from depression, anxiety, fatigue, cognitive impairment, etc., since the surgery.[5] Such plaintiffs seek to have the court limit evidence of alleged depression and accompanying symptoms to those occurring after implantation, as evidence of depression before implantation diminishes claims that silicone caused the depression and limits the damage claims.

Defendants should fully investigate and discover the plaintiff's psychological condition, as psychological and other organic ailments can create mimicking symptoms including chronic anxiety, chronic pain, drug and alcohol abuse, somatoform disorders, and personality disorders. Defendants should argue that by alleging fatigue, depression/psychoses, joint aches and pains, neurologic disorders, attention deficit disorder, mental anguish, and memory loss, the plaintiffs must disclose all medical information relating to those symptoms. The battle over the psychological records and the effect of the patient/psychologist privilege is a significant one that is often fought in pretrial discovery, with the winner generally gaining an advantage at time of trial. Once the psychological records are obtained, an examination and evaluation by a psychiatrist of defendant's choosing should be considered.

An additional defense tactic is a pretrial motion to have the trial heard in phases, first focusing solely on the causation issue. Plaintiffs' counsel, on the other hand, strenuously oppose this concept because a phased trial on causation alone precludes any discussion regarding the conduct of the defendants. In other words, unless and until the plaintiff can establish that her exposure to silicone through her breast implants caused her claimed autoimmune disease, it matters not one wit about the alleged bad conduct of the manufacturers and/or the treating physician. Use of a causation-only trial has been discussed in the bankruptcy court as one potential method to evaluate the claims of the Dow Corning plaintiff creditors. A trial limited to causation would result in a focused, "science only" analysis of this issue. It may well be, however, that the question of whether silicone gel–filled breast implants cause connective tissue disease is not ultimately a matter of opinion or legal argument but rather a matter of biologic fact. Either silicone implants cause connective tissue disease (alone or in conjunction with other factors), or they don't. Medical experts now argue that the only way to answer such questions is through epidemiologic studies, and that anecdotal reports alone do not constitute evidence that the implants cause the disease.[1]

Impact of Anecdotal Case Reports on Causation

The significant impact of anecdotal case reports as evaluated by lay judges and juries cannot be overstated. As the *New York Times* explained after interviewing several nationally recognized experts:

> In the case of silicone breast implants, the courts and much of the scientific world have proceeded on strikingly unparalleled tracks. While the courts have handed down multi-million-dollar awards based on the presumption of a health hazard, . . . the heavy-duty scientific studies now being completed have pointed to exactly the opposite conclusion, that there is no evidence that breast implants are harmful.[6]

The general press articles echoed observations that were the subject of an editorial in the *New England Journal of Medicine* that stated "despite the lack of published epidemiologic studies, the accumulated weight of anecdotes was taken by judges and juries as tantamount proof of causation."[7] The AMA, based on the recommendation of its counsel on scientific affairs, "urges physicians to recognize and address the considerable public anxiety concerning the safety of breast implants. This anxiety is not warranted based on current scientific evidence."[8]

Despite the above observations, judges, juries, and plaintiffs' expert witnesses continue to assert that anecdotal reports are significant. For example, in response to the argument that the disease is so rare that an epidemiologic study is not sufficient, plaintiffs' experts will opine that anecdotal reports are crucial, frequently arguing that "if there was no problem, why are all these women with breast implants presenting with symptoms of disease?"

In addition to the argument that anecdotal case reports and medical device reports are not good science, defendants also argue that there are legal reasons to preclude the introduction of such reports into evidence.

Medical device reports (MDRs) consist of communications to medical device manufacturers from doctors, patients, lawyers, and other laypersons—who are under no obligation to make such reports—that present complaints of serious injury reportedly experienced by the user of a medical device. MDRs vary widely in content, completeness, and form, but almost always are shorter than one page. They can be made in written form or by telephone, either to the manufacturer directly or to the company salespeople in the field. MDRs are maintained by medical device manufacturers in compliance with federal regulations, and forwarded on a routine basis to the FDA for review.[9]

Anecdotal case reports describe isolated instances of typically unexpected medical events occurring coincidentally with the use of a prescription drug or device. Like MDRs, anecdotal case reports tend to be very brief recitals of events, lacking any indicia of the reliability associated with scientific studies and peer-reviewed articles.

Defendants argue that, when offered to establish that the manufacturers knew or should have known that silicone gel breast implants caused rheumatologic disease, MDRs and anecdotal case reports are nothing more than hearsay and should properly be excluded. MDRs and anecdotal case reports are protypical examples of hearsay, evidence of a statement that was made other than by a witness while testifying at the hearing and that has been offered to prove the truth of the matter stated (F.R.E. 800). Such evidence should also be excluded when offered as a basis for expert opinion testimony; because of its inherent unreliability, it is not the type of evidence experts reasonably may rely on in forming an opinion.

Defendants argue that if such MDRs and anecdotal case reports are admitted into evidence, they would have no opportunity to examine the persons who submitted the reports, or the persons from whom such reports originated, as the case may be. As a result, it is impossible to determine whether the subjects of such reports were actually diagnosed with any of the conditions attributed to them; whether they had breast implants identical or even similar to the implants received by the plaintiffs; whether they had any genetic, occupational, or other conditions predisposing them to develop one or more of the conditions reported; or even whether the general circumstances surrounding the reported injuries resemble in any way the plaintiff's own, idiosyncratic set of circumstances.

The manufacturers argue further that they would be deprived of the opportunity to establish or even explore such issues as (1)inaccuracies in the reports; (2) the lack of first-hand knowledge or generally the existence of multiple levels of hearsay; (3) flawed diagnostic criteria; (4) lack of qualification and expertise of the reporter; and (5) potential bias of the patient or the reporter. The denial of a meaningful opportunity for cross-examination with respect to any of the above factors—each of which has a direct bearing on the validity of the conclusions and observations stated in the reports—would be fundamentally unfair to the defendants. Furthermore, defendants argue that nothing about MDRs or anecdotal case reports insures the trustworthiness of their contents. It is therefore argued that the reports do not fall within any exception to the hearsay rule under either the Federal Rules of Evidence or the applicable state rules. Nevertheless, many courts persist in allowing anecdotal case reports to be received into evidence. Courts facing the issues of the admissibility of other types of reports such as drug experience reports have ruled the reports inadmissible hearsay, not subject to exceptions.[10,11]

In addition to the legal argument that MDRs and anecdotal case reports consist of inadmissible hearsay, a further legal argument exists that such reports are irrelevant and any slight probative value they might have is substantially outweighed by the dangers of unfair prejudice, confusion, and undue consumption of time unpresented to the judge or jury. This is based on the fact that a great number of MDRs and anecdotal case reports relating to breast implant patients contain information concerning injuries medically unrelated to the conditions comprising plaintiff's unique symptomatology. In such cases, the defendants argue that the evidence is irrelevant and therefore inadmissible.

Even to the extent that certain MDRs and anecdotal case reports may contain accounts of ailments similar to one or more of those alleged by a plaintiff in a particular case, defendants argue that such evidence remains irrelevant and unfairly prejudicial, and therefore should not be admitted. Evidence of other incidents may be admissible for certain purposes (such as to show notice of a particular problem), but only if the plaintiff first shows that the incidents in question occurred under circumstances substantially similar to those at issue in her own case. Unfortunately, for the most part, it is impossible to determine whether the circumstances surrounding events described in MDRs and anecdotal case reports are even remotely similar to the plaintiff's case; MDRs, for example, often contain no more than a terse statement of the occurrence of a medical event or injury prompting the report, with such highly relevant surrounding circumstances as patient history and treatment left undisclosed. Furthermore, because most of the ailments and diseases described in such reports routinely occur in the population at large, rather than only among women with breast implants, the ideology of such diseases remains largely a function of each individual case history. MDRs, however, shed virtually no light on this point.

Although expert witnesses may properly form an opinion based at least in part on matters otherwise inadmissible, such matters must, at minimum, be of a type that reasonably may be relied on by an expert in forming an opinion on the subject to which the testimony relates. Whether or not an expert has based his or her opinion on unreliable underlying data is a fundamental question. Anecdotal case reports and MDRs are generally considered to lie at the speculative edge of the spectrum of epidemiologic research. The authors of an epidemiologic study of breast implants observed, "Case reports . . . provide the weakest evidence of a cause-and-effect relation."[12] Interestingly, the authors of this study explain that they initiated their population-base, retrospective cohort study in response to these weak case reports and the FDA's partial moratorium on the use of breast implants. Notably, the results of this study bear starkly on the unreliable nature of case reports: "We found no association between breast implants and connective-tissue disease and other disorders that were studied."

Expert Testimony

Because of the complexity of the issues of medical causation, expert witness testimony is critical in breast implant cases. The admissibility of expert opinions, a topic far too broad for this treatise, was directly impacted recently by the United States Supreme Court decision in *Daubert v. Merrill Dow Pharmaceutical, Inc.*[13] In determining the proper standard for the admissibility of expert witnesses, the United States Supreme Court held in *Daubert* that the Federal Rules of Evidence, not a 1923 decision entitled *Frye V. United States,*[14] provides the standard for admitting expert scientific testimony. The court placed appropriate limits on the admissibility of purportedly scientific evidence by assigning to the trial court the task of ensuring that the expert's testimony rests on a reliable foundation and is relevant to the task at hand.

Not all state courts have followed *Daubert,* and there have been many variations on the *Daubert* theme. The United States Court of Appeals for the Ninth Circuit, for example, held that the test under *Daubert* for determining whether an expert may testify is not the correctness of the expert's conclusions, but the soundness of his or her methodology.[15]

Accordingly, the issue of the nature and the extent of the admissibility of anecdotal case reports and MDRs is of paramount importance; the decision by the trial judge as to whether or not to admit, limit, or preclude the introduction of such testimony either directly or through expert witnesses will often be the most important ruling in the trial, as whether one champions the plaintiff or the manufacturers in the breast implant litigation, the causation issue turns on the testimony of the experts.

■ LIABILITY

Certain causes of action have been alleged in nearly every lawsuit that has been filed either in the federal Multi-District Litigation (MDL) proceeding, *In Re: Silicone Gel Breasts Implant Products Liability Litigation* (MDL §926), or in the state courts. These causes of action will vary depending on the status of the defendant as implant manufacturer, bulk supplier of materials to the manufacturer, or a physician, as follows.

Manufacturing Defendants

Generally, a cause of action against a manufacturer will be for strict liability in tort. The theory of strict liability in tort is based on either allegations of manufacturing defect, design defect, or failure to warn.

MANUFACTURING DEFECT

To prevail on a manufacturing defect claim, plaintiff must establish that the implant she received contained a defect before it left the manufacturer that was a proximate or substantial cause of her injury. This theory has not yet proven to be very useful to the plaintiffs' bar in establishing their cases, primarily because of proof problems. Proving this allegation generally requires an unfavorable comparison of the lot history records of the specific implant at issue with the standard specifications of the manufacturer, or an inspection of the implant that shows that the implant does not meet the manufacturer's specifications in such aspects as the thickness of the envelope shell, the constituency of the gel, or the shape and thickness of the envelope patch.

Other methods used in an attempt to establish manufacturing defects have included attacking the manufacturer's entire quality control system at the time of the manufacture of the implant or attempting to identify a particular aspect of the quality control inspection procedure as inadequate. Under this theory, plaintiffs have also attempted to argue that the discovery of an excessive number of "rejects" in a particular lot places the entire lot in jeopardy and that there was a problem with the manufacturing process of that lot.

To prosecute this count successfully, inspection of the plaintiffs's own implant is generally necessary, along with a factual scenario of any unexplained rupture. The plaintiff must retain a credible expert witness who has experience in reviewing lot history records, is familiar with the manufacturing process, and is able to generate and/or interpret visually aided technique results to determine the failure site of the implant. Several of these experts have been former employees of the various manufacturers.

Plaintiff's counsel must also be able to effectively counter the testimony of company representatives regarding its manufacturing and quality control processes. This is often a daunting prospect, as breast implant manufacturers are regulated by the FDA and are thus subject to its good manufacturing procedures (GMP) requirements.

DESIGN DEFECT

The first issue in establishing a design defect claim in a medical device case is to determine whether the device in question is one for which the manufacturer can be held strictly liable, assuming a defect can be shown. The California Supreme Court in *Brown v. Superior Court*[16] held that a drug manufacturer's liability for a defectively designed drug should not be measured by the standards of strict liability. The court addressed the public policy interest in promoting the affordability and availability of pharmaceutical products. In California, at least one appellate court[17] has already agreed with this argument as it relates to breast implants and stated that, although in general product liability litigation a plaintiff may utilize a strict liability design defect theory, the manufacturers of certain "special products," including prescription drugs and implanted medical devices, are exempt from such liability as a matter of law.[17]

Breast implants are clearly implanted medical devices as recognized by the FDA, which has defined "medical device" to include "implants intended to affect the structure of any function of the body."[18] Mammary prostheses are specifically delineated by the FDA as medical devices which are "intended to be implanted to augment or reconstruct the female breast."[19]

Additionally, the sale of mammary implants, the implantation of which requires the skill and expertise of medical professionals, is limited to licensed physicians. In arguing a case outside the jurisdiction of California, the defendant should apprise the court that there is no rational basis on which to distinguish between breast implants and other implanted medical devices for the purpose of adjudicating the strict design liability issue.

Even with the benefit of a court's decision to dismiss the design defect theory of liability as sounding in strict liability, plaintiffs still have available to them the argument of design defect in the negligence context.

One approach used to buoy up the design defect count is to present an expert witness who will indict the entire concept of using silicone gel as a filler of the silicone envelope used in the manufacture of the implant. Examples of this have included experts who have testified that a silicone envelope inflated with saline is a safer and more effective product than a silicone gel implant. Such testimony faces the obstacle of explaining away the self-contained bias, as the expert testifying is usually a designer of such a competitive product.

FAILURE TO WARN

The failure-to-warn theory of liability paraphrases the Watergate refrain: What did the companies know and when did they know it? This theory of liability enables the plaintiff to introduce into evidence the so-called smoking-gun documents and permits certain plaintiffs' experts almost carte blanche as to their scope of testimony.

As discussed above, establishing a causative link between the implants and the claimed autoimmune disease should precede a discussion of the defendants' alleged failure to warn. This reasoning, however, has not generally been followed in the course of the trials. Plaintiffs have opened their trial presentations with frontal attacks on the manufacturer's failure to warn despite the fact that either the plaintiff never reviewed or relied on any literature from the manufacturer (nor did the plastic surgeon, for that matter) or that causation had not yet been established.

Different issues regarding an alleged failure to warn exist for each manufacturer. The following will set forth a few issues commonly seen by three of the major manufacturers and a potential response to each of the claims.

Dow Corning Corporation

- Insufficient premarket testing: For example, plaintiffs have alleged that the silicone fluid that was used to develop the silicone gel was the same fluid that was used in injections to the breasts that were banned by the FDA and various states, including California, and that the breast implant silicone bleed material is the same as the fluids used in the injection. Responses to this argument include the facts that the testing that was performed on the fluids prior to the marketing of the implants was the state of the art at that time, that Dow Corning never recommended direct injection of the fluid into the breast tissue, and that the amount of the fluid to which a recipient may be exposed is in such minimal amounts that it could have no systemic effect.
- Bioincompatibility: Plaintiffs argue that Dow Corning's early 1970s testing allegedly showed silicone was not as inert as supposedly claimed by Dow Corning. A response to this allegation would be that the tests were not related to the type of silicone gel that was used in breast implants, and that the testing protocols were not designed to show what the plaintiffs now claim the tests show. For example, a test often used by the plaintiffs to establish the toxicologic effects of silicone on rats was really a test of dosage effect wherein the rats were poisoned and is not related to the effect of the silicone.[20]
- The Dow Corning "hot documents": Plaintiffs argue that internal memos allegedly regarding the inference of testing when no testing was done establish the alleged bad conduct of Dow Corning. The response to each of these documents is to place them in the proper context as to when and why they were written and who wrote them. Several selected documents over a period of 35 years do not present the complete or accurate picture of Dow Corning's conduct.
- Rupture rates: Plaintiffs argue that the rupture rates are higher than what was originally reported. The response to this is that in fact the reportage of rupture rates was anecdotal and based primarily on the learning curve of the plastic surgeon using new products as each such product was introduced.
- Insufficient warnings in the product literature: The response is that Dow Corning placed warnings in its package literature when appropriate as guided by medical and scientific concerns and not based on anecdotal reportage.

Heyer-Schulte/Baxter

Plaintiffs argue that Heyer-Schulte did not perform any of its own testing but merely relied upon the Dow Corning work that was insufficient. Heyer-Schulte has responded by indicating that it did do some of its own testing, was kept current in the state of the art based on the individuals retained to work on the breast implants, and that it issued other appropriate warnings.

Plaintiffs have also asserted that Heyer-Schulte hired and relied upon Dr. Henry Jenny as a consultant, but then ignored Jenny's warnings. This has particularly become an issue where Dr. Jenny has testified on behalf of the plaintiff. Baxter's response to Dr. Jenny's opinions is that he was wrong and was also very biased as he was attempting to have the company market a different product, and therefore he would, on a regular basis, attempt to denigrate the silicone gel–filled breast implant product for his own benefit. Several cases against Heyer-Schulte/Baxter have recently resulted in verdicts in its favor.

Bristol Myers Squibb

Plaintiffs complain that Bristol Myers purchased a company that made implants from individuals who had no experience and who did no testing on their own. Bristol Myers argues that the testing that it relied on was the state of the art and that there is still no proof that silicone causes any of the diseases alleged by the plaintiffs.

Although not all of the above neatly fit within the failure-to-warn rubric, plaintiffs' counsel have used the broad-brush approach with these claims to establish as much as possible of the so-called bad conduct of the manufacturers.

Defenses to Failure to Warn Claims

A response to the failure-to-warn claim and the plaintiff's standard testimony that "if I had known then what I know now about silicone, I never would have agreed to having the procedure take place" must be developed by both the manufacturing defendants and the defendant plastic surgeons.

Investigation of the plaintiff and her risk-taking propensity is crucial. Such investigation has resulted in extensive discovery disputes that must be resolved by the court prior to trial. Initially, the defendants must convince the court that they are not engaging in a "witch hunt," but rather a systematic approach to determine the propensity of plaintiff's risk-taking in order to rebut the plaintiff's statement of the state of knowledge that would have resulted in her not undergoing the procedure. This analysis necessarily results in determining the smoking habits, alcohol and/or substance abuse history, birth control pill usage, other methods of birth control including but not limited to abortion history, and other examples of the plaintiff taking risks with her body despite knowledge of risks. For example, several plaintiffs have had a history of prior cosmetic surgery, including but not limited to receiving tattoos. Defendants must convince a court that what may appear to be requests for information posited solely for the purpose of harassment are in fact reasonable areas of investigation.

As with the alternative causation theories, plaintiff's counsel should make every effort to limit the scope of inquiry and make the argument that if not a "witch hunt," the defendants are requiring their clients to undergo, at the very least, an interrogation that clearly exceeds the scope of injuries claimed.

Bulk Suppliers of Raw Material Silicone

Suppliers of silicone raw materials to the manufacturers that use the raw material to produce the implant at issue have been named by plaintiffs for several reasons. Including this class of defendants in the action ensures that the manufacturer does not point to an empty chair in the courtroom and blame all of the plaintiff's problems on the absent supplier of the raw material silicone; ensures that a "deep pocket" exists, should a manufacturer not have sufficient assets to cover any adverse verdict; enables the plaintiff's counsel to introduce into evidence "hot" or "bad" documents of the supplier; and/or protects the plaintiff's counsel from a successful claim for legal malpractice should the products liability jury render an adverse verdict to the plaintiff.

Defendant suppliers have argued both in pretrial dispositive motions (for example, the successful motions for summary judgment by General Electric and Rhone Poulenc) and at trial that the bulk suppliers of raw materials or chemicals that are formulated or processed to make finished products bear no responsibility for injuries resulting from alleged defects in the manufacturer's finished product. Additionally, the suppliers of raw materials also claim that they are entitled to rely on the sophisticated manufacturer to determine the risks posed by the medical products the manufacturer made and to communicate those risks to the learned intermediaries, the treating physicians using the products.

Generally, the defendant suppliers provided gel fluid to breast implant manufacturers. The manufacturers used the fluid to make the gel for their own breast implants, a process that involves the cross-linking of silicone chains during which the manufacturer controlled the viscosity and other qualities of the resulting gel by altering, among other things, the mix ratio, cure time, and oven temperature. Additionally, the suppliers generally argue that the manufacturer uses its own sophisticated testing procedures and that the finished product is different from the raw material supplied.

The bankruptcy of Dow Corning has curtailed the analysis of this issue as most if not all of the other suppliers have been successful on pretrial motions, extricating themselves from cases where they have been named as a supplier of raw materials used in the manufacturing of breast implants.

Physicians

The claim against most of the plastic surgeon defendants has sounded in negligence. To prevail, the plaintiff must establish surgical technique negligence, which resulted in undue scarring or a rupture. Issues of informed consent predominate, as most plastic surgeons will argue that they had no specific information regarding the causation issue of silicone and autoimmune disease.

The decision to name a physician as a defendant in these actions and the extent of the role of the physician is controversial. In California, the naming of the physician as a defendant was initially viewed as a procedural tactic to avoid having the case transferred to the federal MDL proceeding, as generally the patient and the physician are citizens of the same state, thereby destroying the diversity grounds for removal to federal court.

As with many malpractice actions, the believability of the treating physician as perceived by the trier of fact is telling. The testimony of the treating plastic surgeon at the trial often sets the tone of the trial. For example, in cases where the treating plastic surgeon has been named as the defendant and he or she cooperates with the manufacturer, both the manufacturer and the plastic surgeon have been successful in defeating the plaintiff's claims.[21] On the other hand, there have been instances where the treating plastic surgeon has not cooperated and the results have been mixed.

Dow Chemical

In 1943 Dow Chemical, Inc. and Corning, Inc., formed Dow Corning Corp. While Dow Chemical has never manufactured implants, a Nevada jury[22] found for the first time Dow Chemical liable in a silicone breast implant case. The jury determined that Dow Chemical had allegedly fraudulently concealed the dangers of liquid silicone, which it had allegedly become aware of more than 30 years ago.

The evidence presented at trial by the plaintiffs focused on Dow Chemical's relationship with Dow Corning, including joint testing conducted by the two companies from the

1950s through the 1980s. Plaintiffs contend that they were able to persuade the Reno jury to find Dow Chemical liable and award the plaintiffs $4.1 million in compensatory damages and $10 million in punitive damages by arguing that the liquid silicone that makes up 85% of the silicone gel in the finished implant migrated throughout the body of the plaintiff to all of the major organs including the heart, liver, lungs, and brain. Plaintiff's counsel also argued that the two companies discovered the liquid silicone affected the immune system and central nervous system. Instead of disclosing this research to the scientific community, according to plaintiff's counsel, Dow Chemical and Dow Corning entered into secret development agreements to develop silicones as drugs attempting to harness their effect on the body's immune system.[23]

Plaintiffs also claim that Dow Chemical, one of the largest pesticide manufacturers in the world, also learned that liquid silicone was effective as an insecticide and secretly attempted to develop it commercially with Dow Corning in the 1980s. The plaintiffs, by arguing such information, were able to persuade a jury to decide that Dow Chemical had exhibited a conscious disregard for safety, thus providing the basis for the punitive damage award.

Interestingly, the successful plaintiff in the Nevada action, who had been implanted in 1985, was not diagnosed with any recognized ACR disease. Her symptoms included chronic fatigue, muscle and joint aches, rashes all over her body, loss of bowel control, and loss of sensation in her extremities.

According to plaintiff's counsel, this case is expected to result in thousands of other cases being filed against Dow Chemical by women who receive Dow Corning implants, which will provide an option for these women in Dow Corning's bankruptcy proceedings.[23]

It remains to be seen whether this case is an aberration or portends the future for Dow Chemical.

■ DAMAGES

The awards of damages in breast implant cases garner the publicity but the type and methods of proof to obtain them are similar to those asserted in most product liability personal injury claims.

Compensatory

A plaintiff's compensatory damages consist of the sum of medical expenses and wage loss claims (sometimes known as "special damages") and damages for pain, suffering, and inconvenience (often known as "general damages").

To establish special damages, the plaintiffs must obtain all billing records from the date of implantation forward that relate to all treatment she received allegedly linked to the breast implants. Questions often arise as to the nature and extent and reasonableness of the treatment and whether it was related to the autoimmune claims being presented.

Issues that arise in the evaluation of wage loss claims often relate to the allegations of a diminished capacity to earn. Several plaintiffs have argued that they were forced to abandon their careers as a result of the effects of their exposure to silicone. Generally, however, the analysis of the amount of special damages is rather straightforward.

The general damages award to the plaintiff is another factor that makes the breast implant litigation unique. For example, this author is not aware of any breast implant case that has gone to a verdict that has not resulted in either a complete defense verdict or an award in the multiples of millions of dollars. Unlike other product liability personal injury cases, the litigation to date appears to be an "all or nothing" proposition. There is no track record of a series of awards that enable parties to assess a verdict that would fall within the parameters of zero and multiple millions of dollars and determine a reasonable settlement value. This fact may be one that has impeded the success in reaching a global settlement of these claims.

Punitive Damages

The headline-grabbing aspect of this litigation, in addition to the numbers of plaintiffs involved, is the fact that juries have awarded damages known as punitive or exemplary (awarded to punish the defendant and deter future conduct) in the multiples of millions of dollars. Punitive damages are not permitted in cases of pure personal injury, but plaintiffs' counsel routinely allege causes of action for intentional misrepresentation, concealment, fraud, and, in some jurisdictions, unfair and deceptive trade practices, to make the plaintiff eligible to receive punitive damages.

Plaintiffs' counsel have been successful in using the "bad conduct" of a company as a theme from the commencement of the trial to posture the defendant as one that deserves a finding of punitive damages, in addition to the compensatory damages discussed above.

In addition to "humanizing" the corporation through use of corporate representatives and illustrating through tests and documents that in fact the manufacturer was acting responsibly, defendants often make use of pretrial motions to avoid punitive damages by attempting to preclude the following: (1) testimony impermissibly characterizing defendant's conduct and "corporate knowledge" as "bad"; (2) evidence of "after-the-fact" conduct of the manufacturer; (3) evidence of representations allegedly made by the manufacturer in support of the plaintiff's fraud and misrepresentation claims, unless and until the plaintiff first shows actual and justifiable reliance upon such representations; (4) evidence of investigations by the FDA or Congress into the breast implant issue. Pretrial and trial motions and appropriate objections are available to preclude and/or control prejudicial remarks made by witnesses and counsel. To date, the success of such attempts in controlling punitive damage awards has been varied.

▪ CONCLUSION

The popular press is replete with stories of how the breast implant litigation has affected thousands of participants. Several plaintiffs have undergone unnecessary surgeries in either removing their implants and/or having breasts removed without medical necessity. Dow Corning Corp., defendant in thousands of civil actions filed across the country, has sought bankruptcy protection under Chapter 11 of United States Bankruptcy Code. The decisions of the FDA regarding this issue have been scrutinized not only by the scientific community but also by the Congress. Pundits, both scientific and otherwise, have commented extensively on the impact and extent of the litigation.

Despite all of the above, once a case proceeds to trial, the matter is assigned a trial judge, and a jury is seated, the issue to be decided rests with the triers of fact. Successful plaintiff's counsel present cogent, well thought out and sympathetic themes that his or her client's exposure to silicone through breast implants has made her sick and she should receive compensation. The defendants, whether they be manufacturers or physicians, respond to these claims with a scientific analysis, with the underlying theme that to date, there is no proof that exposure to silicone causes any disease. Each side presents its case through experts with (at least generally on paper) solid scientific credentials. But the triers of fact alone make the decision.

It has long been the subject of a heated debate as to whether the courtroom is the proper forum to determine science.[24] The breast implant trial adds fuel but not any resolution.

REFERENCES

1. Angell M. Are breast implants actually OK? *New Republic,* September 11, 1995; 18–21.
2. Statement of American College of Rheumatology on Silicone Breast Implants, October 22, 1995.
3. Sanchez-Guerrero J, et al. Silicone breast implants and the risk of connective-tissue diseases and symptoms. *N Engl J Med.* 1995;332:1664–1670.
4. American College of Rheumatology Statement on Silicone Breast Implants, October 22, 1995.
5. Herling DJ, et al. Why breast implant plaintiffs need to supply psychological records. *Medical-Legal Aspects of Breast Implants.* 1994;2(11):1–2.
6. Legal system and science come to different conclusions on silicone. *New York Times,* May 16, 1995;C6.
7. Editorial. *N Engl J Med.* 1994;330:1748–1749.
8. Editorial. *JAMA.* 1994;270:2602.
9. 21 CFR §803.24.
10. *Muilenberg v. UpJohn Co.* (Mich. 1982) 320 N.W.2d 358.
11. *Thomas v. Hoffman-LaRoche, Inc.* (5th Cir. 1992 *rehg-denied*) 949 F.2d 806, 815, M.38 *cert. denied,* 112 S.Ct. 2304.
12. Gabriel SE, et al. Risk of connective-tissue diseases and other disorders after breast implantation. *N Engl J Med.* 330: 1697–1702.
13. 509 U.S. 579, 113 S.Ct. 2786 (1993).
14. *Frye vs United States,* 293 F.1013 (D.C. Cir. 1923).
15. 43 F.2d 1311 (9th Cir. 1995); California, however, has affirmed the *Frye* standard in *People V. Leahy* (1994) 8 Cal.4th 187.
16. (1988) 44 Cal.3d 1049.
17. *Artiglio vs Superior Court* (1994) 22 Cal.App.4th 1388.
18. 21 C.F.R. §321(h).
19. 21 C.F.R. §878.3540.
20. Boley WF, Robert R, LeVier RR. Immunological enhancing activities of organosilicon compounds and non-functional fluids. October 2, 1974.
21. *Turner v. Dow Corning* (1993) County of Denver, State of Colorado, Civil Action No. 92-CV-150.
22. *Mahlum v. Dow Corning Corp.,* CV 93-05941 (2d Jud. Distr. Washoe Cty., Nev.) (Oct. 18, 1995).
23. Ellis FL. How plaintiffs' lawyers beat Dow Chemical in Nevada case. *Medical-Legal Aspects of Breast Implants.* 1994; 3(12):1–2.
24. *Scopes v. State,* 154 Tenn. 105, 289 S.W. 363 (1927).

Glossary

Capsulotomy: a procedure by which the surgeon uses vigorous manual compression to disrupt a hard fibrous capsule. There have been several case reports of capsulotomies causing implant rupture. Capsulotomies are not commonly used today.

Direct silicone injection: an older method of breast augmentation in which silicone oil is directly injected into the breast using a syringe and needle. This method was used most commonly between 1940 and the early 1960s.

Double-lumen implant: has two lumens, most commonly a saline outer chamber surrounding the inner silicone gel lumen. Others may have silicone in the outer chamber and saline within the inner chamber. This type is commonly referred to as expander implants and were commonly used in patients with mastectomies to allow expansion of the skin. The expander implants have a port by which saline can be added to the inner chamber allowing the implant to enlarge and expand the skin.

Extracapsular implant rupture: rupture of both the implant shell and the fibrous capsule, with silicone leakage extending into surrounding tissues.

Fibrous capsule: scar tissue that forms around all implants, which may be soft and impalpable, or hard and resistant. Occasionally, the fibrous capsule can calcify, which can be detected by mammography or computed tomography.

Implant shell (envelope or membrane): a semipermeable membrane of variable thickness constructed of more highly cross-linked polymer chains of silicone to create an elastic solid. The purpose of the soft implant shell is to contain the silicone gel and provide a natural feeling and contour to the augmented breast.

Intracapsular implant rupture: rupture of the implant shell (elastomer envelope) allowing the release of silicone gel, which does not extend beyond the intact fibrous capsule. This is the most common type of implant rupture.

Linguine sign: the MRI finding of multiple curvilinear low signal intensity lines surrounded by the high signal intensity silicone gel. The multiple curvilinear lines represent the collapsed implant shell floating within the silicone gel. This finding is the most reliable sign of either an intracapsular or extracapsular implant rupture. This finding can also be identified on computed tomography and on ultrasonography.

Single-lumen silicone implant: has a smooth or textured outer silicone shell coating that contains the silicone gel.

Silicone: the chemical composition of most medical grade silicones is dimethyl polysiloxane with varying degrees of polymerization or cross-linkages between the methyl groups.

Silicone gel: consists of a mixture of many cross-linked silicone chains immersed in a bath of many non–cross-linked silicone chains. The cross-linked silicone molecules will feel sticky and produce stranding when touched. The non–cross-linked silicone chains are referred to as silicone oil.

Silicone gel bleed: occurs in all silicone implants. The most widely accepted definition is microscopic silicone leakage through an intact implant shell. Some experts consider that a gel bleed is a mixture of cross-linked and non–cross-linked silicone chains (silicone oil). A few experts believe that a gel bleed consists only of silicone oil.

Silicone oil: composed of non–cross-linked silicone chains and will feel slippery when touched. Silicone oil will not form strands when touched as will silicone gel, which has many cross-linkages between the methyl groups.

Snowstorm pattern: an ultrasonographic finding of microglobules of silicone mixed with the tissues of the body. This characteristic highly echogenic pattern of free silicone within the tissues is a reliable sign specific for free silicone mixed with surrounding tissues.

Stacked implants: two or more implants surgically placed within a breast to obtain a larger breast size. Most commonly one will see stacked implants in mastectomy patients.

Stepladder sign: a series of horizontal echogenic straight or curvilinear lines, somewhat parallel, traversing the interior of the implant. This sign represents the collapsed implant shell floating within the silicone gel, and is analogous to the linguine sign seen on MR imaging. The continuity of these echogenic lines is usually not obvious on sonography because of the narrow field of view.

Subglandular implant: describes the location of the implant in respect to the pectoralis major muscle; surgically placed anterior to the pectoralis muscle.

Subpectoral implant: describes the location of the implant in respect to the pectoralis major muscle. The implant is surgically placed posterior to the pectoralis muscle. Although subpectoral implants are technically more difficult to place, they offer the advantages of improved mammography, decrease in capsular contracture, and less obvious surgical scar.

Uncollapsed implant rupture: a ruptured implant shell that does not collapse or only partially collapses. The linguine sign will not be present. The reasons some ruptured implants do not completely collapse is unclear, but one theory is that some of the older implant shells are relatively stiff and some have fixation patches, making collapse less likely.

Index

Figures and tables are indicated by f and t respectively.